AF761059

PUBLIC HEALTH: PRACTICES, METHODS AND POLICIES

SMOKING AND ADOLESCENCE

INTERNATIONAL PUBLIC HEALTH EXPERIENCES

PUBLIC HEALTH: PRACTICES, METHODS AND POLICIES

JOAV MERRICK - SERIES EDITOR –

MEDICAL DIRECTOR, HEALTH SERVICES, DIVISION FOR INTELLECTUAL AND DEVELOPMENTAL DISABILITIES, MINISTRY OF SOCIAL AFFAIRS AND SOCIAL SERVICES, JERUSALEM, ISRAEL

Environment and Public Health: Environmental Health, Law and International Perspectives
I. Leslie Rubin and Joav Merrick (Editors)
2014. ISBN: 978-1-63463-167-9

Tomorrow's Leaders: Service Leadership and Holistic Development in Chinese University Students
Daniel T.L. Shek, Andrew M.H. Siu and Joav Merrick (Editors)
2014. ISBN: 978-1-63321-880-2

Arbovirus: Public Health Experience from Zambia
Seter Siziya, Mazyanga L. Mazaba and Joav Merrick (Editors)
2015. ISBN: 978-1-63463-601-8 (Softcover)

Health Issues in Diverse Cultures
Cecilia Obeng, Samuel Gyasi Obeng and Joav Merrick (Editors)
2015. ISBN: 978-1-63463-613-1

Public Health, Social Work and Health Inequalities
Bruce D. Friedman and Joav Merrick (Editors)
2015. ISBN: 978-1-63482-838-3

Environmental Health Disparities: Costs and Benefits of Breaking the Cycle
I Leslie Rubin and Joav Merrick (Editors)
2016. ISBN: 978-1-63484-211-2

Smoking and Adolescence: International Public Health Experiences
Mazyanga L. Mazabam, Seter Siziya and Joav Merrick (Editors)
2016. ISBN: 978-1-63484-311-9

PUBLIC HEALTH: PRACTICES, METHODS AND POLICIES

SMOKING AND ADOLESCENCE

INTERNATIONAL PUBLIC HEALTH EXPERIENCES

MAZYANGA L. MAZABA
SETER SIZIYA
AND
JOAV MERRICK
EDITORS

nova publishers
New York

Copyright © 2016 by Nova Science Publishers, Inc.

All rights reserved. No part of this book may be reproduced, stored in a retrieval system or transmitted in any form or by any means: electronic, electrostatic, magnetic, tape, mechanical photocopying, recording or otherwise without the written permission of the Publisher.

We have partnered with Copyright Clearance Center to make it easy for you to obtain permissions to reuse content from this publication. Simply navigate to this publication's page on Nova's website and locate the "Get Permission" button below the title description. This button is linked directly to the title's permission page on copyright.com. Alternatively, you can visit copyright.com and search by title, ISBN, or ISSN.

For further questions about using the service on copyright.com, please contact:
Copyright Clearance Center
Phone: +1-(978) 750-8400 Fax: +1-(978) 750-4470 E-mail: info@copyright.com.

NOTICE TO THE READER

The Publisher has taken reasonable care in the preparation of this book, but makes no expressed or implied warranty of any kind and assumes no responsibility for any errors or omissions. No liability is assumed for incidental or consequential damages in connection with or arising out of information contained in this book. The Publisher shall not be liable for any special, consequential, or exemplary damages resulting, in whole or in part, from the readers' use of, or reliance upon, this material. Any parts of this book based on government reports are so indicated and copyright is claimed for those parts to the extent applicable to compilations of such works.

Independent verification should be sought for any data, advice or recommendations contained in this book. In addition, no responsibility is assumed by the publisher for any injury and/or damage to persons or property arising from any methods, products, instructions, ideas or otherwise contained in this publication.

This publication is designed to provide accurate and authoritative information with regard to the subject matter covered herein. It is sold with the clear understanding that the Publisher is not engaged in rendering legal or any other professional services. If legal or any other expert assistance is required, the services of a competent person should be sought. FROM A DECLARATION OF PARTICIPANTS JOINTLY ADOPTED BY A COMMITTEE OF THE AMERICAN BAR ASSOCIATION AND A COMMITTEE OF PUBLISHERS.

Additional color graphics may be available in the e-book version of this book.

Library of Congress Cataloging-in-Publication Data
Names: Mazaba, Mazyanga L. (Mazyanga Lucy) editor.
Title: Smoking and adolescence : international public health experiences / editors, Mazyanga L. Mazaba-Liwewe, Seter Siziya, Ph.D., and Joav Merrick, M.D. (WHO, UN Annex, Lusaka, Zambia, and others).
Description: Hauppauge, N.Y. : Nova Science Publishers, Inc., 2016. | _2014 | Series: Public health: practices, methods and policies | Includes index.
Identifiers: LCCN 2015044866 (print) | LCCN 2015048126 (ebook) | ISBN 9781634843119 (hardcover) | ISBN 9781634843126 ()
Subjects: LCSH: Youth--Tobacco use. | Youth--Social conditions. | Health behavior in adolescence.
Classification: LCC HV5745 .S537 2016 (print) | LCC HV5745 (ebook) | DDC 362.29/620835--dc23
LC record available at http://lccn.loc.gov/2015044866

Published by Nova Science Publishers, Inc. † New York

CONTENTS

INTRODUCTION

In: Smoking and Adolescence ISBN: 978-1-63484-311-9
Editors: M. L. Mazabam, S. Siziya et al. © 2016 Nova Science Publishers, Inc.

Chapter 1

SMOKING AND ADOLESCENCE

***Mazyanga L Mazaba*[1,*]*, Seter Siziya*[2] *and Joav Merrick*[3-7]**

[1]World Health Organization, Lusaka, Zambia
[2]School of Medicine, Copperbelt University, Ndola, Zambia
[3]National Institute of Child Health and Human Development, Jerusalem, Israel
[4]Office of the Medical Director, Health Services, Division for Intellectual and Developmental Disabilities, Ministry of Social Affairs and Social Services, Jerusalem, Israel
[5]Division of Pediatrics, Hadassah Hebrew University Medical Center, Mt Scopus Campus, Jerusalem, Israel
[6]Kentucky Children's Hospital, University of Kentucky College of Medicine, Lexington, Kentucky, USA
[7]Center for Healthy Development, School of Public Health, Georgia State University, Atlanta, USA

INTRODUCTION

Smoking cigarettes starts during adolescence. Some adolescents may stop smoking cigarettes having taken it as an experiment during adolescence but others may continue smoking into adulthood. Most adults who smoke started

* Corresponding author: Mazyanga L Mazaba, BSc, MSc, World Health Organization, Un Annex, Corner Andrew Mwenya/Beit roads, P.O Box 32346, Lusaka, Zambia. E-mail: mazmazli@yahool.com.

smoking during adolescence stage (1, 2) and may have been already addicted to nicotine before the age of 18 years (3, 4), resulting in long-term health consequences. This book compiles and documents the epidemiology and correlates of smoking in adolescents in various regions. It aims to provide critical information that relates to the magnitude of the problem and who is affected so strategies may be identified and implemented to prevent this scourge of public health importance affecting persons not only at the time the smoking habit begins but an influence of the rest of their life.

FACTORS ASSOCIATED WITH ADOLESCENT SMOKING

Various factors associated with smoking in adolescence have been identified and include psychosocial influences, such as peer pressure, biological reasons, surrounding environment, and experimentation. Exposure to cigarette advertising in magazines, billboards, posters, television, and radio is associated with smoking initiation (5, 6). Further, Hunang et al. (7) found that exposure to anti-tobacco materials at school predicted a lower risk of experimentation with smoking. Social influences are strongly associated with Adolescent smoking (8). School- and peer-group influences are important in adolescent life (9) such that other adolescents may provide access, opportunity, and reinforcement for smoking (10, 11). Hunang et al. (7) reported that having a friend who smoked predicted a higher risk of experimentation with smoking. In a study in Greece (12), 40.1% of Greek high school students aged 15-18 years initiated smoking because their friends smoke. Peer smoking has found to be related to adolescent smoking initiation, maintenance and intentions (13, 14). Gilman et al. (15) observed that parental smoking was associated with a significantly higher risk of smoking initiation in adolescent offspring. They also observed that fathers who smoked had a stronger effect on boys than girls initiation of smoking, and a stronger effect of parental smoking before the adolescent was age 13 than afterwards was also observed. Hunang et al. (7) found that seeing a family member smoke predicted a higher risk of experimentation with smoking.

HEALTH EFFECTS OF ADOLESCENT SMOKING

Adolescents' habitual smoking not only leads to all kinds of substance abuse but also causes various health problems. Adolescent smokers suffer from respiratory diseases (16). Gold et al. (17) found that children who took up smoking had higher rates of having had asthma (14%t vs. 10%) and wheezing but not asthma (65% vs. 50%), and concluded that cigarette smoking is associated with evidence of mild airway obstruction and slowed growth of lung function in adolescents. Stress has been associated with initiation to smoking and with maintenance of the behaviour (18-20), although smoking has been cited as a means of dealing with stress among young smokers (21) since nicotine may moderate stress.

Adolescence engage in smoking while searching for identity, new experiences, becoming independence from the parents, and accessing their peers and being accepted by them (22, 23). Whatever it takes, we must ensure that we prevent initiation of smoking or experimental smoking among adolescents because even infrequent experimental smoking in adolescence significantly increases the risk of adult smoking (24). The observation by Gold et al. (17) that the effect of relatively small amounts of cigarette smoke on lung function impairment of children and adolescents further supports the prevention of adolescents to initiate smoking.

Adolescents' smoking is influenced by home and school environment. It is therefore necessary to design preventive education interventions using peer groups at school and engaging homes and communities to protect adolescents' health. These interventions may be guided by the World Health Organization (WHO) Framework Convention on Tobacco Control (FCTC) that addresses the health, social, environmental and economic consequences of tobacco consumption and exposure to tobacco smoke worldwide (http://www.who.int/fctc/text_download/en/). Tobacco control measures include bans on tobacco advertising, promotion and sponsorship, and protection from exposure to second-hand smoke.

REFERENCES

[1] Giovino GA, Henningfield JE, Tomar SL, Escobedo LG, Slade J. Epidemiology of tobacco use and dependence. Epidemiol Rev1995; 17: 48–65.

[2] Gilpin EA, Lee L, Evans N, Pierce JP. Smoking initiation rates in adults and minors: United States, 1944-1988. Am J Epidemiol 1994; 140: 535–43.

[3] Lamkin L, Houston TP. Nicotine dependency and adolescents: Preventing and treating. Prim Care 1998; 25: 123-35.
[4] Houston TP, Kolbe LJ, Eriksen MP. Tobacco-use cessation in the 90s- not "adults only" anymore. Prev Med 1998; 27: A1-A2.
[5] Hanewinkel R, Isensee B, Sargent JD, Morgenstern M. Cigarette advertising and teen smoking initiation. Pediatrics. 2011; 127: e271–8.
[6] Henriksen L, Schleicher NC, Feighery EC, Fortmann SP. A longitudinal study of exposure to retail cigarette advertising and smoking initiation. Pediatrics 2010; 126: 232–8.
[7] Huang C, Koplan J, Yu S, Li C, Guo C, Liu J, et al. Smoking experimentation among elementary school students in China: Influences from peers, families, and the school environment. PLoS One 2013; 8: e73048.
[8] Kobus K. Peers and adolescent smoking. Addiction 2003; 98: 37–55.
[9] Steinberg L, Monahan KC. Age differences in resistance to peer influence. Dev Psychol 2007; 43: 1531–43.
[10] Kirke DM. Chain reactions in adolescents' cigarette, alcohol, and drug use: similarity through peer influence or the patterning of ties in peer networks. Soc Networks. 2004; 26: 3–28.
[11] O'Loughlin J, Paradis G, Renaud L, Gomez LS. One-year predictors of smoking initiation and of continued smoking among elementary schoolchildren in multiethnic, low-income, inner-city neighbourhoods. Tobacco Control 1998; 7: 268–75.
[12] Sichletidis LT, Chloros DA, Tsiotsios AI, Spyratos DG. Prevalence and risk factors for initiation of smoking in Greek high-school students. Int J Environ Res Public Health 2009; 6: 971-9.
[13] Botvin GJ, Baker E, Goldberg CJ, Dusenbury L, Botvin EM. Correlates and predictors of smoking among Black adolescents. Addict Behav 1992; 17: 97–103.
[14] Biglan A, Duncan TE, Ary DV, Smolkowski K. Peer and parental influences on adolescent tobacco use. J Behav Med 1995; 18: 315-30.
[15] Gilman SE, Rende R, Boergers J, Abrams DB, Buka SL, Clark MA, et al. Parental smoking and adolescent smoking initiation: an intergenerational perspective on tobacco control. Pediatrics 2009; 123: e274–81.
[16] Myers MG, Brown SA. Smoking and health in substance-abusing adolescents: a two-year follow-up. Pediatrics 1994; 93: 561–6.
[17] Gold DR, Wang X Wypij D, Speizer FE, Ware JH, Dockery DW. Effects of cigarette smoking on lung function in adolescent boys and girls. N Engl J Med 1996; 335: 931-7.
[18] Bonaguro JA, Bonaguro EW. Self-concept, stress symptomatology, and tobacco use. J Sch Health 1987; 57: 56–8.
[19] Reppucci JD, Revenson TA, Aber M, Dickon Reppucci N. Unrealistic optimism among adolescent smokers and nonsmokers. J Primary Prev 1991; 11: 227–36.
[20] Byrne DG, Byrne AE, Reinhart MI. Personality, stress and the decision to commence cigarette smoking in adolescence. J Psychosom Res 1995; 39: 53–62.
[21] Mates D, Allison KR. Sources of stress and coping responses of high school students. Adolescence 1992; 27: 461–74.

[22] McDermott RJ, Sarvela PD, Hoalt PN, Bajracharya SM, Marty PJ, Emery EM. Multiple correlates of cigarette use among high school students. J Sch Health 1992; 62: 146-50.

[23] Sperber AD, Peleg A, Friger M, Shvartzman P. Factors associated with daily smoking among Israeli adolescents; a prospective cohort study with a 3-year follow-up. Prev Med 2001; 33: 73-81.

[24] Chassin L, Presson CC, Sherman SJ, Edwards DA. The natural history of cigarette smoking: predicting young-adult smoking outcomes from adolescent smoking patterns. Health Psychol 1990; 9: 701–16.

Section one: Smoking

In: Smoking and Adolescence ISBN: 978-1-63484-311-9
Editors: M. L. Mazabam, S. Siziya et al. © 2016 Nova Science Publishers, Inc.

Chapter 2

PREVALENCE AND CORRELATES FOR CIGARETTE SMOKING AMONG SCHOOL-GOING ADOLESCENTS: AN INTERNATIONAL PERSPECTIVE FROM THE GLOBAL YOUTH TOBACCO SURVEYS

Mazyanga L Mazaba*[*] *and Seter Siziya
World Health Organization, Lusaka,
Zambia and Department of Clinical Sciences,
School of Medicine, Copperbelt University, Ndola, Zambia

Smoking cigarettes is a growing epidemic globally. The Global Tobacco Surveillance System (GTSS) was developed to assist World Health Organization (WHO) member countries to collect data to prevent and control tobacco use. The GTSS includes collection of data through three surveys. The Global Youth Tobacco Survey (GYTS), a school-based adolescents' survey, is one of the three surveys used in the collection of data. The objectives of this review were to determine the prevalence of cigarette smoking and its correlates across the World Health Organization regions in order to inform policy on what factors may be considered in designing interventions to curtail the epidemic of cigarette smoking. Overall prevalence of smoking ranged from 4.9% in East Mediterranean region to 19.2% in European region with a median (Q1, Q3) prevalence

[*] Corresponding author: Mazyanga L Mazaba, BSc, MSc, World Health Organization, Lusaka, Zambia. E-mail: mazmazli@yahoo.com; liwewema@who.int.

of 10.7 (5.7, 15.5)%. The lowest median of overall prevalence of smoking was in East Mediterranean region (6.3%) and highest in European region (17.6%). Girls were less likely to smoke cigarettes than boys in the regions of Africa, Eastern Mediterranean, South-East Asia, and Western Pacific; yet in the Americas girls were more likely than boys to smoke cigarettes. No significant gender differences were observed in the Americas and Europe. Prevalence and correlates for smoking varied within and between regions. Site specific interventions must be designed considering site specific correlates for smoking in order to curtail the epidemic of cigarette smoking.

INTRODUCTION

Cigarette smoking in adolescents is a global public health problem. Among adolescents who smoke cigarettes, about 25% smoked their first cigarette before the age of 10 years, and become addicted to smoking, leading to ill health (1). Smoking cigarettes is a growing epidemic globally. In response to curtail or prevent the epidemic in some regions, the World Health Organization (WHO), Centers for Disease Control and Prevention (CDC), and Canadian Public Health Association (CPHA) developed the Global Tobacco Surveillance System (GTSS) to assist WHO Member countries to collect data to prevent and control tobacco use. The GTSS includes collection of data through three surveys. The Global Youth Tobacco Survey (GYTS), a school-based adolescents' survey, is one of the three surveys used in the collection of data. The other two surveys being: the Global School Personnel Survey (GSPS) and the Global Health Professional Survey (GHPS) for adults (2).

Prior to the commencement of the GTYS system, there were a few cross-country systems such as the Health Behaviour in School Aged Children [HBSC] and the European School Survey Project on Alcohol and Drugs [ESPAD] in Western Europe. The GYTS was initiated in December 1998 and by 2005, the GYTS had achieved broad global coverage in 140 WHO member across all six WHO Regions countries and 11 territories. The surveys were repeated every 4-5 years and more than 40 countries had conducted a second round of the GYTS by 2005 (3-5).

For most sample designs, a minimum of 1500 completed student interviews was needed to obtain a precision level of ±5% for a given estimate. The desired sample size was then adjusted for anticipated non-response at the school, class, and student levels. GYTS used a standard methodology for sampling schools and classes in which most students aged 13-15 years were found. Schools were selected in two stages: in the first stage, schools were selected with probability proportional to school enrolment size, and then classes were systematically sampled. All students in the selected classes, regardless of their ages, were eligible to participate in the surveys.

The GYTS questionnaire was a self-administered anonymously in one class period, consisting of a "core" set of questions that were used by all countries. Some of the core questions were not relevant in some countries and were rephrased or omitted entirely. There was an optional set of questions that countries could use depending on their needs. The 2001 core questionnaire consisted of 56 questions and included questions on: prevalence of tobacco use, age of initiation, exposure to tobacco advertising, perceptions and attitudes towards tobacco use, media and advertising, and environmental tobacco smoke. Valladolid-Lopez et al. [6] evaluated the validity of self-reported smoking in Mexican adolescents and concluded that self-reported current smoking (having smoked even a puff in the past 30 days) used in the GYTS was a valid and stable indicator of current smoking behavior that could be used for public health research and surveillance. The completed questionnaires were computerized using an optical reader scanner. Consistency and out-of-range checks were performed to ensure high quality data. Before the surveys were conducted approval was sought from ethical research committees and permission obtained from relevant authorities. During the analysis, the data was weighted using the following formula:

$$W = W1 * W2 * f1 * f2 * f3 * f4$$

where

W1 =the inverse of the probability of selection for each school

W2 = the inverse of the probability of selection of each classroom within each selected school

f1 = a school level, non-response adjustment calculated by school enrolment size category (small, medium, large); school non-response is calculated within each tertile

f2 = a class level, non-response adjustment factor calculated for each school

f3 = a student level, non-response adjustment factor calculated by class

f4 = a post-stratification adjustment factor calculated by gender and grade.

The objectives of this review were to determine the prevalence of cigarette smoking and its correlates across the World Health Organization regions in order to inform policy on what factors may be considered in designing interventions to curtail the epidemic of cigarette smoking.

Table 1. Participating WHO member states in the GTYS between 2000 and 2007

WHO region	Number of states and territories in WHO region*	Number of states and territories who participated in GTYS (%)
Africa	47	29 (61.7)
Americas	47	38 (80.9)
East Mediterranean	23	23 (100)
European	54	29 (53.7)
South East Asia	11	10 (90.9)
Western Pacific	37	22 (59.5)

* http://www.who.int/countries/en/.

FINDINGS

The prevalence of smoking across WHO regions and territories (4) was reviewed. A total of 29 WHO member states and territories in Africa, 38 in Americas, 23 in East Mediterranean, 29 in European, 10 in South East Asia and 22 in West Pacific region participated in the GTYS between 2000 and 2007. European, Western Pacific and Africa regions were under sampled (see Table 1).

Table 2. Median prevalence of smoking by WHO region

WHO region	Median (Q_1, Q_3)
Africa	7.2 (3.9, 12.3)
Americas	13.0 (7.2, 18.0)
East Mediterranean	6.3 (4.6, 8.6)
European	17.6 (8.1, 26.5)
South East Asia	9.2 (3.8, 11.9)
Western Pacific	17.0 (6.5, 26.6)

Overall prevalence of smoking ranged from 4.9% in East Mediterranean region to 19.2% in European region with a median (Q_1, Q_3) prevalence of 10.7 (5.7, 15.5)%. The lowest median of overall prevalence of smoking (see Table 2) was in East Mediterranean region (6.3%) and highest in European region (17.6%).

Gender difference in prevalence of smoking

Surveys were conducted in 25 European countries between 2002-2005. In 17 of these 25 countries, current cigarette smoking did not differ between boys and girls (7). In another study involving 151 sites, Warren et al. (4) reported that the level of cigarette smoking between boys and girls was similar in many sites. Specifically, girls were less likely to smoke cigarettes than boys in the regions of Africa, Eastern Mediterranean, South-East Asia, and Western Pacific; yet in the Americas girls were more likely than boys to smoke cigarettes. No significant gender differences were observed in the Americas and Europe (8).

Correlates of cigarettes smoking

Apart from gender being associated with smoking in some sites, The Global Youth Tobacco Survey Collaborative Group (1) observed other correlates for tobacco use that varied between sites. These included: cultural and religious norms, availability of different types of tobacco products, tobacco control strategies, and tobacco industry behaviour to promote tobacco use.

Changes in prevalence of smoking observed in GTYS

Warren et al. (9) observed that of the 100 sites surveyed, 61 reported no change over time in prevalence of cigarette smoking. In another study, El-Awa et al. (10) reporting using data from 13 EMR countries and the areas administered by the Palestinian Authority found that between the initial survey and the repeat survey, the level of smoking decreased significantly in two sites, increased significantly in one site, but did not change significantly in the other sites. Even in the absence of an intervention, GYTS may act as an intervention.

Conclusion

The prevalence of and correlates for smoking varied within and between WHO regions. Site specific interventions must be designed considering site specific correlates for smoking in order to curtail the epidemic of cigarette smoking.

References

[1] The Global Youth Tobacco Survey Collaborative Group. Tobacco use among youth: a cross country comparison. Tob Control 2002; 11: 252–70.

[2] Global Tobacco Surveillance System Collaborating Group. Global Tobacco Surveillance System (GTSS): purpose, production, and potential. J Sch Health. 2005; 75: 15-24.

[3] The GTSS Collaborative Group. The Global Tobacco Surveillance System. Tob Control 2006; 15(Suppl II): ii1–ii3.

[4] Warren CW, Jones NR, Peruga A, Chauvin J, Baptiste J-P, de Silva VC, et al. Global Youth Tobacco Surveillance, 2000-2007. MMWR Surveill Summ 2008; 57: 1-28.

[5] Warren CW, Lee J, Lea V, Goding A, O'Hara B, Carlberg M, et al. Evolution of the Global Tobacco Surveillance System (GTSS) 1998–2008. Glob Health Promot 2009; 16(Supp 2):4-37.

[6] Valladolid-Lopez MC, Barrientos-Gutierrez T, Reynales-Shigematsu LM, Thrasher JF, Pelaez-Ballestas I, Lazcano-Ponce E, et al. Evaluating the validity of self-reported smoking in Mexican adolescents. BMJ Open 2015; 5: e007485.

[7] Baska T, Warren CW, Baskova M, Jones NR. Prevalence of youth cigarette smoking and selected social factors in 25 European countries: findings from the Global Youth Tobacco Surveys. Int J Public Health 2009; 54: 439-45.

[8] The GTSS Atlas: Part Three: Global Youth Tobacco Survey. URL: http://www.cdc.gov/tobacco/global/gtss/tobacco_atlas/pdfs/part3.pdf.

[9] Warren CW, Lea V, Lee J, Jones NR, Asma S, McKenna M. Change in tobacco use among 13–15 year olds between 1999 and 2008: findings from the Global Youth Tobacco Survey. Glob Health Promot 2009 (Supp 2):38-90.

[10] El-Awa F, Warren CW, Jones NR. Changes in tobacco use among 13–15-year-olds between 1999 and 2007: findings from the Eastern Mediterranean Region. East Mediterr Health J 2010; 16: 266-73.

In: Smoking and Adolescence ISBN: 978-1-63484-311-9
Editors: M. L. Mazabam, S. Siziya et al. © 2016 Nova Science Publishers, Inc.

Chapter 3

ADOLESCENT SMOKING IN RURAL AND URBAN AREAS IN THE LUSAKA PROVINCE, ZAMBIA

Seter Siziya *

Department of Community Medicine, School of Medicine,
University of Zambia, Lusaka, Zambia

Results on the association between smoking and urbanization have not been consistent. In this chapter the prevalence rates of smoking in school-going adolescents among urban, peri-urban, and rural districts in Lusaka province of Zambia is compared. Secondary analysis was conducted on the Zambia Global Youth tobacco Survey (GTYS) data that was collected in 2007. A total of 2,378 adolescents in Lusaka urban, 1,756 in Kafue per-urban, and 1,386 in Chongwe/Luangwa rural districts were enrolled into the study. Smoking rates were 10.5% in urban, 11.1% in peri-urban, and 13.5% in rural districts. After adjusting for age, gender, grade, parental and best friend smoking status, and knowing that smoking is harmful to health, compared to adolescents in Lusaka urban districts were 17% (AOR = 1.17; 95%CI [1.10, 1.23]) more likely to smoke cigarettes. No significant difference in smoking rates was observed between adolescents in urban and peri-urban districts. The prevalence rate of smoking among adolescents was higher in rural than urban district.

* Corresponding author: Professor Seter Siziya, Clinical Sciences Department, School of Medicine, Copperbelt University, Ndola Central Hospital, 6th Floor, P.O. Box 71191, Ndola, Zambia. E-mail: ssiziya@gmail.com.

Antismoking interventions should be more targeted to adolescents in rural than urban areas.

INTRODUCTION

Tobacco smoking is increasing in developing countries, and is linked to an increase in socioeconomic status despite the fact that it causes cancer and other diseases (1). However, the results on the association between smoking and urbanization have not been consistent. While there was no significant difference in tobacco use between urban and rural children in Cameroon (2) Steyn et al. (3) found that smoking patterns were influenced by the degree of urbanization in women of the Cape Peninsula, tobacco consumption in the urban than rural Tongans population was reported by Finau et al. (4).

With limited resources available for tobacco control, it is important that targeted interventions are conducted in areas with higher prevalence of tobacco smoking. And only in such areas would the impact of the intervention be easily evaluated. A pilot tobacco intervention is underway in Lusaka urban district, and a roll-out of the intervention should be in areas with high prevalence of smoking. The current study was conducted to compare smoking prevalence rates among urban, peri-urban and rural districts in the Lusaka province.

OUR STUDY

Data from the Lusaka-Zambia GYTS conducted in 2007 was used in the current study. A two stage cluster sampling design was used. A total of 25 schools were selected first with probability proportional to their student enrolment size, and 24 (96.0%) participated. In the second stage of sampling, classes were randomly selected and 2,678 students were sampled, out of whom 2,378 (88.8%) eventually participated in the survey.

A standard GYTS questionnaire with a few country-specific data was administered to students in their classrooms during one class period. A comprehensive description of the GYTS methodology has been reported elsewhere (5, 6). Students were asked the following question, among others: During the past 30 days (1 month), on how many days did you smoke cigarettes? Do your parents smoke? And do any of your friends smoke cigarettes?

The project coordinator for the Zambia 2007 GTYS provided the data for analysis. The GYTS data were analyzed in SPSS 11.5 (Chicago, IL, United States of America). As is the convention in the Global Tobacco Surveillance System (GTSS), current cigarette smoking was defined as having smoked a cigarette, even a single puff, within the last 30 days prior to the survey (5-7). A weighted analysis was conducted to obtain the prevalence of current cigarette smoking, as well as other relevant characteristics.

We report results of bivariate logistic regression analysis as unadjusted odds ratios (ORs), while the results from multivariate analysis are reported as adjusted odds ratio (AOR) together with their 95% confidence intervals (CI).

FINDINGS IN THIS STUDY

Totals of 2,378 students in Lusaka urban, 1,756 in Kafue peri-urban, and 1,386 in Chongwe/Luangwa rural districts participated in the survey. The prevalence rates for tobacco smoking were 10.5%, 11.1% and 13.5% in urban, peri-urban and rural districts respectively.

Table 1. Identification of confounding factors

Factor	**Exposure (District)**			
	Urban	**Peri-urban**	**Rural**	**Outcome (Smoking)**
	n (%)	**n (%)**	**n (%)**	**OR[1] (95% CI[2])**
Age (year)	$p < 0.001$			$p < 0.001$
≤11	151 (6.1)	125 (7.0)	86 (6.4)	1
12	256 (10.6)	148 (7.8)	114 (6.9)	1.00 (0.93,1.09)
13	404 (16.7)	249 (12.6)	167 (11.0)	0.49 (0.45, 0.53)
14	517 (22.3)	364 (19.7)	260 (17.1)	0.61 (057, 0.65)
15	441 (19.1)	333 (19.9)	271 (21.3)	0.85 (0.80, 0.90)
16	343 (15.1)	283 (17.8)	251 (20.3)	1.03 (0.97, 1.09)
17+	250 (10.0)	236 (15.2)	217 (16.9)	2.03 (1.92, 2.15)
Gender	$p < 0.001$			$p < 0.001$
Male	1281 (43.2)	818 (45.8)	661 (45.3)	1
Female	1093 (56.8)	936 (54.2)	714 (54.7)	0.85 (0.83, 087)
Grade	$P < 0.001$			$P < 0.001$
7	1030 (44.1)	696 (34.6)	576 (36.0)	1
8	686 (22.5)	475 (24.1)	557 (26.5)	0.81 (0.77, 0.86)

Table 1. (Continued)

Factor	Exposure (District)			
	Urban	Peri-urban	Rural	Outcome (Smoking)
	n (%)	n (%)	n (%)	OR[1] (95% CI[2])
9	660 (33.4)	1756 (41.3)	244 (37.6)	0.90 (0.86, 0.93)
Parental smoking status	P < 0.001			P < 0.001
None	1591 (77.2)	1060 (72.3)	846 (71.3)	1
Both	74 (3.4)	83 (5.6)	69 (5.0)	0.74.(1.59, 1.92)
Father only	354 (17.3)	286 (19.6)	286 (22.1)	0.89 (0.83, 0.95)
Mother only	41 (2.0)	40 (2.5)	25 (1.6)	2.32 (2.04, 2.63)
Best friends' smoking status	P < 0.001			P < 0.001
None	1613(69.4)	1054 (60.6)	921 (69.8)	1
Some	533 (22.0)	487 (28.3)	319 (21.8)	0.85 (0.81, 0.89)
Most	120 (4.70	126 (7.0)	88 (5.7)	1.67 (1.55, 1.79)
All	90 (3.9)	76 (4.2)	48 (2.8)	3.89 (3.59, 4.22)
Smoking is harmful to health	P < 0.001			P < 0.001
Definite not	786 (33.8)	628 (36.8)	459 (31.4)	1
Probably not	245 (10.0)	226 (12.5)	147 (10.2)	1.38 (1.31, 1.47)
Probably yes	194 (7.9)	162 (9.1)	138 (10.5)	1.48 (1.39, 1.15)
Definite yes	1141 (48.3)	719 (41.6)	635 (47.9)	0.66 (0.63, 0.69)

OR[1] Odds ratio CI[2] Confidence interval.

Table 1 shows that all the factors considered in the analysis were confounding the relationship between district (urban, peri-urban, and rural) and tobacco smoking.

In bivariate analysis (see Table 1), while respondents in a peri-urban district were less likely to smoke compared to respondents in an urban district, respondents in a rural district were more likely to smoke.

After adjusting for age, gender, grade, smoking status for parents and best friends, and knowing that smoking is harmful to health, the results did not significantly change. Compared to respondents in an urban district, respondents in a peri-urban district were 13% less likely to smoke; and respondents in a rural district were 20% more likely to smoke (see Table 2).

Table 2. Relationship between district (urban, peri-urban, and rural) and smoking status

District	Total	Smoker (%)	OR[1] (95% CI[2])	AOR[3] (95% CI)
Urban	2378	10.5	1	1
Peri-urban	1756	11.1	0.95 (0.91,1.00)	0.87 (0.83, 0.92)
Rural	1386	13.5	1.19 (1.13, 1.24)	1.20 (1.14, 1.26)

OR[1] Odds ratio; CI[2] confidence interval; AOR[3] Adjusted odds ratio.

DISCUSSION

A significant relationship between district (urban, peri-urban, and rural) and smoking status was observed in the current study. Respondents in a rural district were more likely to smoke cigarettes. This finding contradicts the results of Walker (1) who reported that the prevalence of smoking was linked to an increase in socioeconomic status; and of Finau et al. (4) who found significantly higher total tobacco consumption in the urban than rural Tongans population. It further contradicts the findings by Proctor et al. (2) who found no significant difference in tobacco use between urban and rural children in Cameroon.

While it has been generally reported that the prevalence of smoking is higher in developed than in developing countries, our finding suggests that this observation may not hold in other populations. Differences in smoking rates may be related to local cultural and social determinants, and not only to economic development. It is important to determine local smoking prevalence rates so that informed interventions may be instituted in areas of high prevalence rates. Factors driving the smoking epidemic should be considered in designing interventions for a targeted population.

There are limitations for the current study. For example, as in any cross sectional study, we cannot ascribe causation to the relationship between district and smoking. Further, the factors were self reported, and bias may have been introduced in our finding to the extent that the mis-reporting by the respondents differed among districts. There is no reason why the rate of mis-reporting should be different among districts. Although it is not possible to determine the magnitude and direction of the bias, it is believed that the effect of bias on the study finding may have been non-significant.

In conclusion, the finding that the prevalence rate of smoking was higher in rural than urban districts suggests that most antismoking interventions should be targeted to rural populations in the Lusaka province.

ACKNOWLEDGMENTS

The efforts by the research team and the students are gratefully acknowledged for making the survey a success.

This paper is a revised version of an original publication in Medical Journal of Zambia (Siziya S. Higher prevalence rates of smoking in rural than urban areas among school-going adolescents in the Lusaka province, Zambia. Med J Zambia 2009; 36:107-109) and the author have obtained the permission from Medical Journal of Zambia to use this material.

REFERENCES

[1] Walker AR Urbanisation of developing populations: what are the health/illhealth prospects regarding diseases of prosperity? Urban Health Newslett 1996; 30: 20-8.
[2] Proctor MH, Moore LL, Singer MR, Hood MY, Nguyen US, Ellison RC. Risk profile for non-communicable diseases in rural and urban school children in the Republic of Cameroon. Ethn Dis 1996; 6: 235-43.
[3] Steyn K, Kazenellenbogen JM, Lombard CJ, Bourne LT. Urbanization and the risk for chronic diseases of lifestyle in the black population of the Cape Peninsula, South Africa. J Cardiovasc Risk 1997, 4. 135-42.
[4] Finau SA, Stanhope JM, Prior IA. Kava, alcohol and tobacco consumption among Tongans with urbanization. Soc Sci Med 1982; 16: 35-41.
[5] The GTSS Collaborative Group. The global tobacco surveillance system. Top Control 2006; 15: ii1-3.
[6] Global Tobacco Surveillance System Collaborating Group. Global Tobacco Surveillance System (GTSS): Purpose, production, and potentional. J Sch Health 2005; 75: 15-24.
[7] Yang T, Wu Y, Abdullah ASM, Dai D, Fuzhong L, Wu J, et al. Attitudes and behavioral response toward key tobacco control measures from the FCTC among Chinese urban residents. BMC Public Health 2007; 7: 248.

In: Smoking and Adolescence ISBN: 978-1-63484-311-9
Editors: M. L. Mazabam, S. Siziya et al. © 2016 Nova Science Publishers, Inc.

Chapter 4

TOBACCO SMOKING PREVALENCE AMONG IN-SCHOOL ADOLESCENTS AGED 13-15 YEARS IN ZAMBIA

Richard Zulu[1], BA, MPhil,
Seter Siziya[2,*], BA(Ed), MSc, PhD,
and Selestine H Nzala[2], MBChB, MPH
[1]Institute of Economic and Social Research,
University of Zambia, Lusaka
[2]Department of Community Medicine, School of Medicine,
University of Zambia, Lusaka, Zambia

Zambia has been controlling tobacco use in terms of legislative interventions, and acceding to the World Health organization (WHO) Framework Convention on Tobacco Control (FCTC). In this chapter we aimed to determine the baseline prevalence of current smoking to be used in the evaluation of the implementation of the WHO FCTC. Survey data from the 2002 and 2007 Global Youth Tobacco Surveys (GYTS) were used to estimate the prevalence of tobacco use. The standard protocol for GYTS was used in the surveys, and only data for students aged 13 to 15 years was used in the analysis. Data were analyzed using SUDAAN (Research Triangle institute), and SPSS (version 11.5) software packages.

[*] Corresponding author: Professor Seter Siziya, Clinical Sciences Department, School of Medicine, Copperbelt University, Ndola Central Hospital, 6th Floor, P.O. Box 71191, Ndola, Zambia. E-mail: ssiziya@gmail.com.

Weighted analysis was used to produce estimates together with their 95% confidence intervals (CI). The current cigarette smokers were 9.2% in 2002 and 6.8% in 2007 ($p > 0.05$), with an overall rate of 7.4% (95%CI [7.1, 7.7]). No significant difference in current cigarette smoking rates was observed between gender. However, compared to students of age 15 years, those of ages 13 and 14 years were less likely to be current smokers (AOR = 0.82, 95%CI [0.77, 0.88]) for 13 years, and AOR = 0.90, 95% CI [0.85, 0.96] for 14 years). The results showed that the Lusaka district is in the first stage of the tobacco epidemic. There is urgent need, guided by the WHO FCTC, for effective interventions to be put in place before the epidemic becomes unmanageable.

INTRODUCTION

Tobacco use is one of the major preventable causes of death in the world. The World Health Organization (WHO) attributes some 4 million deaths a year to tobacco use, a figure which is expected to rise to 8.4 deaths a year by 2020 (1). Developing countries are in the first stage of the tobacco epidemic (2). The initiation of tobacco smoking by most adults occurs early in life as adolescents or young adults. However, comprehensive tobacco prevention and control information on young people has been rare until recently when the Global Youth Tobacco Surveys (GYTS) started conducting surveys among in-school adolescents targeting those of ages 13-15 years (3). To address the problem of lack of information on tobacco use in Zambia, the Global Youth Tobacco Survey (GYTS) was conducted in 2002 and a repeat GYTS in 2007. GYTS is an international surveillance project that generates comparisons of tobacco use between countries with the aim to enhance the capacity of countries to monitor tobacco use and to evaluate preventive programs.

The aim of the GYTS is to enhance the capacity of a country to design, implement and evaluate comprehensive tobacco control programs. It is a school-based survey that focuses on adolescents aged 13 to 15 years. The specific objectives of the survey are: (a) To assess knowledge, attitudes and practices related to tobacco smoking, exposure, prevention, community programs and media interventions; (b) To make comparison over time between the initial GYTS and the repeat GYTS; and (c) To give suggestions to local partners on the best modalities for implementing and up-scaling of tobacco control programs.

Since the surveys in Zambia were conducted before Zambia accented to the WHO Framework Convention on Tobacco Control (FCTC), the current study aims to determine the prevalence of tobacco use as baseline to which the implementation of the WHO FCTC would be evaluated. Another objective of the current study was to compare these rates to determine if there were changes in the rates of tobacco smoking in the absence of tangible interventions.

OUR STUDY

The GYTS were school-based cross sectional surveys of students in grades 7 to 9, conducted in 2002 and 2007, to mainly enroll 13-15 years old adolescents in the surveys. Detailed descriptions of the purpose and methodology for GYTS have been described elsewhere (4). In collaboration with the Ministry of Education (MOE), it was decided to conduct the survey in the Lusaka province in which the capital city, Lusaka, is located. The province has four districts namely: Lusaka, Kafue, Chongwe, and Luangwa districts. The present study was limited to the Lusaka district.

A two-stage cluster sample design was used to produce representative data for the district. At the first stage, schools were selected with probability proportional to enrolment size. At the second stage, classes were randomly selected and all students in selected classes were eligible to participate. The response rate in 2002 for schools was 96.0%, 87.5% for students, with an overall response rate of 84% (5). Meanwhile the response rates in 2007 for schools, students, and overall were 96%, 88.8%, and 85.3%, respectively (Zambia, Lusaka 2007 fact sheet, unpublished).

A self-administered structured questionnaire was used to collect data. The questionnaire was completed within one class session. Students recorded their responses directly on answer sheets that were later scanned by computer for data entry. Although the questionnaire included questions on age, gender, history of ever smoked cigarettes, current cigarette smoking status, having parents or friends who smoked cigarettes, exposure to environmental tobacco smoke, and perceptions on cigarette smoking, the current study only used data on ever smoked cigarettes and current smoking status.

Although data was collected from all the adolescents irrespective of their ages in grades 7 to 9, for the purpose of comparison, only data from 13-15 year olds were analyzed. Data were analyzed using SUDAAN (Research Triangle institute), and SPSS (version 11.5) software packages. Tobacco rates were stratified by gender. Percents and their 95% confidence intervals are presented. The analysis was weighted in order to adjust for varying non response rate and probability of selection at the school, grade and student levels. The weight use has been described by The GYTS Collaborating Group 7, and given as:

Table 1. Descriptions of the samples

Factor	2002	2007
	n* (%)**	n* (%)**
Grade		
7	779 (83.0)	613 (45.8)
8	259 (8.5)	447 (25.7)
9	200 (8.4)	301 (28.5)
Age		
13	363 (32.7)	404 (28.7)
14	487 (38.6)	517 (38.4)
15	391 (28.7)	441 (32.9)
Gender		
Male	568 (50.7)	681 (40.3)
Female	660 (49.3)	681 (59.7)

* Unweighted frequency ** weighted percent.

$$W = W1*W2*f1*f2*f3*f4$$

where:

W1 = the inverse of the probability of selecting a school
W2 = the inverse of the probability of selecting a grade within a school
f1 = a school-level non response adjustment factor calculated by school size category (small, medium, large)
f2 = a grade-level non response adjustment factor calculated for each school
f3 = a student level non response adjustment factor calculated by grade
f4 = a post stratification adjustment factor calculated by grade

Informed consent was obtained from the respondents before data collection. For this purpose, an information sheet was read to respondents so that they were informed about the study. The survey procedures were designed to protect students' privacy by allowing for anonymous and voluntary participation.

OUR FINDINGS

Totals of 1,241 adolescents in 2002, and 1,362 in 2007 aged 13-15 years participated in the surveys. The samples comprised of 50.7% males in 2002 and 40.3% males in 2007. The sample in 2007 tended to be in higher grades, and older than the sample in 2002. Table 1 shows the descriptions of the samples.

Overall, 28.0% of the students had ever smoked cigarettes in 2002 compared to 22.3% in 2007. The current cigarette smokers were 9.2% in 2002 and 6.8% in 2007. The above comparisons were not significant ($p > 0.05$) as shown in Table 2. The overall current smoking prevalence was 7.4% (95% CI [7.1, 7.7]).

Table 3 shows comparisons of rates for ever smoked cigarettes and current cigarette smoking. Students in 2002 were 8% (AOR = 1.08, 95% CI [1.05, 1.11]) more likely to have ever smoked cigarettes compared to students in 2007. Compared to students of age 15 years, those of age 13 years were 21% (AOR = 0.79, 95% CI [0.76, 0.82]) less likely to have ever smoked cigarettes. Meanwhile, students of age 14 years were 4% (AOR = 1.04, 95% CI [1.01, 1.08]) more like to have ever smoked cigarettes compared to students of age 15 years. Male students were 21% (AOR = 1.21, 95% CI [1.18, 1.32]) more likely to have ever smoked cigarettes than female students.

No significant differences in current smoking rates were observed between 2002 and 2007, and between gender. However, compared to students of age 15 years, those of ages 13 and 14 years were less likely to be current smokers (AOR = 0.82, 95% CI [0.77, 0.88]) for 13 years, and AOR = 0.90, 95% CI [0.85, 0.96] for 14 years).

Table 2. Prevalence rates of tobacco use among in-school adolescents in 2002 and 2007

Year/Factor	Total OR* (95% CI**)	Males OR* (95% CI**)	Females OR* (95% CI**)
2002			
Ever smoked cigarettes	28.0 (21.7, 35.3)	32.9 (23.0, 44.6)	22.8 (17.2, 29.6)
Current cigarette smoker	9.2 (6.7, 12.6)	9.4 (6.3, 13.9)	8.7 (4.6, 15.9)
2007			
Ever smoked cigarettes	22.3 (17.0, 28.8)	25.3 (19.9, 31.5)	20.4 (14.4, 28.0)
Current cigarette smoker	6.8 (4.3, 10.5)	6.7 (4.0, 11.1)	6.8 (4.0, 11.3)

* Unadjusted odds ratio ** confidence interval.

Table 3. Comparison of ever smoked and current smoking prevalence rates between 2002 and 2007 adjusted for age, gender, and grade

	Ever smoked	Current smoker
Factor	**AOR* (95% CI**)**	**AOR* (95% CI**)**
Year		
2002	1.08 (1.05, 1.11)	1.01 (0.96, 1.06)
2007	1	1
Age		
13	0.79 (9.76, 0.82)	0.82 (0.77, 0.88)
14	1.04 (1.01, 1.08)	0.90 (0.85, 0.960
15	1	1
gender		
Male	1.21 (1.18, 1.32)	0.99 (0.95, 1.03)
Female	1	1
Grade		
7	1.27 (1.22, 1.32)	1.80 (1.68, 1.93)
8	0.63 (0.60, 0.66)	0.70 (0.64, 0.76)
9	1	1

* Adjusted odds ratio ** confidence interval.

DISCUSSION

We found no significant difference in the rates of current cigarette smokers between 2002 and 2007. The overall combined rate of current cigarette smokers was 7.4%. This rate compares very well with what has been reported in neighboring countries for males of 4.2 (+4.8)% in Blantyre, and 9.5 (+3.1)% in Lilongwe in Malawi; similar to that reported in Manicaland, Zimbabwe of 10.3% (+3.9)%; and in Mozambique of 5.0 (+2.5)% in Maputo and 5.0 (+3.9)% in Gaza, Inhambe; lower than that observed in Harare of 11.6% (+3.0)%; and higher than that reported in Botswana of 3.9 (+1.6)% (6). Compared to other rates observed in the neighboring countries for females, our rate was higher than that observed in Botswana (2.1 [+1.3])%, Malawi (0.9 [+0.5]% in Blantyre, and 3.1 [+2.1]% in Lilongwe), and in Mozambique (1.4 [+1.1])% in Maputo, and 3.2 [+2.3])% in Gaza Inhambe), but comparable to those obtained in Zimbabwe (9.9 [+5.0])% in Harare, and 8.7 [+4.2])% in Manicaland) (7).

Considering the tobacco epidemic model proposed by Lopez et al. (2), the above rates are lower than 20%, suggesting that the tobacco epidemic is in its infancy in Zambia, and in its neighboring countries. The time to act to control this epidemic in is now. However, before Zambia accented to the WHO FCTC on 28th May 2008, she had already started the campaign against tobacco. It 1992, It banned cigarette sales to minors who are less than 16 years of age (The Public Health (Tobacco) Regulation, 1992), and free products (The Public Health (Tobacco) Regulation, 1992; Health regulation-Statutory Instrument No. 163 of 1992; dated 7 December 1992). It also banned tobacco advertisement in mass media (Statutory Instrument No. 163, 1992), smoking in government buildings (The Public Health (Tobacco) Regulation, 1992; Health regulation-Statutory Instrument No. 163 of 1992; dated 7 December 1992), private worksites (Factory Act), educational facilities, health care facilities, and public transport, and other public places (The Public Health (Tobacco) Regulation, 1992; Health regulation-Statutory Instrument No. 163 of 1992; dated 7 December 1992). There is a further restriction on the label design on packaging. Advertisements must display the warning "Warning: Tobacco is harmful to health" (The Public Health (Tobacco) Regulation, 1992). Each tobacco product pack must display the following warning "WARNING: TOBACCO IS HARMFUL TO HEALTH" (The Public Health (Tobacco) Regulation, 1992, Regulation 3). The warning must be printed on both sides of the larger surface area of the pack in bold letters against a contrasting background (The Public Health (Tobacco) Regulation, 1992, Regulation 3). More recently the Local government (Prohibition of Smoking in public Places) regulations, 2008 (The Local Government Act, Laws, Volume 16, Cap 281) has come into force. These pieces of tobacco control legislation will now be backed by the newly ratified WHO FCTC to make them more effective. The success of the implementation of the WHO FCTC in Zambia would depend on the maintenance or reduction of the 7.4% current smoking rate. Since most adults who smoke may have started the habit when they were adolescents, a feasible intervention would be to control or prevent tobacco smoking among in-school adolescents. This is the target for the current study. Inclusion of tobacco control in primary and secondary school syllabi should be considered. Interventions targeting out-of-school adolescents should also be explored. Generally, Zambia should be guided by the WHO FCTC to formulate effective intervention policies and programs.

We observed no gender difference in the current cigarette smoking rates. This finding confirms what has been reported in Zimbabwe, and contradicts findings from Botswana, Malawi, and in Maputo in which more males than females were current cigarette smokers (6).

Our finding of no gender difference in current smoking rate may be explained as follows: female adolescents may perceive smoking to be fashionable as equally as male adolescents do. Communities may also tolerate adolescent smoking without respect to gender. On the contrary, gender differences in adolescent smoking may be due to differential perceptions communities have towards male and female adolescent smokers. Communities may be more tolerant to male than female smoking.

Younger age groups were less likely to smoke because the fewer who smoked may have been experimenting. Smoking even a single puff should be discouraged among the adolescents because this experimentation may develop into a habit.

Data collection was limited to school-going adolescents and so may not be representative of all adolescents in Lusaka district, Zambia. Our results may be biased to the extent non respondents differed from the participants. Non respondents were not followed up to obtain information that could have been used to compare respondents and non respondents in order to determine the magnitude and direction of bias due to non respondents. Also the data were self-reported and so mis-reporting is possible whether deliberate or inadvertent. We are unable to determine the direction of bias that might have arisen in our results. However, we feel that the magnitude of bias that may have been introduced is not significant because of high response rates achieved in the surveys, and that most of the adolescents of school-going age were attending schools.

In conclusion, the results of this study show that the Lusaka district is in the first stage of the tobacco epidemic. There is urgent need, guided by the WHO FCTC, for effective interventions to be put in place before the epidemic becomes unmanageable.

ACKNOWLEDGMENTS

We thank all the study participants for their involvement in the study. We are also grateful to the Centers for Disease Control and Prevention (CDC) for making the 2002 GYTS available to us for analysis. The 2007 GYTS data set was availed by the first author, Richard Zulu who coordinated both surveys. The CDC had no influence regarding the analysis that we conducted, nor the decision to have these findings published.

This chapter is a revised version of an original paper published in the Medical Journal of Zambia (Zulu R, Siziya S, Nzala SH. Tobacco smoking prevalence among in-school adolescents aged 13-15 years: baseline for evaluation of the implementation of the FTCTC in Lusaka district, Zambia. Med J Zambia 2008; 35: 100-4) and the authors have obtained the permission from Medical Journal of Zambia to use this material.

REFERENCES

[1] WHO Report on the Global Tobacco Epidemic 2008, The MPOWER Package. Geneva, World Health Organization, 2008.

[2] Lopez AD, Collishaw NE, Piha T. A descriptive model of the cigarette epidemic in developed countries. Tob Control 1994; 3: 242-7.

[3] The Global Youth Tobacco Survey Collaborating Group: Tobacco use among youth: a cross country comparison. Tob Control 2002; 11: 252-70.

[4] Global Tobacco Surveillance System Collaborating Group. Global Tobacco Surveillance System (GTSS): purpose, production, and potential. J Sch Health 2005; 75: 15-24.

[5] Warren CW, Jones NR, Peruga A, Chauvin J, Baptiste JP, Costa de Silva V, et al. Global youth tobacco surveillance, 2000-2007. MMWR Surveill Summ 2008; 57: 1-28.

[6] Global Youth Tobacco Survey Collaborating Group. Differences in worldwide tobacco use by gender: findings from the Global Youth Tobacco Survey. J Sch Health 2003; 73: 207-15.

In: Smoking and Adolescence ISBN: 978-1-63484-311-9
Editors: M. L. Mazabam, S. Siziya et al. © 2016 Nova Science Publishers, Inc.

Chapter 5

CIGARETTE SMOKING AMONG SCHOOL-GOING ADOLESCENTS

Seter Siziya[1,*], BA(Ed), MSc, PhD, Emmanuel Rudatsikira[2], MD, MPH, DrPH, and Adamson S Muula[3], MBBS, MPH, PhD

[1]Department of Community Medicine, University of Zambia, Medical School, Lusaka, Zambia
[2]Departments of Epidemiology and Biostatistics and Global Health, Loma Linda University, School of Public Health, Loma Linda, California, USA
[3]Department of Community Health, University of Malawi, College of Medicine, Blantyre, Malawi

Cigarette smoking is a leading cause of global morbidity and mortality. Interest in developing countries smoking prevalence has been growing since 1999. In this chapter we estimate the prevalence of current cigarette smoking and associated factors among school-age adolescents in Kafue, Zambia. A cross sectional study was conducted using standard Global Youth Tobacco Survey (GYTS) methodology. Odds ratios were obtained to assess the association between selected factors and current cigarette smoking. Data on current smoking was available for 1872 adolescents, of

* Corresponding author: Professor Seter Siziya, Clinical Sciences Department, School of Medicine, Copperbelt University, Ndola Central Hospital, 6th Floor, P.O. Box 71191, Ndola, Zambia. E-mail: ssiziya@gmail.com.

whom 891 (47.6%) were males and 981 females. Overall 154 (8.2%) adolescents were current cigarette smokers, while 93 (10.4%) males and 61 (6.2%) females were current smokers ($p < 0.001$). The majority of the smokers usually smoked at own home or at a friends' house. Having some pocket money, friends or parents who are smokers, exposed to pro-tobacco advertisements at social gatherings were associated with being a current cigarette smoker. The traditional factors associated with smoking among adolescent elsewhere are also associated with smoking among adolescents in Kafue, Zambia. Public health interventions aimed to reduce adolescent smoking should be designed with these identified associations in mind.

INTRODUCTION

Tobacco is the single most important cause of chronic morbidity in the developed world (1-4). Although the bulk of morbidity and mortality in the sub-Saharan Africa arises from communicable diseases, overall the contribution of tobacco use to ill-health in the developing world has been growing. Tobacco is the leading cause of cancers, chronic obstructive airways diseases and cardiovascular mortality (1-7).

Cigarette smoking among adolescents is of public health importance as many adult smokers started smoking as adolescents or young adults. Smoking among adolescents has also been reported to be associated with other unhealthy life styles such as alcohol consumption, illicit drug use and pre-marital gender. Adolescent smokers are also likely to be truant from school, an experience that may further jeopardise their future life chances in life (8-10).

Since 1999, there has been growing interest in estimating the prevalence of adolescent tobacco use and associated social and political environmental factors. This impetus has largely been spearheaded by the Global Youth Tobacco Survey Collaborative Group (11-14).

In this chapter we use data from the Global Youth Tobacco Survey (GYTS) conducted in Kafue, Zambia to estimate the prevalence of current cigarette smoking and associated factors. This information is important in the design, implementation of public health interventions aimed to prevent adolescents' tobacco use in particular and overall health promotion among this population group.

OUR STUDY

The study was conducted in Kafue district, which is situated in Lusaka province, 45 km south of the Lusaka capital city of Zambia. The district had 77001 males and 73216 females (15). Major crops that are produced in the district were cotton and maize. Tobacco was only marginally produced.

Table 1. Variables considered in the analyses of factors associated with smoking

Dependent variable

Have you ever smoked cigarettes, even a single puff, in the last 30 days? Yes/no

Independent variables

Demographic, social and economic

1. Age (11 or 12, 13, 14, 15, 16 or 17)
2. Grade (7, 8 or 9)
3. Received pocket money (yes or no)

Parent and friends smoking status

4. Parents smoked cigarettes (yes or no)
5. Closest friends smoked cigarettes (yes or no)

Advertisements and campaigns against smoking

6. Had seen anti-smoking media messages during the past 30 days (yes or no)
7. Had seen anti-smoking messages at social gatherings (yes or no)
8. Had seen actors smoking on TV, videos or movies (yes or no)
9. Had something such as a t-shirt or pen with a cigarette brand logo on it (yes or no)
10. Had seen cigarette brand names on TV during the past 30 days (yes or no)
11. Had seen advertisements for cigarettes on billboards during the past 30 days (yes or no)
12. Had seen advertisements for cigarettes in newspapers or magazines during the past 30 days (yes or no)
13. Had seen advertisements for cigarettes at social gatherings (yes or no)

Effects of smoking on health

14. Smoking cigarettes is less dangerous for young people because they can always stop later (yes or no)
15. Cigarette smoking is harmful to health (yes or no)

Table 2. Number of cigarettes usually smoked per day during the past 30 days

Number of cigarettes usually smoked per day	Males Total = 92 n (%)	Females Total = 60 n (%)
<1	33 (35.9)	20 (33.3)
1	28 (30.4)	21 (35.0)
2-5	20 (21.7)	4 (6.7)
6+	11 (12.0)	15 (25.0)

Basic schools cater for grades 1 to 7 and secondary schools cater for grades 8 to 12. The district had 60 basic schools and 7 secondary schools by the year 2003. Totals of 4525, 645 and 746 adolescents were grades 7 to 9, respectively, in the male: female ratios of 1:0.9, 1:0.6 and 1:0.6, respectively (16).

The Kafue GYTS was conducted in 2002 as a cross sectional study, aimed to estimate the prevalence of tobacco use and associated personal and social environmental factors. School-going adolescents in grades 7 to 9 were recruited using a two-stage probability sampling technique. In the first stage of sampling, primary sampling units were schools which were selected with a probability of being selected proportional to their enrolment size. In the second step, a random sample of classes in the selected school was obtained. All students in the selected classes were eligible to participate. A self administered questionnaire was used and included core GYTS questions as has been described elsewhere regarding the GYTS methodology (11-14). Permission to conduct the study was obtained from the Ministry of Education. For the purposes of this study we aimed to estimate the prevalence of current cigarette smoking, assess whether there were any gender differences in the number of cigarettes smoked per day, and assess other social environmental factors associated with current cigarette smoking. The variables assessed in this study are outlined in Table 1. Current smoking was defined as having smoked, even a single puff in the past 30 days preceding the day of questionnaire completion. Data were analysed using SPSS 11.5 (Chicago, Illinois, United States). Upon considering all factors that were significant in bivariate analyses, we conducted Backward logistic regression analysis to determine independent predictors of current cigarette smoking.

FINDINGS

Information on smoking status and gender was available from 1872 adolescents. There were 891 (47.6%) males and 981 females. Overall 154 (8.2%) adolescents were current cigarette smokers. Of the 891 males, 93 (10.4%) were current smokers, while 61 (6.2%) of 981 females were current smokers ($p < 0.001$). Table 2 shows the frequency of smoking in the previous 30 days to the survey. Female respondents tended to smoke more cigarettes per day than males ($p = 0.027$).

Table 3 shows the places where the respondents usually smoked. Most respondents smoked at home (males 29.9%, females 23.5%) and at friends' houses (males 27.3%, females 29.4%).

Table 1 shows the variables that were considered in the analyses of factors associated with smoking status. Only the significant factors In bivariate analyses were further analysed in multivariate logistic regression.

Table 3. Places where respondents usually smoked

Place	**Males Total = 77 n (%)**	**Females Total = 51 n (%)**
At own home	23 (29.9)	12 (23.5)
At friend's house	21 (27.3)	15 (29.4)
At school	10 (13.0)	7 (13.7)
At work	7 (9.1)	2 (3.9)
At social events	9 (11.7)	7 (13.7)
In public places*	4 (5.2)	3 (5.9)
Other	3 (3.9)	5 (9.8)

* Public places included parks, shopping centres and street corners.

Factors associated with smoking among males

Significant factors associated with smoking among males are shown in Table 4. Compared to boys in grade 9, boys in grade 8 were 43% (OR = 0.57, 95% CI [0.38, 0.86]) less likely to have been smokers. Boys who received pocket money were 2.30 (95% CI [1.75, 3.03]) times more likely to have been smokers compared with those who did not receive pocket money.

Table 4. Factors associated with smoking among males

Factor	Total	n (%)	OR (95% CI)
Grade			
7	317	40 (12.6)	1.31 (0.92, 1.89)
8	292	18 (6.2)	0.57 (0.38, 0.86)
9	277	33 (11.9)	1
Received pocket money			
Yes	143	45 (31.5)	2.30 (1.75, 3.03)
No	736	47 (6.4)	1
Had seen advertisements for cigarettes on billboards			
Yes	470	62 (13.2)	-
No	378	28 (7.4)	
Had something such as a t-shirt or pen with a cigarette brand logo on it			
Yes	155	29 (18.7)	1.47 (1.10, 1.98)
No	692	56 (8.1)	1
Had seen anti-smoking messages at social gatherings			
Yes	362	58 (16.0)	1.34 (1.03, 1.75)
No	516	34 (6.6)	1
Had seen anti-smoking media messages during the past 30 days			
Yes	599	72 (12.0)	-
No	279	18 (6.5)	
Parents smoked cigarettes			
Yes	267	49 (18.4)	1.51 (1.15, 1.97)
No	621	42 (6.8)	1
Closest friends smoked cigarettes			
Yes	256	58 (22.7)	1.74 (1.34, 2.27)
No	626	35 (5.6)	1
Smoking cigarettes makes boys look more or less attractive			
Yes	209	26 (12.4)	-
No	484	39 (8.1)	
Smoking cigarettes is less dangerous for young people because they can always stop later			
Yes	367	52 (14.2)	-
No	507	39 (7.7)	

Boys who had something like a t-shirt or a pen with a cigarette brand logo on it were 47% (OR = 1.47, 95% CI [1.10, 1.98]) more likely to have been smokers compared with those who had no such things. Compared with boys who had not seen anti-smoking messages at social gatherings, boys who had seen such messages at social gatherings were 34% (OR = 1.34, 95% CI [1.03, 1.75]) more likely to have been smokers. Boys whose parents who smoked were 51% (OR = 1.51, 95% CI [1.15, 1.97]) more likely to have been smokers than boys whose parents did not smoke. Boys who had closest friends who smoked were 74% (OR = 1.74, 95% CI [1.34, 2.27]) more likely to smoke than boys who did not have closest friends who smoked.

Table 5. Factors associated with smoking among females

Factor	Total	n (%)	OR (95% CI)
Grade			
7	386	39 (10.1)	1.94 (1.26, 2.99)
8	303	10 (3.3)	0.66 (0.38, 1.15)
9	281	12 (4.3)	1
Received pocket money			
Yes	120	29 (24.2)	2.41 (1.72, 3.37)
No	848	30 (3.5)	1
Had seen advertisements for cigarettes at social gatherings			
Yes	352	38 (10.8)	1.52 (1.10, 2.09)
No	612	23 (3.8)	1
Had something such as a t-shirt or pen with a cigarette brand logo on it			
Yes	150	21 (14.0)	-
No	799	38 (4.8)	
Had seen anti-smoking messages at social gatherings			
Yes	399	39 (9.8)	-
No	573	21 (3.7)	
Smoking makes one gain or lose weight			
Gain weight	112	11 (9.8)	-
Lose weight	664	31 (4.7)	
No difference	189	16 (8.5)	
Parents smoked cigarettes			
Yes	269	37 (13.8)	1.63 (1.17, 2.27)
No	710	24 (3.4)	1
Closest friends smoked cigarettes			
Yes	239	37 (15.5)	1.72 (1.23, 2.40)
No	733	22 (3.0)	1

Factors associated with smoking among females

Significant factors associated with smoking among females are shown in table 5. Compared to girls in grade 9, girls in grade 7 were 94% (OR = 1.94, 95% CI [1.26, 2.99]) more likely to have been smokers. Girls who received pocket money were 2.41 (95% CI [1.72, 3.37]) times more likely to have been smokers compared with girls who did not receive pocket money. Girls who had seen advertisements for cigarettes at social gatherings were 52% (OR = 1.52, 95% CI [1.10, 2.09]) more likely to have been smokers compared with girls who had not seen such advertisements at social gatherings. Compared with girls whose parents smoked, girls whose parents did not smoke were 63% (OR = 1.63, 95% CI [1.17, 2.27]) more likely to have been smokers. Girls who had closest friends who smoked were 72% (OR = 1.72, 95% CI [1.23, 2.40]) more likely to have been smokers.

The overall prevalence estimate obtained from our study is higher than the 5.3% prevalence reported by Mpabulungi and Muula for school-going adolescents in the Kampala, Global Youth Tobacco Survey conducted in 2002 (16). However, the Kafue estimates are much lower than the 21.9% current cigarette smoking prevalence estimated in Arua, Uganda in 2002 (18). Arua is in the tobacco growing region in Uganda, so it has been suggested that society is more tolerant of adolescent smoking than may be the case in Kampala. Tobacco was marginally grown in Kafue and its population may not have been tolerant of adolescent smoking.

The proportion of girls smoking more than 6 cigarettes per day was higher than the percentage in males. The reasons for such gender disparity is currently unclear to us.

We found that the majority of adolescent smokers smoked either at home or at a friends' house. This suggests the potential influence of the home environment and peer factors in supporting adolescent smokers. Interventions to prevent adolescent smoking should seriously consider the locations at which adolescents smoke.

The odds of smoking among adolescents who reported having some pocket money was 2.3 compared to those who reported none. Mohan et al. who studied adolescent boys in Kerala, India have also reported a higher likelihood of being a smoker among those receiving pocket money compared to those not receiving any pocket money (19). It is likely that having some disposable cash influences adolescents to spend the money on tobacco.

As has been consistently demonstrated elsewhere, parental and peer smoking were associated with current smoking status among adolescents (19-

23). Due to the cross sectional nature of this study however, we were unable to determine whether having a friend acted as an influence to initiate smoking or whether an adolescent smoker selects other adolescents who smoke as friends (24). We suspect though that both mechanisms are plausible.

We also found that both girls and boys who reported having seen pro-tobacco advertisements at social gatherings were more likely to be current smokers than those who had not seen such advertisements. The role of pro-tobacco advertisements has been studied extensively (25-26). Evidence suggests that having been exposed to favourable tobacco advertisements is an important risk factor for adolescent smoking. Interestingly also, exposure to anti-tobacco television programs sponsored by tobacco firms have been identified as a risk factor for adolescent smoking (28). The programming of either anti- or pro-tobacco advertisements is especially a delicate issue in the tobacco prevention arena.

Our study has several limitations. Firstly, due to the cross sectional nature of the design, the factors that have been identified as associated with current cigarette smoking cannot be described in causative terms (29-31). The study also recruited only school going adolescents in the study area. The findings may therefore be representative of the in-school adolescents in Kafue but not those out of school adolescents. Also, history of current smoking was by self-report. We did not validate the self-reports with biomarkers such as exhaled carbon monoxide or hair or blood cotinine level to assess exposure to cigarettes (32-34). However, the study utilised standardised methodology that has been used to estimate the prevalence of tobacco use across the globe. This fact allows for meaningful comparisons to be made between different settings both within the same country and without.

ACKNOWLEDGMENTS

The data for this study was obtained from the Zambia Global Youth Survey Collaborative Group that jointly worked with the Institute of Economic and Social Research (INESOR), University of Zambia. We are especially grateful to Richard Zulu who coordinated data collection for the Zambia GYTS.

This chapter is a revised version of an original paper published in the Malawi Medical Journal (Siziya S, Rudatsikira E, Muula AS. Cigarette smoking among school-going adolescents in Kafue, Zambia. Malawi Med J 2007; 19: 75-78) and the authors have obtained the permission from Malawi Medical Journal to use this material.

REFERENCES

[1] Laber DA. Risk factors, classification, and staging of renal cell carcinoma. Med Oncol 2006; 23: 443-54.

[2] Greenwald P. A favourable view: progress in cancer prevention and screening. Recent Results Cancer Res 2007; 174: 3-17.

[3] Subramanian J, Govindan R. Lung cancer in never smokers. J Clin Oncol 2007; 25: 561-70.

[4] Lopez AD, Mathers CD, Ezzati M, Jamison DT, Murray CJ. Global and regional burden of disease and risk factors, 2001: systematic analysis of population health data. Lancet 2006; 367: 1747-57.

[5] McKenna MT, Michaud CM, Murray CJ, Marks JS. Assessing the burden of disease in the United States using disability-adjusted life years. Am J Prev Med 2005; 28: 215-23.

[6] Carter S, Percival T, Paterson J, Williams M. Maternal smoking: risks related to maternal asthma and reduced birth weight in a Pacific Island birth cohort in New Zealand. NZ Med J 2006; 119: U2081.

[7] Steyn K, de Wet T, Saloojee Y, Nel H, Yach D. The influence of maternal smoking, snuff use and passive smoking on pregnancy outcomes: The Birth To Ten Study. Pediatr Perinat Epidemiol 2006; 20: 90-9.

[8] Myers MG, Kelly JF. Cigarette smoking among adolescents with alcohol and other drug problems. Alcohol Res Health 2006; 29: 221-7.

[9] Tosh AK, Simmons PS. Sexual activity and other risk-taking behaviours among Asian-American adolescents. J Pediatr Adolesc Gynecol 2007; 20: 29-34.

[10] Upadhyaya HP, Deas D, Brady KT, Kruesi M. Cigarette smoking and psychiatric comorbidity in children and adolescents. J Am Acad Child Adolesc Psychiatry 2002; 41: 1294-305.

[11] Arora M, Peddy KS. Global Youth Tobacco Survey-Dehli. Indian Pediatr 2005; 42: 850-1.

[12] Global Youth Tobacco Survey Collaborative Group. Tobacco use among youth: A cross country comparison. Tob Control 2002; 11: 252-70.

[13] Kyrlesi A, Soteriades ES, Warren CW, Kremastinou J, Papastergiou P, Jones NR, et al. Tobacco use among students 13-15 years in Greece: the GYTS project. BMC Public Health 2007; 7: 3.

[14] Global Youth Tobacco Survey Collaborating Group. Differences in worldwide tobacco use by gender: findings from the Global Youth Tobacco Survey. J Sch Health 2003; 73: 207-15.

[15] Central Statistical Office [Zambia]. Census of population and housing 2000 (Summary). Lusaka: Central Statistical Office, 2003.

[16] Ministry of Education [Zambia]. Zambia annual schools census 2003. Lusaka: Ministry of Education, 2003.

[17] Mpabulungi L, Muula AS. Tobacco use among high school students in Kampala: questionnaire study. Croat Med J 2004; 45: 80-3.

[18] Mpabulungi L, Muula AS. Tobacco use among high school students in a remote district of Arua, Uganda. Rural Remote Health 2006; 6: 609.

[19] Mohan S, Sankara Sarma P, Thankappan KR. Access to pocket money and low educational performance predict tobacco use among adolescent boys in Kerala, India. Prev Med 2005; 41: 685-92.

[20] Oqwell AE, Astrom AN, Haugejorden O. Sociodemographic factors of pupils who use tobacco in randomly-selected primary schools in Nairobi Province, Kenya. East Afr Med J 2003; 80: 235-41.

[21] Brook JS, Morojele NK, Brook DW, Rosen Z. Predictors of cigarette use among South African adolescents. Int J Behav Med 2005; 12: 2007-17.

[22] Kobus K. Peers and adolescent smoking. Addiction. 2003; 98(Suppl 1): 37-55.

[23] Alexander C, Piazza M, Mekos D, Valente T. Peers, schools, and adolescent smoking. J Adolesc Health 2001; 29: 22-30.

[24] de Vries H, Candel M, Engels R, Mercken L. Challenges to the peer influencer paradigm: results from 12-13 year olds from six European countries from the European Smoking Prevention Framework Approach Study. Tob Control 2006; 15: 83-9.

[25] Charlesworth A, Glantz SA. Smoking in the movies increases adolescent smoking: a review. Pediatrics 2005; 116: 1516-28.

[26] Auger N, Raynault MF. The future of tobacco marketing in Canada. Can J Public Health 2005; 96: 278-80.

[27] McGee R, Ketchel J. Tobacco imagery on New Zealand Television, 2002-2004. Tob Control 2006; 15: 412-14.

[28] Wakefield M, Terry-McElrath Y, Emery S, Saffer H, Chaloupka FJ, Szczypka G, Flay B, O'Malley PM, Johnston LD. Effect of televised tobacco company-funded smoking prevention advertising on youth smoking-related beliefs, intentions, and behaviour. Am J Public Health 2006; 96: 2154-60.

[29] Hofler M. Causal inference based on counterfactuals. BMC Med Res Methodol 2005; 5: 8.

[30] Kaufman JS, Cooper RS. Seeking explanations in social epidemiology. Am J Epidemiol 1999; 150: 113-20.

[31] Kaufman JS, Kaufman S, Poole C. Causal inference from randomised trials in social epidemiology. Soc Sci Med 2003; 57: 2397-409.

[32] Breland AB, Kleykamp BA, Eissenberg BA. Clinical laboratory evaluation of potential reduced exposure products for smokers. Nicotine Tob Res 2006; 8: 727-38.

[33] Hobbs SD, Adam DJ, Bradbury AW. Assessment of smoking status in patients with peripheral artery disease. J Vasc Surg 2005; 41: 451-6.

[34] Ismail AA, Gill GV, Lawton K, Houghton GM, MacFarlane IA. Comparison of questionnaire, breath carbon monoxide and urine cotinine in assessing the smoking habits of Type 2 diabetic patients. Diabet Med 2000; 17: 119-23.

In: Smoking and Adolescence ISBN: 978-1-63484-311-9
Editors: M. L. Mazabam, S. Siziya et al. © 2016 Nova Science Publishers, Inc.

Chapter 6

PREDICTORS OF CIGARETTE SMOKING AMONG ADOLESCENTS

Seter Siziya[1,*], BA(Ed), MSc, PhD, Emmanuel Rudatsikira[2], MD, MPH, DrPH, Adamson S Muula[3,4], MBBS, MPH, PhD, and Pierson RT Ntata[3], BA, MA, PhD

[1]Department of Community Medicine, University of Zambia, Medical School, Lusaka, Zambia

[2]Departments of Epidemiology and Biostatistics and Global Health, Loma Linda University, School of Public Health, Loma Linda, California, USA

[3]Department of Community Health, University of Malawi, College of Medicine, Blantyre, Malawi

[4]Department of Epidemiology, University of North Carolina at Chapel Hill, North Carolina, USA

Cigarette smoking is a leading cause of morbidity and mortality globally. There are limited data on the prevalence of and factors associated with smoking among in-school adolescents in developing countries. Th objectives of the study were to estimate prevalence of those who have

* Corresponding author: Professor Seter Siziya, Clinical Sciences Department, School of Medicine, Copperbelt University, Ndola Central Hospital, 6th Floor, P.O. Box 71191, Ndola, Zambia. E-mail: ssiziya@gmail.com.

smoked cigarettes and to identify associated socio-demographic factors among adolescents in Chongwe district, Lusaka Province, Zambia. Data used was from the Zambia Global Youth Tobacco Survey, which was conducted using standardized methodology among in-school adolescents in 2002. Data were analysis to assess if selected socio-demographic variables were associated with having smoked cigarettes. Bivariate and multivariate logistic regression analysis was used to assess the associations. A history of having smoked cigarettes ranged from 20.5% among 15 year olds to 37.2% among males younger than 12 years old. In females, 20.7% of 13 year olds and 37.7% of those less than 12 years old had smoked. Parental smoking, friends smoking, a lack of perception that smoking was harmful, and exposure to pro-tobacco advertisements were associated with having smoked cigarettes. Adolescents who had smoked cigarettes were more likely to allow others to smoke in their presence. Many adolescents in rural Chongwe, Zambia had tried cigarette smoking. The identification of predictors for smoking should guide the design and implementation of programs aimed to prevent initiation and maintenance of tobacco use among adolescents.

INTRODUCTION

Cigarette smoking is the single most common cause of preventable morbidity and mortality globally. It is estimated that by 2020 tobacco-related deaths will be the leading cause of deaths in the developing countries (1, 2). While smoking is an important disease risk factor on its own, many adolescents who smoke also have unhealthy lifestyle clusters such as smoking, alcohol and illicit drug use (3). Smoking may, therefore, be a marker of other harmful adolescents behaviours.

Research into adolescent cigarette smoking has mostly been conducted with current smoking status as the main outcome. However, history of previous smoking is an important predictor of current or future smoking (4). Also, studies into adolescent cigarette smoking have generally reported on the prevalence of smoking without considerations of relevant potential associations with socio-demographic factors. However, the identification of such factors can best inform the design and implementation of public health interventions aimed to reduce adolescent tobacco use. We report a study aimed to estimate the prevalence of having smoked cigarettes, and its association with relevant socio-demographic characteristics.

OUR STUDY

The data were obtained in a cross sectional school-based survey conducted under the Zambia Global Youth Tobacco Survey (GYTS) in 2002. The GYTS aimed to enroll students aged 13–15 years in order to estimate the prevalence of various forms of tobacco use and relevant socio-demographic variables. School grades likely to have students within the selected age range (13-15 years) were identified. For Zambia, these were students in grades 7 to 9. Identification of study participants was conducted through probability sampling using a multistage sample design. Schools were the primary sampling units, while classes were the secondary sampling units. All the students within the selected classes were eligible to participate regardless of their actual ages, therefore some students participated although they were outside the selected age range. The school response rate was 100% while the student response rate was 78.3%. A standardised questionnaire was self-completed anonymously by the students and this it took between 30 to 40 min. The GYTS core questionnaire collected information on: cigarette smoking (current and ever); knowledge and attitudes of young people towards cigarette smoking; exposure to various media and advertisements on tobacco, access to cigarettes; tobacco-related school curriculum; exposure to environmental tobacco smoke (ETS); and cessation of cigarette smoking. For the purpose of this study, however, only data related to a history of having smoked cigarettes and associated factors were analyzed. A comprehensive description of GYTS methodology has been reported by Warren et al. (5) and the Global Youth Tobacco Surveillance Collaborative Group (6).

Chongwe district is a rural area and spans for about 100 km from the outskirts of Lusaka, Zambia's capital city. Chongwe's population is approximately 148 000. Agriculture and charcoal production are the main sources of livelihoods, with the Chongwe district being the largest source of charcoal for Lusaka. The district is served by 15 health centers and a mission hospital; some of the health centers are located over 40 km from main roads (7). Data were analysed using SPSS v 14.0 (SPSS Inc; Chicago, IL, USA). It was aimed to assess the prevalence of having smoked cigarettes, stratified by gender. Bivariate logistic regression analyses were conducted to obtained unadjusted odd ratio between having smoked and explanatory variables of interest (Model 1). Model 2 was multivariate analysis with the explanatory variables of interest as main exposures controlling for the other variables.

Permission to conduct this study was obtained from the Zambian Ministry of Education. Parents and guardians were informed of the study. Parents who did not want their children to participate were asked to inform their children not to participate. All students were informed that they were free not to participate or not answer any questions on the questionnaire. The questionnaire was completed in class time. Students who did not want to participate remained in class but could submit an uncompleted questionnaire, because excluding them from class was potentially stigmatizing. To preserve individual confidentiality, the questionnaire was self-completed anonymously by students. School teachers were not in the classrooms at the time of questionnaire completion.

OUR FINDINGS

The prevalence of a history of having smoked cigarettes - even a single puff – was assessed. The results are presented in Table 1. Overall, the proportion of adolescents who reported having smoked was 27.0%. Generally all age groups had a prevalence exceeding 20%. However, the extremes of the age group had the highest history of having smoked. A similar distribution was observed for class grades where the lowest and highest grades had higher prevalence than the middle grade. Adolescents whose parents were smokers or whose friends were smokers were themselves more likely to have smoked.

Attitudes towards smoking

It was also aimed to assess attitudes towards smoking. In general, study participants had negative attitudes towards tobacco or smoking. There were, however, exceptions: for instance, the finding that favouring banning smoking in public and the perception that environmental exposure was harmful were all associated with having smoked. The other results are presented in Table 2.

Tobacco advertisement and smoking

It was also aimed to determine if having smoked was associated with exposure to different forms of tobacco advertisements, owning a cigarette-logo branded item, and exposure to pro-tobacco advertisements at sports or social events. Exposure to both forms of exposure to advertisements were associated with having been a smoker. The detailed results are presented in Table 3.

Table 1. Demographic factors associated with ever tried cigarette smoking among school going adolescents in Chongwe and Luangwa districts, Zambia

Factor	Male				Female			
	Total	n (%)	Model 1 OR (95% CI)	Model 2 OR (95% CI)	Total	n (%)	Model 1 OR (95% CI)	Model 2 OR (95% CI)
Age (years)		P = 0.015				P = 0.079		
<12	78	29 (37.2)	1.38 (0.91, 2.09)	-	77	29 (37.7)	1.74 (1.14, 2.64)	-
12	77	25 (32.5)	1.12 (0.73, 1.72)		95	24 (25.3)	0.97 (0.64, 1.48)	
13	115	34 (29.6)	0.98 (0.68, 1.41)		140	29 (20.7)	0.75 (0.51, 1.10)	
14	133	34 (25.6)	0.80 (0.56, 1.15)		152	35 (23.0)	0.86 (0.60, 1.23)	
15	176	36 (20.5)	0.60 (0.43, 0.84)		147	34 (23.1)	0.87 (0.60, 1.24)	
16	191	58 (30.4)	1.02 (0.75, 1.37)		141	31 (22.0)	0.81 (0.56, 1.18)	
17+	209	77 (36.8)	1		141	31 (31.3)	1	
Grade		P = 0.379				P < 0.001		
7	416	125 (30.0)	1.00 (0.84, 1.21)	-	383	125 (32.6)	1.52 (1.28, 1.94)	1.63 (1.24, 2.14)
8	322	88 (27.3)	0.88 (0.72, 1.07)		283	45 (15.9)	0.61 (0.48, 0.79)	0.62 (0.45, 0.86)
9	251	82 (32.7)	1		190	46 (24.2)	1	1
Parents smoked		P < 0.001						

Table 1. (Continued)

Factor	Male				Female			
	Total	n (%)	Model 1 OR (95% CI)	Model 2 OR (95% CI)	Total	n (%)	Model 1 OR (95% CI)	Model 2 OR (95% CI)
None	593	144 (24.3)	0.72 (0.62, 0.84)	-	548	88 (16.1)	0.50 (0.42, 0.60)	0.58 (0.47, 0.72)
Either parent smoked	286	109 (38.1)	1		227	98 (43.2)	1	1
Closest friends smoked		P < 0.001				P<0.001		
None	610	120 (19.7)	0.38 (0.31, 0.48)	0.45 (0.34, 0.58)	585	104 (17.8)	0.42 (0.34, 0.53)	0.47 (0.35, 0.64)
Some of them	126	126 (43.4)	1.20 (0.96, 1.51)	1.09 (0.83, 1.43)	184	64 (34.8)	1.04 (0.81, 1.35)	1.02 (0.72, 1.43)
Most or all of them	81	47 (58.0)	1	1	82	44 (53.7)	1	1

Table 2. Attitudes towards and factors associated with ever tried cigarette smoking among school going adolescents in Chongwe and Luangwa districts, Zambia

Factor	Male				Female			
	Total	n (%)	Model 1 OR (95% CI)	Model 2 OR (95% CI)	Total	n (%)	Model 1 OR (95% CI)	Model 2 OR (95% CI)
Cigarette smoking is harmful to health		$P = 0.040$				$P < 0.001$		
Definitely not	307	95 (30.9)	1.00 (0.80, 1.25)	1.40 (1.03, 1.90)	301	75 (24.9)	0.99 (0.77, 1.26)	1.48 (1.06, 2.06)
Probably not	135	45 (33.3)	1.11 (0.83, 1.49)	1.06 (0.71, 1.58)	128	40 (31.3)	1.35 (0.99, 1.84)	0.99 (0.64, 1.54)
Probably yes	143	51 (35.7)	1.23 (0.93, 1.64)	0.96 (0.65, 1.40)	135	30 (22.2)	0.85 (0.61, 1.18)	0.59 (0.36, 0.97)
Definitely yes	397	98 (24.7)	1	1	282	65 (23.0)	1	1
Smoking makes people comfortable		$P = 0.132$				$P = 0.350$		
More comfortable	386	124 (32.1)	1.10 (0.91, 1.33)	-	308	68 (22.1)	0.85 (0.68, 1.07)	-
Less comfortable	409	107 (26.2)	0.83 (0.68, 1.00)		359	90 (25.1)	1.01 (0.81, 1.25)	
No difference from non-smokers	187	60 (32.1)	1		176	49 (27.8)	1	
Smoke from other people's cigarettes is harmful to health		$P = 0.016$						
Definitely not	367	88 (24.0)	0.69 (0.55, 0.87)	0.57 (0.42, 0.77)	341	78 (22.9)	0.84 (0.66, 1.07)	-

Table 2. (Continued)

Factor	Male				Female			
	Total	n (%)	Model 1 OR (95% CI)	Model 2 OR (95% CI)	Total	n (%)	Model 1 OR (95% CI)	Model 2 OR (95% CI)
Probably not	156	54 (34.6)	1.16 (0.88, 1.53)	1.00 (0.68, 1.47)	166	44 (26.5)	1.02 (0.76, 1.37)	
Probably yes	132	47 (35.6)	1.22 (0.91, 1.63)	1.14 (0.78, 1.67)	124	41 (33.1)	1.40 (1.03, 1.91)	
Definitely yes	331	105 (31.7)	1	1	221	50 (22.6)	1	
Would let someone smoke in their presence		P < 0.001				P = 0.054		
Yes	224	95 (38.9)	1.36 (1.17, 1.59)	1.31 (1.08, 1.58)	211	62 (29.4)	1.28 (1.14, 1.44)	-
No	721	185 (25.7)	1	1	627	141 (22.5)	1	
Favours public smoking ban								
Yes	353	119 (33.7)	1.16 (1.01, 1.34)	-	350	100 (28.6)	1.19 (1.01, 1.39)	1
No	624	171 (27.4)	1		496	110 (22.2)	1	

Table 3. Associations between advertisements and ever tried cigarette smoking among school going adolescents in Chongwe and Luangwa districts, Zambia

Factor	Male				Female			
	Total	n (%)	Model 1 OR (95% CI)	Model 2 OR (95% CI)	Total	n (%)	Model 1 OR (95% CI)	Model 2 OR (95% CI)
Had an item with a cigarette brand logo		P < 0.001				P < 0.001		
Yes	209	108 (51.7)	1.87 (1.59, 2.19)	1.61 (1.32, 1.96)	193	79 (40.9)	1.72 (1.44, 2.04)	1.54 (1.24, 1.92)
No	759	177 (23.5)	1	1	630	120 (19.0)	1	1
Exposed to cigarette advertisements at sports or at other social events								
Never attend the events	290	73 (25.2)	0.77 (0.61, 0.97)	0.68 (0.51, 0.92)	262	58 (22.1)	0.84 (0.64, 1.08)	-
A lot	196	74 (37.8)	1.38 (1.08, 1.77)	1.47 (1.07, 2.00)	197	62 (31.5)	1.35 (1.04, 1.76)	
Sometimes	187	66 (35.3)	1.24 (0.96, 1.60)	1.08 (0.79, 1.48)	152	46 (30.3)	1.28 (0.95, 1.71)	
Never	298	75 (25.2)	1	1	230	44 (19.1)	1	

DISCUSSION

Our study found that the prevalence of having smoked cigarettes among in-school adolescents in Chongwe district, Zambia was 27%. This prevalence is lower than 31% reported by Mpabulungi and Muula for Arua, rural Uganda (8), and the reason for this is unknown. One possible explanation is that Arua's economy largely depends on tobacco farming, while Chongwe's does not, and so there may be a greater tolerance of tobacco use in Arua. Other unknown country-level factors may account for the differences between the two districts (e.g., in the Greek GYTS, Kyrlesi et al. (9) reported a 32.2% prevalence of having smoked among 13-15 year-old adolescents). While the present study revealed no gender differences, another study of Zambian adults identified a higher prevalence among males (10).

Our study identified that having a parent who smoked was associated with the adolescent having smoked. Ornelas et al. (11) in their US study on parental influence on adolescent physical activity, found that parental-child communication and family cohesiveness were important influencing factors. Although that study found that parental monitoring was not a good predictor of adolescent physical activity, Arredondo et al. (12) reported that parental monitoring was a good predictor of adolescent healthy eating and physical activity. Factors involved in parental influencing adolescents' smoking may include permissiveness, the availability of cigarettes in the home and role modeling, ant this should be investigated further.

Thomas et al. in their systematic review of family-based tobacco-control programs aimed at preventing adolescent smoking (13), suggested that well-conducted programs were effective. School-based programs may also be effective (14).

In our study, adolescents who perceived tobacco smoke to be harmful to their health were less likely to have smoked than those who were not concerned about the harmful effects of tobacco. This was also reported by Rodriguez et al. (15). This suggests an opportunity to change adolescents' beliefs about smoking, by using the media to reduce smoking behaviour.

It has been established that tobacco promotion directed at adolescents encourages the uptake and maintenance of smoking (16, 17). Gritz et al. reported that exposure to pro-tobacco advertisements was a strong predictor of being a smoker among US adolescents (18). Our study supports this trend among adolescents in Chongwe.

Many previous studies have reported about the association between adolescent smoking and having a friend who smokes. Bricker et al. found that smoking among adolescents' friends could influence both the initiation of smoking and maintenance of the habit (19). Our results suggested that adolescents who had smoked were likely to have had friends who were smokers. Whether friends influenced the initiation of smoking, or whether adolescent smokers are more likely to choose other smokers as friends requires further study.

In our study, 15 year olds had the lowest prevalence of smoking (20.5%), compared with younger and older adolescents. This was an unexpected finding and the reasons should be explored further.

Limitations to the present study include that participants may have under-report their smoking status, as was demonstrated in a Tanzania adult-smoking study (20). And, in our study, as the sample was drawn from schools, the findings may not be appropriate to out of school adolescents.

In conclusion, many adolescents in rural Chongwe, Zambia, have tried cigarette smoking, and associated factors among in-school adolescents in Chongwe have been identified. The identification of predictors of smoking should guide the design and implementation of programs aimed to prevent the initiation and maintenance of tobacco use among adolescents.

ACKNOWLEDGMENTS

We are grateful to Mr. Richard Zulu who coordinated data collection. The data used in this study were obtained from the Global Youth Tobacco Survey (GYTS).

This chapter is a revised version of an original paper published in the journal Rural and Remote Health (Siziya S, Rudatsikira E, Muula AS, Ntata PRT. Predictors of cigarette smoking among adolescents in rural Zambia: results from a cross sectional study from Chongwe district. Rural Remote Health 2007; 7: 728) and the authors have obtained the permission from Rural and Remote Health to use this material.

REFERENCES

[1] Mathers CD, Loncar D. Projections of global mortality burden from 2002 to 2030. PLoS Med 2006; 3: e442.

[2] Lopez AD, Mathers CD, Ezzati M, Jamison DT, Murray CJ. Global and regional burden of disease and risk factor, 2001: systematic analyses of population health data. Lancet 2006; 367: 1747-57.

[3] Faeh D, Viswanathan B, Chiolero A, Warren W, Bovet P. Clustering of smoking, alcohol drinking and cannabis use in adolescents in a rapidly developing country. BMC Public Health 2006; 6: 169.

[4] Silva MA, Rivera IR, Carvalho AC, Guerra Ade H Jr. The prevalence of and variables associated with smoking in children and adolescents. J Pediatrics (Rio de Janiero) 2006; 82: 365-70.

[5] Warren CW, Riley L, Asma S, Eriksen MP, Green L, Blanton C, et al. Tobacco use by youth: a surveillance report from the Global Youth Tobacco Survey Project. Bull World Health Organ 2000; 78: 868-76.

[6] Global Youth Surveillance Collaborative Group. Tobacco use among youth: a cross country comparison. Tob Control 2002; 11: 252-70.

[7] Furth R. Zambia Performance-based incentives pilot study. Final report. United States Agency for International Development and the Government of Zambia. (Online) 2006. URL: http://www.qaproject.org/news/PDFs/ZambiaPerformance PilotStudyInitiatives.pdf

[8] Mpabulungi L, Muula AS. Tobacco use among high school students in a remote district of Arua, Uganda. Rural Remote Health 2006; 6: 609.

[9] Kyrlesi A, Soteriades ES, Warren CW, Kremastinou J, Papastergiou P, Jones NR, et al. Tobacco use among students aged 13-15 years in Greece: the GYTS project. BMC Public Health 2007; 7: 3.

[10] Pampel FC. Patterns of tobacco use in the early epidemic stages: Malawi and Zambia. Am J PublicHealth 2005; 95(6): 1009-15.

[11] Orenelas IJ, Perreira KM, Ayala GX. Parental influences on adolescent physical activity: a longitudinal study. Int J Behav Nutr Phys Activity 2007; 4: 3.

[12] Arredondo EM, Elder JP, Ayala GX, Campbell N, Baquero B, Duerksen S. Is parenting style related to children's healthy eating and physical activity in Latino families. Health Educ Res 2006; 21: 862-71.

[13] Thomas RE, Baker P, Lorenzetti D. Family-based programmes for preventing smoking by children and adolescents. Cochrane Database Syst Rev 2007; 1: CD004493. doi: 10.1002/14651858.CD004493.pub2.

[14] Thomas R, Perera R. School-based programmes for preventing smoking. Cochrane Database Syst Rev 2006; 3: CD001293. doi: 10.1002/14651858.CD001293.pub2.

[15] Rodriguez D, Romer D, Audrain-McGovern J. Beliefs about the risks of smoking mediate the relationship between exposure to smoking and smoking. Psychosomat Med 2007; 69: 106-3.

[16] Lovato C, Linn G, Stead LF, Best A. Impact of tobacco advertising and promotion on increasing adolescent smoking behaviours. Cochrane Database Syst Rev 2003; 3: CD003439. doi: 10.1002/14651858.CD003439.

[17] Sargent JD, Dalton M, Beach M, Bernhardt A, Heatherton T, Stevens M. Effect of cigarette promotions on smoking uptake among adolescents. Prev Med 2000; 30: 320-7.

[18] Gritz ER, Prokhorov AV, Hudmon KS, Mullin Jones M, Rosenblum C, Chang CC, et al. Predictors of susceptibility of smoking and ever-smoking: longitudinal study of a triethnic sample of adolescents. Nicotine Tob Res 2003; 5: 493-506.

[19] Bricker JB, Peterson AV Jr, Andersen MR, Rajan KB, Leroux BG, Sarason IG. Childhood friends who smoke: do they influence adolescents to make smoking transitions? Addict Behav 2006; 31: 889-900.

[20] Jagoe K, Edwards R, Mugusi F, Whiting D, Unwin N. Tobacco smoking in Tanzania, East Africa: population based smoking prevalence using expired alveolar carbon monoxide as a validation tool. Tob Control 2002; 11: 210-304.

In: Smoking and Adolescence ISBN: 978-1-63484-311-9
Editors: M. L. Mazabam, S. Siziya et al. © 2016 Nova Science Publishers, Inc.

Chapter 7

CIGARETTE SMOKING, SCHOOL AGE ADOLESCENTS AND ADVERTISEMENT-PROMOTION-SPONSORSHIP ISSUES

Richard Zulu[1], BA, MPhil,
Seter Siziya[2,*], BA(Ed), MSc, PhD,
Adamson S Muula[3], MBBS, MPH, PhD,
and Emmanuel Rudatsikira[4], MD, MPH, DrPH
[1]University of Zambia, Institute of Economic and Social and Research, Lusaka, Zambia
[2]Department of Community Medicine, University of Zambia, Medical School, Lusaka, Zambia
[3]Department of Community Health, University of Malawi, College of Medicine, Blantyre, Malawi
[4]Division of Epidemiology and Biostatistics, Graduate School of Public Health, San Diego State University, San Diego, California, USA

Tobacco use is the leading cause of non-communicable disease morbidity and mortality. Most smokers initiate the smoking habit as adolescents or young adults. Survey data from the 2007 Lusaka (Zambia) Global Youth

[*] Corresponding author: Professor Seter Siziya, Clinical Sciences Department, School of Medicine, Copperbelt University, Ndola Central Hospital, 6th Floor, P.O. Box 71191, Ndola, Zambia. E-mail: ssiziya@gmail.com.

Tobacco Survey were used to estimate the prevalence of current cigarette smoking and assess whether exposure to pro-tobacco media and perception of the potential harm of second hand smoke are associated with adolescents' smoking. Logistic regression analysis was used to estimate the associations. Altogether, 2,378 students of whom 56.8% were females participated in the study. Overall, 10.5% of the students (9.3% among males, and 12.1% among females) smoked cigarettes in the past 30 days to the survey. Students who favoured banning smoking in public places were 33% (OR = 0.67, 95%CI [0.47, 0.96]) less likely to smoke cigarettes compared to those who were not in favour of the ban. Seeing actors smoking on TV, videos, or movies was positively associated with smoking (OR = 1.90, 95%CI [1.26, 2.88]). However, having an item with a cigarette brand logo on it, seeing advertisements for cigarettes on billboards, and ever offered a free cigarette by a cigarette representative were negatively associated with smoking (OR = 0.39, 95%CI [0.26, 0.58], OR = 0.63, 95%CI [0.43, 0.92], and OR = 0.43, 95%CI [0.29, 0.65], respectively). Findings from this study indicate that TV advertisement-promotion-sponsorship was positively associated with smoking while it was the opposite with other forms of advertisement; there is a need for further studies.

INTRODUCTION

Tobacco smoking, especially cigarette smoking, is the leading cause of preventable deaths and disability from non-communicable diseases. While cigarette smoking has stabilised or is in decline in many developed nations, there is evidence to suggest of a growing epidemic in low and middle-income countries (1, 2). In these settings (middle and low-income countries), there is a growing recognition that there is need for significant investment to be devoted to the fight against the growing burden of non-communicable diseases arising from among others, tobacco use, just as resources are being provided towards major and neglected communicable diseases (3, 4). In fact, Kengne and Anderson have described stroke as a neglected disease in Africa (5).

On 28th May 2008, Zambia acceded to the Framework Convention on Tobacco Control (FTCT). Among other things, the convention requires that governments control tobacco adverting, promoting and sponsorship. Even before Zambia acceded to FTCT, it had passed the following regulations on tobacco control in 1992 by banning sale of tobacco to persons below the age of 16 years; tobacco advertisement in mass media; and smoking in government buildings, private worksites, education and health facilities, public transport, and other public places. However, these regulations were not strictly enforced, as can be noted in a previous report (6). With the accession of the country to the FCTC, however, there is an expectation that enforcement of regulations will be stricter and access to tobacco and exposure to various pro-tobacco media will be restricted for adolescents. Information on the Framework Convention on Tobacco Control has been published elsewhere (7-9). We therefore conducted this analysis of the Lusaka Global Youth Tobacco Survey (GYTS) 2007 for the following reasons: i) To assess the baseline exposure to pro-tobacco (cigarette) advertisements among adolescents within the 12 months preceding accession to the FCTC; ii) Assess if exposure to pro-tobacco media and advertisements is associated with current cigarette smoking.

Our study

We used data from the Lusaka-Zambia GYTS conducted in 2007, a second wave of the GYTS conducted in Zambia after the 2002 survey. Following the standard protocol of the GYTS, only schools and classes with students of ages 13 to 15 years were eligible to participate. The 2007 GTYS for Lusaka, Zambia included grades 7, 8 and 9 students. Grade 7 students were in primary school, while grades 8 and 9 consisted of secondary students. These grades were selected because they contained the majority of 13 to 15-year-old adolescents in the country. A two-stage cluster sampling design was used to produce representative data for the country. In the first stage of sampling, schools were selected with probability proportional to their student enrolment size. At the second stage, classes were randomly selected and all students in selected classes were eligible to participate, regardless of their actual ages. A total of 25 schools were selected to participate and 24 (96.0%) participated. Of the 2,678 students who were sampled, 2,378 (88.8%) eventually participated. Hence an overall response rate of 85.3% (product of school and student response rates) was achieved.

A standard GYTS questionnaire with a few country-specific data was administered to students in their classrooms during one subject session. The questionnaire was administered only to students who were present on the day a particular school was visited. No effort was made to follow-up any of the students who were not present. Questionnaires were self-completed anonymously on computer-scannable survey sheets.

Students were asked the following questions, among others: During the past 30 days (1 month), on how many days did you smoke cigarettes? Has anyone in your family discussed the harmful effects of smoking with you? During the past 30 days (1 month), how many anti-smoking media messages (e.g., television, radio, billboards, posters, newspapers, magazines, movies) have you seen or heard? When you go to sports events, fairs, concerts, community events or social gatherings, how often do you see anti-smoking messages? Responses to the questions were all pre-coded. A comprehensive description of the GYTS methodology has been reported elsewhere (10, 11).

The following questions were used for variable derivation for this study: Do you think the smoke from other people's cigarettes is harmful to you? Are you in favor of banning smoking in public places and public transport (such as in streetcars, schools, and sports arenas)? When you watch TV, videos, or movies, how often do you see actors smoking? Do you have something (T-shirt, pen, backpack, etc.) with a cigarette brand logo on it? During the past 30 days (1 month), when you watched sports events or other programs on TV, how often did you see cigarette brand names? During the past 30 days (1 month), how many advertisements for cigarettes have you seen on billboards? During the past 30 days (1 month), how many advertisements or promotions for cigarettes have you seen in newspapers or magazines? When you go for sports events, fairs, concerts or community events, how often do you see advertisements for cigarettes? Has a cigarette representative ever offered you a free cigarette? How old are you? What is your sex?

Permission to conduct the study was obtained from the Ministry of Education. All eligible students were also informed that participation was voluntary. Data collection was conducted in school by trained assistants without the presence of the teacher.

The GYTS data were analyzed in SPSS 11.5 (Chicago, IL, United States of America). As is the convention in the Global Tobacco Surveillance System (GTSS), current cigarette smoking was defined as having smoked a cigarette, even a single puff, within the last 30 days prior to the survey (9-11). A weighted analysis was conducted to obtain the prevalence of current cigarette smoking, as well as other relevant characteristics. We assessed associations between current smoking and the following: sex; age; and whether the student had reported the following: seen advertisements for cigarettes at sports events, fairs, concerts or community events; ever offered a free cigarette by a cigarette representative; possessed an item with a cigarette brand logo on it; seen actors smoking on TV shows, videos or movies; seen advertisements for cigarettes on billboards; seen advertisements or promotions for cigarettes in newspapers or magazines; seen cigarette brand names at sports events or other programmes on TV.

Table 1. Sample description of adolescents in the Zambia GYTS 2007

Factors	Males	Females	Total
	n (%)	n (%)	n (%)
Age group (years)			
≤12	185 (15.2)	220 (18.5)	407 (16.7)
13	199 (16.8)	205 (16.7)	404 (16.7)
14	278 (24.7)	239 (19.2)	517 (22.3)
15	204 (19.6)	237 (18.7)	441 (19.1)
16+	224 (23.8)	368 (26.9)	593 (25.1)
Sex			
Female	-	-	1093 (56.8)
Male	-	-	1281 (43.2)
Knew that smoke from other people's cigarettes is harmful			
No	539 (48.8)	576 (47.1)	1115 (48.0)
Yes	539 (51.2)	689 (52.9)	1232 (52.0)
Favored banning smoking in public places			
No	688 (63.2)	713 (57.6)	1405 (60.9)
Yes	379 (36.8)	532 (42.4)	911 (39.1)
Had seen actors smoking in TV shows, videos or movies			
No	233 (20.4)	256 (21.0)	489 (20.6)
Yes	844 (79.6)	1009 (79.0)	1857 (79.4)
Possessed something with a cigarette brand logo on it			
No	826 (79.8)	993 (79.2)	1822 (79.5)
Yes	229 (20.2)	253 (20.8)	483 (20.5)
Had seen cigarette brand names at sports events or other programs on TV			
No	402 (37.2)	467 (36.7)	870 (36.9)
Yes	679 (62.8)	803 (63.3)	1485 (63.1)
Had seen advertisements for cigarettes on billboards			
No	478 (45.1)	499 (41.0)	979 (43.3)
Yes	583 (54.9)	732 (59.0)	1317 (56.7)
Had seen advertisements or promotions for cigarettes in newspapers or magazines			
No	432 (41.2)	561 (44.0)	994 (42.4)
Yes	632 (58.8)	691 (56.0)	1326 (57.6)
Had seen advertisements for cigarettes at sports events, fairs, concerts or community events			
No	585 (54.5)	703 (55.6)	1290 (55.0)
Yes	498 (45.5)	556 (44.4)	1056 (45.0)
Had been ever offered a free cigarette by a cigarette sales representative			
No	839 (83.1)	988 (81.7)	1829 (82.4)
Yes	174 (16.9)	218 (18.3)	394 (17.6)
Smoked cigarettes in the 30 days prior to the survey			
No	802 (90.7)	912 (87.9)	1717 (89.5)
Yes	89 (9.3)	125 (12.1)	214 (10.5)

Other variables were also created from individual perceptions towards the following: Favoured banning smoking in public places; and believed that smoke from other people's cigarettes (i.e., second hand smoke) is harmful. A cut off point for statistical significance was set at the 5% level. We report results of bivariate logistic regression analysis as unadjusted odds ratio (OR) while the results from multivariable analysis are reported as adjusted odds ratios (AORs) together with 95% confidence intervals (CI).

FINDINGS

Altogether, 2,378 students participated in the Lusaka-Zambia GTYS. A description of the sample is elaborated in table 1. The sample comprised of mostly females (56.8%), 16 years or older (25.1%), and 39.1% favoured banning smoking in public places. About half (52.0%) of the students reported that smoke from cigarettes being smoked by other people is harmful. Overall, 10.5% of the students (9.3% among males, and 12.1% among females) smoked cigarettes in the 30 days prior to the survey.

Table 2 shows unadjusted and adjusted odds ratios for factors considered in the study with smoking status as the outcome. All the factors were significantly associated with smoking at bivariate analyses except the following: Seeing actors smoke on TV shows, video or movies; seeing cigarette brand names at sports events or other programs on TV; and reporting that smoke from other people's cigarettes is harmful. However, in multivariate analysis, factors that were significantly associated with smoking were: age; favouring banning smoking in public places; seeing actors smoking on TV, videos or movies; having something with a cigarette logo on it; seeing advertisements for cigarettes on TV; and having ever been offered a free cigarette by a cigarette representative.

Compared to students of age 12 years or less, older children were less likely to smoke cigarettes (OR = 0.51, 95% CI [0.31, 0.84] for 13 year-olds, OR = 0.16, 95% CI [0.08, 0.31] for 14 year-olds, OR = 0.24, 95% CI [0.14, 0.41] for 15 year-olds, OR = 0.47, 95% CI [0.29, 0.75] for 16+ year-olds). Students who favoured banning smoking in public places were 33% (OR = 0.67, 95% CI [0.47, 0.96]) less likely to smoke cigarettes compared to those who were not in favour of the ban. Seeing actors smoking on TV shows, videos or movies was positively associated with smoking (OR = 1.90, 95% CI [1.26, 2.88]). However, possessing an item with a cigarette brand logo on it; seeing advertisements for cigarettes on billboards and ever offered a free cigarette by a cigarette sales representative were negatively associated with smoking (OR = 0.39, 95% CI [0.26, 0.58]; OR = 0.63, 95% CI [0.43, 0.92]; and OR = 0.43, 95% CI [0.29, 0.65], respectively).

Table 2. Associations of advertisement-promotion-sponsorship-related factors with cigarette smoking

Factors	OR (95% CI)	AOR (95% CI)
Age group (years)		
≤12	1	1
13	0.39 (0.25, 0.63)	0.51 (0.31, 0.84)
14	0.65 (0.46, 0.92)	0.16 (0.08, 0.31)
15	1.07 (0.79, 1.47)	0.24 (0.14, 0.41)
16+	2.22 (1.73, 2.84)	0.47 (0.29, 0.75)
Sex		
Female	1	-
Male	1.24 (0.93, 1.65)	
Knew that smoke from other people's cigarettes is harmful		
No	1	-
Yes	0.82 (0.71, 0.95)	
Favored banning smoking in public places		
No	1	1
Yes	1.29 (1.12, 1.50)	0.67 (0.47, 0.96)
Had seen actors smoking in TV shows, videos or movies		
No	1	1
Yes	0.61 (0.52, 0.71)	1.90 (1.26, 2.88)
Possessed something with a cigarette brand logo on it		
No	1	1
Yes	1.99 (1.70, 2.33)	0.39 (0.26, 0.58)
Had seen cigarette brand names at sports events or other programs on TV		
No	1	-
Yes	0.87 (0.75, 1.01)	
Had seen advertisements for cigarettes on billboards		
No	1	1
Yes	1.35 (1.16, 1.58)	0.63 (0.43, 0.92)
Had seen advertisements or promotions for cigarettes in newspapers or magazines		
No	1	-
Yes	1.29 (1.11, 1.50)	
Had seen advertisements for cigarettes at sports events, fairs, concerts or community events		
No	1	-
Yes	1.30 (1.12, 1.50)	
Had been ever offered a free cigarette by a cigarette sales representative		
No	1	1
Yes	2.05 (1.74, 2.52)	0.43 (0.29, 0.65)

DISCUSSION

Overall, 10.5% of the students (9.3% among males, and 12.1% among females) smoked cigarettes in the 30 days prior to the survey. In a 1999 Kafue (Zambia) GYTS reported by Siziya et al., 8.2% of the adolescents were current cigarette smokers, while 93 (10.4%) males and 61 (6.2%) females were current smokers ($p < 0.001$) (6).

We have assessed proportions of adolescents who remembered to have been exposed to pro-tobacco advertisements and also perceptions of second hand tobacco smoke exposure among this sample. It is of interest that just about half (52%) perceived that second hand smoke (SHS) is harmful to health. This may suggest that education programs in Zambia may not have emphasised the fact that SHS is a health hazard. As the country implements the FCTC, this is an aspect that may have to be emphasised.

Perhaps as a consequence of limited knowledge of the potential harms of SHS, only 39.1% of respondents favoured a ban on smoking in public spaces. It can be argued that as long as adolescents are unaware of the health hazard of exposure to SHS, many may dislike exposure just as a nuisance or for other reasons but not for preventing harm to health. Again, we emphasise our expectation that as more and more adolescents become apprised about the harmful effects of SHS, there will be an increasing number of adolescents who will find smoking in public spaces offensive. Although there have been various regulations to restrict children's exposure to tobacco advertisement, many adolescents reported being exposed to information on tobacco products in magazines, billboards, television and videos. About a quarter (20.5%) possessed an item with a cigarette brand logo on it, and 17.6% had been offered free cigarettes by a tobacco sales representative.

When we assessed whether there was any association between the explanatory variables and current cigarette smoking, we found that adolescents who were males/or, aged $\leq$ 12 years and/or who had seen movie actors smoking in a video were more likely to be current cigarette smokers. Paradoxically, we found favouring a ban on public smoking, possessing an item with a cigarette brand logo on it, having had exposure to pro-tobacco advertisements and having ever been offered free cigarettes were negatively associated with being a current cigarette smoker.

The predominance of smoking among males has been reported in many studies (6). This has been explained as a consequence of the cultural tolerance that societies have towards male smoking. However, male predominance is not universal; as in some settings (12), such as the United States, adolescent girls and boys have similar smoking prevalence (13). That younger adolescents were more likely to smoke may be a reflection of smoking debut within this population. Younger adolescents may be more likely to smoke, but quit smoking as they grow older. The reasons behind this transition may be suggested and may include acquisition of health information in terms of the harmful effects of smoking. We suggest that studies be conducted to assess why younger adolescents seem more likely to be smokers compared to older peers.

While previous reports have suggested that exposure to tobacco advertisements (14-17) through the media, having ever been offered a free cigarette, and possessing an item with a cigarette brand logo on it were associated with smoking, we found that adolescents in Zambia seemed to behave differently. While this study was not designed to answer why this may have been the case, there are possible explanations. One of the explanations was that these promotion efforts were actually in place because tobacco firms had realised that adolescents were not smoking as much as they would have liked. In such a setting, we would find promotion efforts are in place but are yet to "bear dividends" for the tobacco firms.

This study has several limitations, which have been previously reported (13, 18). The sampling frame comprised of schools only in Lusaka, which means that only students were eligible to be included in the survey. The findings therefore, although representative of students in Lusaka, may not be representative of all adolescents in Lusaka, let alone in Zambia. Furthermore, even students who were eligible to participate but were not in school on the day that their school was surveyed were not followed up. However with a response rate of 85.3%, the findings can be described as representative enough.

We also assessed history of current cigarette smoking, which was defined as having smoked, even a single puff, within the 30 days prior to the survey. No bio-specimens for assessment of cotinine, exhaled carbon monoxide and for other relevant tests were collected and assessed to validate self-reports of smoking. Finally, as cross sectional data were collected, there is the limitation that we cannot ascribe causation to any of the variables assessed. We therefore report associations between the variables and current smoking and not causes.

In conclusion, findings from this study indicate that TV advertisement-promotion-sponsorship was positively associated with smoking, while it was the opposite with other forms of advertisement; there is a need for further studies.

ACKNOWLEDGMENTS

We thank the Centers for Disease Control and Prevention, as well as the Global Tobacco Surveillance System (GTSS), for technical assistance. This study would not have been possible without the participation of the students.

This chapter is a revised version of an original paper published in the Annals of African Medicine (Zulu R, Siziya S, Muula AS, Rudatsikira E. Associations of advertisement-promotion-sponsorship-related factors with current cigarette smoking among in-school adolescents in Zambia. Ann Afr Med 2009; 8:2 29-245) and the authors have obtained the permission from Annals of African Medicine to use this material.

REFERENCES

[1] Mathers CD, Loncar D. Projections of global mortality and burden of disease from 2002 to 2030. PLoS Med 2006; 3: e442.

[2] Murray CJ, Lopez AD. Mortality by cause for eight regions of the world: Global Burden of Disease Study. Lancet 1997; 349: 1269-76.

[3] Snow RW, Guerra CA, Mutheu JJ, Hay SI. International funding for malaria control in relation to populations at risk of stable Plasmodium falciparum transmission. PLoS Med 2008; 5: e142.

[4] Gruskin S, Tarantola D. Universal Access to HIV prevention, treatment and care: assessing the inclusion of human rights in international and national strategic plans. AIDS 2008; 22(Suppl 2): S123-S132.

[5] Kengne AP, Anderson CS. The neglected burden of stroke in Sub-Saharan Africa. Int J Stroke 2006; 1: 180-90.

[6] Siziya S, Rudatsikira E, Muula AS. Cigarette smoking among school-going adolescents in Kafue, Zambia. Malawi Med J 2007; 19: 75-8.

[7] Warner KE. The Framework Convention on Tobacco Control: opportunities and issues. Salud Publica Mex 2008; 50(Suppl 3):S283-S291.

[8] Wakefield M, Liberman J. Back to the future: tobacco industry interference, evidence and the Framework Convention on Tobacco Control. Tob Control 2008; 17: 145-6.

[9] Yang T, Wu Y, Abdullah AS, Dai D, Li F, Wu J, Xiang H. Attitudes and behavioral response toward key tobacco control measures from the FCTC among Chinese urban residents. BMC Public Health 2007; 7: 248.

[10] The GTSS Collaborative Group. The global tobacco surveillance system. Tob Control 2006; 15(Suppl 2):ii1-ii3.

[11] Global Tobacco Surveillance System Collaborating Group. Global Tobacco Surveillance System (GTSS): purpose, production, and potential. J Sch Health 2005; 75: 15-24.

[12] Global Youth Tobacco Survey Collaborating Group. Differences in worldwide tobacco use by gender: findings from the Global Youth Tobacco Survey. J Sch Health 2003; 73: 207-15.
[13] Warren CW, Jones NR, Peruga A, Chauvin J, Baptiste JP, Costa de Silva V, et al. Global youth tobacco surveillance,2000-2007. MMWR Surveill Summ 2008; 57:1-28.
[14] Siziya S, Rudatsikira E, Muula AS. Antismoking messages and current cigarette smoking status in Somaliland: results from the Global Youth Tobacco Survey 2004. Confl Health 2008; 2: 6.
[15] Osungbade KO, Oshiname FO. Determinants of cigarette smoking among senior secondary school students in a rural community of southwest Nigeria. Niger J Med 2008; 17: 40-4.
[16] Guindon GE, Georgiades K, Boyle MH. Susceptibility to smoking among South East Asian youth: a multilevel analysis. Tob Control 2008; 17: 190-7.
[17] St Romain T, Hawley SR, Ablah E, Kabler BS, Molgaard CA. Tobacco use in silent film: precedents of modern-day substance use portrayals. J Commun Health 2007; 32: 413-8.
[18] Muula AS, Siziya S, Rudatsikira E. Cigarette smoking and associated factors among in-school adolescents in Jamaica: comparison of the Global Youth Tobacco Surveys 2000 and 2006. BMC Res Notes 2008; 1: 55.

In: Smoking and Adolescence ISBN: 978-1-63484-311-9
Editors: M. L. Mazabam, S. Siziya et al. © 2016 Nova Science Publishers, Inc.

Chapter 8

GENDER DIFFERENCES IN PREVALENCE RATES AND PREDICTORS OF CIGARETTE SMOKING IN ADOLESCENCE

Seter Siziya[1,*], BA(Ed), MSc, PhD,
Pierson RT Ntata[2], BA, MA,
Emmanuel Rudatsikira[3], MD, MPH, DrPH,
Cecilia M Makupe[4], BA, MA, Eric Umar[5] BA, MA,
and Adamson S Muula[5], MBBS, MPH, PhD

[1]Department of Community Medicine, School of Medicine, University of Zambia, Lusaka, Zambia
[2]Department of Sociology, Chancellor College, University of Malawi, Zomba, Malawi
[3]Departments of Epidemiology and Biostatistics and Global Health, School of Public Health, Loma Linda University, Loma Linda, California, USA
[4]Department of Demography and Population Studies, Chancellor College, University of Malawi, Zomba, Malawi
[5]Department of Community Health, College of Medicine, University of Malawi, Blantyre, Malawi

[*] Corresponding author: Professor Seter Siziya, Clinical Sciences Department, School of Medicine, Copperbelt University, Ndola Central Hospital, 6th Floor, P.O. Box 71191, Ndola, Zambia. E-mail: ssiziya@gmail.com.

An analysis of the Global Youth Tobacco Survey for Kilimanjaro, Tanzania was carried out to assess gender differences in the prevalence rates and predictors of current cigarette smoking among in-school adolescents. A total of 2,323 adolescents, participated in the study of whom 53% were females and 47% males. The prevalence of current cigarette smoking was 3.0% and 1.4% among males and females, respectively. The common factors that were significantly positively associated with cigarette smoking between genders were: having more pocket money, closest friend smoked cigarettes, seeing actors smoke on TV, videos or movies, and seeing advertisements for cigarettes at social gatherings. Seeing anti-smoking messages at social gatherings were negatively associated with smoking among both gender. While having had something such as a t-shirt or pen with a cigarette brand logo on it was positively associated with cigarette smoking among males, it was negatively associated with cigarette smoking among females. Male adolescents older than 15 years, those in their 9th year of schooling, and those who had seen cigarette brand names on TV were more likely to smoke. Meanwhile, male respondents who were in their 8th year of schooling, had seen anti-smoking media messages, and advertisements for cigarettes in newspapers or magazines were less likely to smoke. Among female adolescents, those who had parents who smoked, and surprisingly those who perceived that cigarette smoking as harmful were more likely to smoke. Interestingly, seeing advertisement for cigarettes on billboards was negatively associated with smoking among female adolescents. Interventions aimed to reduce adolescent smoking need to be designed and implemented with due consideration of gender differences in these associated factors.

INTRODUCTION

Cigarette smoking is the leading cause of morbidity and mortality in the world. Total tobacco-attributable deaths are projected to rise from 5.4 million in 2005 to 6.4 million in 2015 and 8.3 million in 2030 (1). Many adult smokers initiate smoking either as young adults or adolescents (2, 3). Adolescent smoking is also of public health interest as it is associated with immediate or short-term consequences such as exacerbation of asthma and increased risk for respiratory infections (4). Adolescent smokers are also likely to engage in other unhealthy or harmful lifestyles such as illicit drug use, teen sex, alcohol use and truancy (5-7). An association between adolescent smoking and peer and/or parental smoking has been previously reported (8, 9). Studies on cigarette smoking among adolescents in sub-Saharan Africa have reported on the prevalence of exposure to both pro- and anti-tobacco smoking (10, 11). Tobacco use among adolescents is a growing problem in the region, and in Kilimanjaro in particular.

In order to inform the targeting of at risk individuals in the design and implementation of anti-smoking intervention efforts, there is need to assess whether there exists associations between selected socio-demographic variables and adolescent smoking in Africa. No previous studies on cigarette smoking we are aware of have ever been done in the region, and in particular to assess gender differences in smoking prevalence rates and associated factors. This study was therefore carried out to estimate the prevalence rates of current cigarette smoking and the associated factors between gender among in-school adolescents in Kilimanjaro, Tanzania in 2003.

OUR STUDY

The study was conducted in Kilimanjaro region in northern Tanzania. All schools in the region with classes 6 and 7 and forms 1 and 2 (6 to 9 years of schooling) were eligible to take part in the study. This study involved secondary analysis of data from the Global Youth Tobacco (GYTS) conducted in the region in 2003 The GYTS is an in-school survey that uses a standard methodology for constructing the sampling frame, selecting schools and classes, preparing questionnaires, following consistent field procedures, and using consistent data management procedures for data processing and analysis (12).

Data were collected in a survey that used a two-stage probability sampling technique. Primary sampling units were schools which were selected with a probability proportional to their enrolment size. In the second step of sampling, a systematic sample of classes in the selected school was obtained. All students in the selected classes were eligible to participate. A self-completed questionnaire was used. Completion of question occurred within one class period and trained research assistants supervised the process.

The main outcome variable was current cigarette smoking defined as having smoked a cigarette, even a single puff, within 30 days preceding the survey. Study participants were asked on how many days they smoked cigarettes. A response of zero days was recoded as ‘not a current smoker’ while a response of any number of days of smoking was recoded as a yes for current smoking.

Independent variables included age, year of schooling, whether the adolescent usually had pocket money, smoking status of parents and close friends. Other variables were whether study participants had seen anti-smoking media messages; seen anti-smoking messages at social gatherings; seen actors smoking on television (TV), videos or movies; had item such as a t-shirt or pen with a cigarette brand logo on it; seen cigarette brand names on TV; seen advertisements for cigarettes on billboards; seen advertisements for cigarettes in newspapers or magazines; and seen advertisements for cigarettes at social gatherings. Study participants were also asked whether they perceived cigarette smoking as harmful to health.

Data was analysis to determine the prevalence and associated factors of cigarette smoking between gender. A weighting factor was used in the analysis to reflect the likelihood of sampling each student and to reduce bias by compensating for differing patterns of non response. The weight used for estimation is given by the following formula as described by The GTSS Collaborative Group (13):

$$W = W1 * W2 * f1 * f2 * f3 * f4$$

where:

W1 = the inverse of the probability of selecting the school

W2 = the inverse of the probability of selecting the classroom within the school

f1 = a school-level non response adjustment factor calculated by school size category (small, medium, large)

f2 = a class-level non response adjustment factor calculated for each school

f3 = a student-level non response adjustment factor calculated by class

f4 = a post stratification adjustment factor calculated by grade

Backward logistic regression analyses to estimate the associations between relevant predictor variables and cigarette smoking within the last 30 days prior to the survey were done for each gender. Results for multivariate analysis (adjusted odds ratios) for the factors found significantly associated with the outcome are reported.

Permission for the data collection was obtained from the Ministry of Education. All eligible students were invited to participate. They were however free not to participate or not to complete any segments of the questionnaire if they so desired. Questionnaires were completed anonymously.

OUR FINDINGS

A total of 2,323 adolescents, 47% males and 53% females, participated in the survey. Overall prevalence of smoking was 3.0% and 1.4% among males and females, respectively. Table 1 shows socio-demographic correlates for cigarette smoking between gender among adolescents in Kilimanjaro.

Table 1. Prevalence and associated socio-demographic factors of cigarette smoking adolescents in Kilimanjaro

Factor	Males		Female	
	n (%)[a]	OR (95%CI)[b]	n (%)[a]	OR (95%CI)[b]
Age (years)				
<13	123 (2.3)	1	173 (2.9)	-
13	165 (1.9)	0.64 (0.51, 0.81)	243 (1.3)	
14	186 (2.6)	0.56 (0.45, 0.69)	264 (0)	
15	195 (3.5)	0.84 (0.70, 1.02)	221 (0.9)	
>15	300 (4.6)	2.02 (1.72, 2.38)	201 (2.0)	
Schooling (years)				
6	300 (2.6)	1	376 (1.1)	-
7	330 (2.9)	1.10 (0.95, 1.27)	447 (0.6)	
8	186 (2.7)	0.46 (0.37, 0.57)	164 (1.3)	
9	157 (5.6)	1.74 (1.51, 2.02)	116 (3.7)	
Pocket money received				
None	795 (1.8)	1	982 (0.5)	1
<1000	100 (7.0)	0.87 (0.75, 1.02)	75 (5.0)	0.83 (0.64, 1.08)
1000+	68 (11.4)	2.22 (1.93, 2.55)	34 (15.6)	14.24 (10.84,18.70)
Parent smoked cigarettes				
No	729 (2.7)	-	802 (0.6)	1
Yes	216 (4.1)		255 (3.2)	1.79 (1.49, 2.14)
Closest friend smoked cigarettes				
No	676 (0.9)	1	805 (0.1)	1
Yes	288 (8.5)	2.62 (2.39, 2.87)	279 (3.9)	2.95 (2.35, 3.70)

[a] % - Weighted percentage.

n - Unweighted number of respondents for the entire sample and not for complete case analysis in the multivariate analyses.

[b] OR (95%CI) - adjusted odds ratios for all the factors in tables 1 to 3 in a Backward logistic regression analysis.

Table 2. Prevalence and associated anti-smoking factors of cigarette smoking adolescents in Kilimanjaro

Factor	Males		Females	
	n (%)[a]	OR (95%CI)[b]	n (%)[a]	OR (95%CI)[b]
Seen anti-smoking media messages				
No	214 (5.4)	1	245 (0.9)	-
Yes	735 (2.3)	0.51 (0.47, 0.56)	844 (1.2)	
Seen anti-smoking messages at social gatherings				
No	508 (3.1)	1	625 (0.7)	1
Yes	447 (3.5)	0.89 (0.80, 0.98)	452 (0.9)	0.46 (0.37, 0.56)
Cigarette smoking is harmful to health				
No	937 (2.9)	-	1043 (0.9)	1
Yes	27 (11.5)		41 (7.2)	1.64 (1.27, 2.12)

[a] % - weighted percentage.

n - un-weighted number of respondents for the entire sample and not for complete case analysis in the multivariate analyses.

[b] OR (95%CI) - adjusted odds ratios for all the factors in Tables 1 to 3 in a Backward logistic regression analysis.

The common socio-demographic factors associated with cigarette smoking between gender were having more pocket money, and closest friend smoked cigarettes. Among the male respondents alone, adolescents of age more than 15 years were more likely to smoke cigarettes than younger ones. Compared to male adolescents in their 6th year of schooling, those in their 8th and 9th years of schooling were less and more likely, respectively, to smoke cigarettes. Parental smoking was significantly associated with cigarette smoking among only female respondents.

Seeing anti-smoking messages at social gatherings was negatively associated with cigarette smoking among both male and female respondents. Furthermore, seeing anti-smoking media messages was negatively associated with cigarette smoking among only male adolescents. Perception of cigarette smoking as harmful to health was positively associated with cigarette smoking among only female adolescents. Anti-smoking correlates for cigarette smoking among adolescents in Kilimanjaro are shown in Table 2.

Table 3 shows factors related to advertisements that were associated with cigarette smoking. Seeing advertisements for cigarettes at social gatherings, and seeing actors smoking on TV, videos or movies were positively associated with cigarette smoking among both gender. While having had something such as a t-shirt or pen with a cigarette brand logo on it was positively associated with cigarette smoking among males, it was, surprisingly, negatively associated with cigarette smoking among females. Seeing cigarette brand names on TV, videos or movies was positively associated with cigarette smoking among only males. Interestingly, seeing advertisements for cigarettes in newspapers or magazines was negatively associated with cigarette smoking among only male adolescents, and seeing advertisements for cigarettes on billboards was negatively associated with cigarette smoking among only female adolescents.

DISCUSSION

Our study has found that the prevalence of smoking was higher among males compared to females. The prevalence of current cigarette smoking in Kilimanjaro is much lower than the 16.2% reported by Kyrlesi et al. (14) for Greek adolescent and 12.2% to 25.5% for Ugandan ones (11). The finding that males were more likely to be smokers than females has been reported in other studies in diverse settings across the globe. However, an assessment of the GYTS surveys also has reported that males and females were equally likely to be smokers (13). In the current study, males were more likely to be smokers than females partly because more males than females were more likely to be outgoing to social gatherings, where temptations to smoke are great.

Pressure of examinations may have contributed to adolescents in their 9th year of schooling to be more likely to smoke. The 8th year of schooling is a non-examination year in Tanzania and in-school adolescents may be less likely to smoke. However, although examinations are held in the 9th year of schooling in Tanzania, at worst if a student fails, he/she can only repeat the year of schooling. Students are not dropped from school for failing examinations in the 9th year of schooling.

Our study also found that having closest friends as smoker and parental smoking were all associated with current smoking in the study participant. Due to the cross sectional nature of the study design and the questions asked in the survey we are unable to determine whether being a smoker attracts friends who are themselves smokers or rather that smokers preferentially select other smokers as their closest friends. It is possible that both mechanisms may be operational. The findings suggest that smoking cessation interventions targeting adolescents should be designed in such a way that the smoker's closest friends are also targeted.

Table 3. Prevalence and associated advertisement factors of cigarette smoking adolescents in Kilimanjaro

	Males		Females	
Factor	**n (%)[a]**	**OR (95%CI)[b]**	**n (%)[a]**	**OR (95%CI)[b]**
Seen actors smoking on TV, videos or movies				
No	536 (1.4)	1	711 (0.7)	1
Yes	430 (4.8)	1.64 (1.49, 1.82)	386 (1.6)	1.38 (1.12, 1.69)
Had something such as a t-shirt or pen with a cigarette brand logo on it				
No	743 (2.7)	1	877 (0.8)	1
Yes	198 (4.9)	1.16 (1.05, 1.27)	199 (1.1)	0.68 (0.55, 0.84)
Seen cigarette brand names on TV				
No	532 (2.2)	1	702 (0.6)	-
Yes	419 (4.5)	1.48 (1.33, 1.65)	377 (2.1)	
Seen advertisements for cigarettes on billboards				
No	345 (3.2)	-	446 (0.5)	1
Yes	606 (3.2)		633 (1.2)	0.75 (0.60, 0.94)
Seen advertisements for cigarettes in newspapers or magazines				
No	464 (2.6)	1	587 (0.7)	-
Yes	485 (3.8)	0.71 (0.64, 0.78)	497 (1.2)	
Seen advertisements for cigarettes at social gatherings				
No	617 (2.2)	1	741 (0.5)	1
Yes	346 (4.8)	1.19 (1.08, 1.31)	355 (2.5)	4.60 (3.60, 5.88)

[a] % - Weighted percentage.

n - Unweighted number of respondents for the entire sample and not for complete case analysis in the multivariate analyses.

[b] OR (95%CI) - adjusted odds ratios for all the factors in Tables 1 to 3 in a Backward logistic regression analysis.

The odds of being a current smoker among adolescents were higher if they reported parental smoking. Parental smoking may mean that the adolescent has assured access to cigarettes within the home. Also parents who smoke may not be committed to discourage adolescent smoking. Our findings demonstrate that in general exposure to pro-tobacco media is associated with being a smoker. Exposure to anti-tobacco media was associated with less likelihood of being a smoker. Other workers have reported similar findings elsewhere (15). The harmful effects of anti-tobacco advertisements from tobacco firms on adolescent smoking have been reported recently (16). These authors found that anti-tobacco messages directed at parents and guardians from tobacco firms in fact had the opposite effect of encouraging adolescent smoking. This suggests to us that public health policy makers should be vigilant and not just get satisfied with awareness campaigns without assessing their impact.

The finding that adolescents who believed that smoking was harmful to health were likely to be smokers themselves is interesting. This probably suggest that adolescent smokers are aware of the harmful effects of smoking but continue to smoke. A similar finding was reported by Young et al. (17) who has reported that Australian smokers strongly support more regulatory control of tobacco.

Adolescents who reported having pocket money were more likely to be smokers than those who reported never having money. Having money could accord the adolescent purchasing power which may not be available when one does not have the money. The policy implication of this finding is not clear though. Probably, parental monitoring of how adolescents use their money may be useful.

While this study only aimed to assess adolescent smoking, it is also important to recognise that adolescents who engage in one unhealthy life style are also likely to engage in many other harmful lifestyles. Lee et al. (18) have reported that adolescent smokers were more likely to be involved in physical fights, use of illicit drugs and carrying of weapons to schools.

This study had a number of limitations. The study design was cross sectional so it is not possible to assign causation to any of the factors identified as associated with adolescent smoking. Since the data were self-reported by the study participants, it is possible that some participants may have intentionally misreported or inadvertently misreported. Inadvertent misreporting could also occur when the study participants does not remember whether they had smoked within the 30 days period that the study questionnaire asked. Another limitation was that the study design did not incorporate verification of current smoking status by using biomarkers for assessment of nicotine metabolites or exhaled carbon monoxide (19, 20). In the case of blood or hair cotinine however, it has to be recognised too that environmental exposure to smoking may also produce a positive result (21). Furthermore, our study only recruited in-school adolescents and therefore these findings may not be applicable to out-of-school adolescents. The data used in the current study were collected before Tanzania committed itself to the World Health Organization's Framework Convention on Tobacco Control (FCTC) in April 2007. It will be important to assess adolescent smoking patterns in a few years' time so as to estimate the possible impact of the FCTC on Tanzania.

ACKNOWLEDGMENTS

This study was conducted as part of the Global Youth Tobacco Survey. The data used for the study were obtained from the Centers of Disease Control and Prevention CDC), Atlanta, Georgia, United States. The views expressed in the manuscript belong to the authors and not the CDC. Adamson S. Muula is the guarantor of the study.

This chapter is a revised version of an original paper published in the Tanzania Health Research Bulletin (Siziya S, Ntata PRT, Rudatsikira E, Makupe CM, Umar E, Muula AS. Gender differences in prevalence rates and predictors of cigarette smoking among in-school adolescents in Kilimanjaro, Tanzania. Tanzan Health Res Bull 2007; 9:190-195) and the authors have obtained the permission from the Tanzania Health Research Bulletin to use this material.

REFERENCES

[1] Mathers CD, Loncar D. Projections of global mortality and burden of disease from 2002 to 2030. PLoS Med 2006; 3: e442.

[2] Centers for Disease Control and Prevention (CDC). Use of cessation methods among smokers aged 16-24 years--United States, 2003. MMWR 2006; 55: 1351-4.

[3] Patton GC, Coffey C, Carlin JB, Sawyer SM, Wakefield M. Teen smokers reach their mid twenties. J Adolesc Health 2006; 39: 214-20.

[4] Gilliland FD, Islam T, Berhane K, Gauderman WJ, McConnell R, Avol E, Peters JM. Regular smoking and asthma incidence in adolescents. Am J Respir Crit Care Med 2006; 174:1094-100.

[5] Weden MM, Zabin LS. Gender and ethnic differences in the co-occurrence of adolescent risk behaviors. Ethn Health 2005; 10: 213-34.

[6] Kokkevi A, Richardson C, Florescu S, Kuzman M, Stergar E. Psychosocial correlates of substance use in adolescence: a cross-national study in six European countries. Drug Alcohol Depend 2007; 86: 67-74.

[7] Myers MG, Doran NM, Brown SA. Is cigarette smoking related to alcohol use during the 8 years following treatment for adolescent alcohol and other drug abuse? Alcohol Alcohol 2007; 42: 226-33.

[8] Brook JS, Pahl K, Ning Y. Peer and parental influences on longitudinal trajectories of smoking among African Americans and Puerto Ricans. Nicotine Tob Res 2006; 8: 639-51.

[9] Bricker JB, Peterson AV Jr, Sarason IG, Andersen MR, Rajan KB. Changes in the influence of parents' and close friends' smoking on adolescent smoking transitions. Addict Behav 2007; 32: 740-57.

[10] Mpabulungi L, Muula AS. Tobacco use among high school students in Kampala, Uganda: questionnaire study. Croat Med J 2004; 45: 80-3.

[11] Mpabulungi L, Muula AS. Tobacco use among high school students in a remote district of Arua, Uganda. Rural Remote Health 2006; 6: 609.

[12] Warren CW, Riley L, Asma S, Eriksen MP, Green L, Blanton C, et al. Tobacco use by youth: a surveillance report from the Global Youth Tobacco Survey project. Bull World Health Organ 2000; 78: 868-76.

[13] Global Youth Tobacco Survey Collaborating Group. Differences in worldwide tobacco use by gender: findings from the Global Youth Tobacco Survey. J Sch Health 2003; 73: 207-15.

[14] Kyrlesi A, Soteriades ES, Warren CW, Kremastinou J, Papastergiou P, Jones NR, et al. Tobacco use among students aged 13-15 years in Greece: the GYTS project. BMC Public Health 2007; 7: 3.

[15] Primack BA, Gold MA, Land SR, Fine MJ. Association of cigarette smoking and media literacy about smoking among adolescents. J Adolesc Health 2006;39:465-72.

[16] Wakefield M, Terry-McElrath Y, Emery S, Saffer H, Chaloupka FJ, Szczypka G, et al. Effect of televised, tobacco company-funded smoking prevention advertising on youth smoking-related beliefs, intentions, and behaviour. Am J Public Health 2006; 96: 2154-60.

[17] Young D, Borland R, Siahpush M, Hastings G, Fong GT, Cummings KM. Australian smokers support stronger regulatory controls on tobacco: findings from the ITC Four-Country Survey. Aust NZ J Public Health 2007; 31: 164-9.

[18] Lee LK, Chen PC, Lee KK, Kaur J. Violence-related behaviours among Malaysian adolescents: a cross sectional survey among secondary school students in Negeri Sembilan. Ann Acad Med Singapore 2007; 36: 169-74.

[19] Al-Delaimy WK. Hair as a biomarker for exposure to tobacco smoke. Tob Control 2002; 11: 176-82.

[20] Chetiyanukornkul T, Toriba A, Kizu R, Kimura K, Hayakawa K. Hair analysis of nicotine and cotinine for evaluating tobacco smoke exposure by liquid chromatography-mass spectrometry. Biomed Chromatogr 2004; 18: 655-61.

[21] Sorensen M, Bisgaard H, Stage M, Loft S. Biomarkers of exposure to environmental tobacco smoke in infants. Biomarkers 2007; 12: 38-46.

In: Smoking and Adolescence ISBN: 978-1-63484-311-9
Editors: M. L. Mazabam, S. Siziya et al. © 2016 Nova Science Publishers, Inc.

Chapter 9

CIGARETTE SMOKING AMONG ADOLESCENTS IN MALAWI

Adamson S Muula[1], MBBS, MPH, PhD,
Seter Siziya[2,*], BA(Ed), MSc, PhD,
and Emmanuel Rudatsikira[3], MD, MPH, DrPH

[1]Department of Community Health, University of Malawi, College of Medicine, Blantyre, Malawi,
[2]Department of Community Medicine, University of Zambia, School of Medicine, University Teaching Hospital Grounds, Lusaka, Zambia
[3]Department of Global Health
[4]Department of Epidemiology and Biostatistics, Loma Linda University, School of Public Health, Loma Linda, California, USA

The majority of adults who smoke cigarettes initiated the habit when they were adolescents or young adults. While rates of smoking and associated factors are known among 13-15 year olds in Malawi, correlates of cigarette smoking among adolescents in a national representative sample in Malawi have not been studied. We, therefore, carried out this study to estimate the prevalence of current smoking and determine its correlates in

* Corresponding author: Professor Seter Siziya, Clinical Sciences Department, School of Medicine, Copperbelt University, Ndola Central Hospital, 6th Floor, P.O. Box 71191, Ndola, Zambia. E-mail: ssiziya@gmail.com.

a nationally representative sample of in-school adolescents in Malawi. An analysis of the Malawi Global Youth Tobacco Survey (GYTS) 2005 was conducted. Using logistic regression analysis, we estimated the association between current cigarette smoking and potential explanatory variables. Overall, 2.5% of adolescents (3.2% among males, and 1.8% among females) were current cigarette smokers. Smoking among parents was 9.6% with no significant difference between males and females (10.3% versus 10.1%). Stronger associations with smoking were observed for friends smoking status (AOR = 3.07, 95% CI [2.99, 3.16]), receiving pocket money (AOR = 3.06, 95% CI [2.98, 3.14]), and perception that smoking increases body weight (AOR=2.98, 95% CI [2.81, 3.16]). Students who thought that cigarette smoking is harmful to health were 56% (AOR = 0.44, 95% CI [0.43, 0.45]) less likely to smoke than students who thought otherwise. Despite being the world's second leading grower of tobacco, prevalence of cigarette smoking among adolescent is lower than has been reported elsewhere.

INTRODUCTION

Tobacco is a leading cause of preventable non-communicable deaths. Mathers and Loncar (1) projected the total tobacco-attributable deaths to rise from 5.4 million in 2005 to 6.4 million in 2015. Furthermore, tobacco was projected to kill 50% more people in 2015 than HIV/AIDS, and to be responsible for 10% of all deaths globally.

Recently, Pampel (2) using data from the Malawi Demographic and Health Survey of 2000, reported the prevalence of cigarette smoking at 16–18% for men and 1% for women. Muula and Mpabulungi (3) and Muula (4) have reported the prevalence of current cigarette smoking among in-school adolescents at 6.2% in Lilongwe and 3.0% in Blantyre in Malawi using data obtained from the Global Youth Tobacco Survey (GYTS) of 2001. Before the 2005 Malawi GYTS, there was paucity of data on a national representative sample of adolescents in Malawi. Following the 2005 survey, a fact sheet (5) has been published outlining rates of a limited list of tobacco use and associated factors. However, the possible associations of any explanatory variables to cigarette smoking have not been reported at a national level.

The majority of adult smokers initiated the habit as adolescents or young adults. This therefore makes the monitoring and prevention of adolescent smokers a critical public health exercise. Our understanding of adolescent smoking is enriched when we also explore the socio-demographic variables that are associated with smoking at both the personal and the societal level.

We therefore carried out this study to estimate the prevalence of current smoking and associated variables in a nationally representative sample of in-school adolescents in Malawi. We also assessed associations between relevant explanatory variables and current cigarette smoking among the adolescents.

OUR STUDY

This study was based on a secondary analysis of data from the 2005 Malawi Global Youth Tobacco Survey. A comprehensive description of the GYTS purpose and methodology has been reported elsewhere (6). In brief however, the GYTS uses a questionnaire survey, recruits in-school adolescents from classes and the majority of students are aged between 13-15 years. A two-stage cluster sampling approach is used in which the primary sampling units are schools. In the second stage of sampling, classes within the school are randomly selected. All students within the selected classes are eligible to participate in the study, regardless of their actual ages. However, students are free not to participate although identified as eligible for participation.

Study participants self-complete a questionnaire that has standard "core" questions, and a few other country-specific questions that are included by the specific country team. The core questions enable meaningful comparisons on responses between countries. Completion of the questionnaire is estimated to take about 40 minutes, and is done within a class session. There is no recording of student names or any person identifiers on the questionnaire. Questions are asked to collect information on the following variables: age, history of having ever smoked, gender, current smoking status, parental smoking, having friends who smoked, exposure to environmental tobacco smoke and tobacco advertisements, perception that smoking is harmful to health and amount of pocket money usually received per month.

In the Malawi GYTS, permission to conduct the study was obtained from the Ministry of Education. Completed questionnaires were scanned by computer and a data file was generated in Access. Overall response rate was 92.5%. As per GYTS methodology, current cigarette smoking was defined as having smoked even a single puff of cigarette within the last 30 days preceding the survey (7). Data were analysed using SPSS software version 14.0 (Chicago, Illinois, United States). To assess associations between variables that were identified from the literature as possibly associated with current cigarette smoking, logistic regression analysis was conducted both at bivariate and multivariate level (8, 9). Backward logistic regression analysis was conducted to identify variables that are independently associated with smoking. Associations of cigarette advertisement or promotion factors with the outcome were adjusted for age and gender in addition to the other factors in the model. Messages against cigarette smoking were also adjusted for age and gender in addition to factors in the model. We report crude odds ratios (OR) and adjusted odds ratios (AOR) together with their 95% confidence intervals (CI).

FINDINGS

A total of 5,135 students participated in the Malawi GYTS 2005. However, data on gender were available for 5119 students of whom 46.0% were male, and 54.0% were female students. About a third (32.0%) of the students was aged 13 years. The proportions of participants whose parents and friends smoked were 10.3% and 15.5%, respectively. The overall prevalence of current smoking was 2.5% (1.8% among females, and 3.2% among males). The majority (86.0%) of the students felt that smoking makes one lose weight. One in five (19.5%) of the students recently received pocket money. Distributions of these factors by gender are shown in Table 1.

Overall, a third (31.8% and 30.8%) of the respondents had seen actors smoking on television (TV), video or movies, and saw cigarette brand names when watching sports events or other programs on TV, respectively. About half (54.2% of the students had heard about cigarette brand names on radio, 53.2% had seen advertisements for cigarette on billboards, and 50.3% had seen advertisements for cigarettes in newspapers or magazines) were subjected to smoking advertisements through the media. About a quarter (26.0%) of the students had seen advertisements for cigarettes at sports events, fairs, concerts or community events (see Table 2).

Main sources of antismoking messages were media (84.8%), youth groups (73.1%), religious organizations (73.0%), and family members (71.8%). The majority of the respondents (82.2%) thought cigarette smoking is harmful (see Table 3). Between 22.3% and 54.2% of the participants had seen actors smoking on television, had an item with a tobacco brand logo on it, seen tobacco brands while watching games, heard about tobacco brand names on radio, seen tobacco advertisements in magazines and newspapers, and had seen adverts at sports or community events. About 17.3% and 13.2% had attended a concert promoted by a tobacco company and offered a free cigarette by a tobacco company sales representative, respectively.

Table 1. Social demographic description of the study participants in the Malawi GYTS 2005

Factor	Total	Male	Female
	n* (%)**	n* (%)**	n* (%)**
Age			
≤12	1591 (32.0)	679 (31.1)	912 (33.0)
13	1171 (20.7)	480 (18.0)	691 (23.4)
14	1098 (21.3)	471 (19.4)	625 (23.1)
15+	1253 (26.0)	724 (31.5)	527 (20.5)
Gender			
Male	2357 (49.9)	-	-
Female	2762 (50.1)	-	-
Parents smoked			
Yes	474 (9.6)	232 (10.3)	241 (10.1)
No	4466 (90.4)	2041 (89.7)	2411 (89.9)
Friends smoked			
Yes	761 (15.5)	452 (20.0)	306 (11.0)
No	4307 (84.5)	1876 (80.0)	2419 (89.0)
Received pocket money			
Yes	1045 (19.5)	480 (19.9)	561 (18.9)
No	4058 (80.5)	1862 (80.1)	2184 (81.1)
Changes in body weight due to smoking			
Gain weight	199 (3.9)	99 (4.4)	100 (3.5)
Lose weight	4089 (81.7)	1835 (78.8)	2243 (83.3)
Weight unchanged	778 (15.4)	393 (16.8)	381 (13.2)

* Unweighted frequency.
** Weighted percent.

Table 2. Prevalence of exposure to pro-smoking advertisements stratified by gender among study participants in the Malawi GYTS 2005

Factor	Total	Male	Female
	n* (%)**	n* (%)**	n* (%)**
Seen actors smoking on TV, video, or movies			
Yes	1820 (35.9)	935 (34.9)	882 (28.8)
No	1067 (21.1)	417 (21.4)	647 (25.1)
Did not watch TV	2177 (43.0)	967 (43.7)	1202 (46.1)

Table 2. (Continued)

Factor	Total	Male	Female
	n* (%)**	n* (%)**	n* (%)**
Had something with a cigarette logo on it			
Yes	1133 (22.3)	563 (23.6)	564 (21.1)
No	3872 (77.7)	1730 (76.4)	2133 (78.9)
Saw cigarette brand names when watching sports events or other programs on TV			
Yes	1734 (30.3)	820 (31.2)	907 (29.2)
No	1489 (30.8)	701 (30.8)	784 (31.9)
Never watched TV	1860 (38.9)	813 (38.0)	1042 (38.9)
Heard cigarette brand names on radio			
Yes	2877 (54.2)	1358 (54.1)	1511 (54.4)
No	1276 (26.2)	536 (25.9)	737 (26.5)
Never listened to radio	908 (19.6)	429 (20.0)	475 (19.1)
Seen advertisements for cigarettes on billboards			
Yes	2787 (53.2)	1395 (57.1)	1384 (49.3)
No	2198 (46.8)	880 (42.9)	1310 (50.7)
Seen advertisements for cigarettes in newspapers or magazines			
Yes	2549 (50.3)	1278 (54.9)	1261 (45.7)
No	2358 (49.7)	967 (45.1)	1386 (54.3)
Seen advertisements for cigarettes at sports events, fairs, concert or community events			
Yes	1337 (26.0)	664 (28.3)	665 (23.6)
No	2095 (41.0)	968 (41.5)	1122 (40.5)
Never attended public gatherings	1636 (33.0)	691 (30.2)	942 (35.9)
Attended concert sponsored by a cigarette brand			
Yes	821 (17.3)	419 (17.2)	397 (17.2)
No	4254 (82.7)	1903 (82.8)	2340 (82.8)
Cigarette representative ever offered a free cigarette			
Yes	633 (13.2)	338 (13.8)	292 (12.6)
No	4390 (86.8)	1956 (86.2)	2422 (87.4)

* Unweighted frequency.

** Weighted percent.

Table 3. Prevalence of exposure to anti-smoking stratified by gender among study participants in the Malawi GYTS 2005

Factor	Total	Male	Female
	n* (%)**	n* (%)**	n* (%)**
Taught dangers of smoking			
Yes	3097 (61.7)	1485 (64.8)	1601 (58.5)
No	1878 (38.3)	794 (35.2)	1080 (41.5)
Seen or heard antismoking media messages			
Yes	4290 (84.9)	1999 (86.2)	2277 (83.6)
No	782 (15.1)	333 (13.8)	447 (16.4)
Seen antismoking messages at sports events, fairs, concert, community gathering or social gathering			
Yes	2052 (39.0)	973 (40.9)	1071 (37.0)
No	799 (14.3)	344 (14.3)	452 (14.4)
Never attended social gatherings	2226 (46.7)	1014 (44.8)	1207 (48.6)
Taught effects of smoking like yellowing of teeth, causes wrinkles, or makes one smell badly			
Yes	3173 (64.0)	1517 (67.0)	1648 (61.0)
No	1898 (36.0)	804 (33.0)	1086 (39.0)
Heard from youth groups discouraging young people from smoking			
Yes	3704 (73.1)	1694 (73.5)	1997 (72.6)
No	1301 (26.9)	598 (26.5)	701 (27.4)
Health professionals explained why smoking is dangerous to health			
Yes	2956 (58.8)	1384 (61.8)	1561 (55.7)
No	2064 (41.2)	920 (38.2)	1140 (44.3)
Religious organizations discouraged young people from smoking			
Yes	3626 (73.0)	1664 (74.8)	1951 (71.1)
No	1315 (27.0)	607 (25.2)	707 (28.9)
Family members discussed harmful effects of smoking			
Yes	3740 (71.8)	1739 (73.4)	1987 (70.1)
No	1326 (28.2)	595 (26.6)	729 (29.9)
Thought cigarette smoking is harmful to health			
Yes	4208 (82.2)	1888 (81.8)	2307 (82.5)
No	776 (17.8)	404 (18.2)	371 (17.5)

* Unweighted frequency.

** Weighted percent.

Social, demographic, and economic correlates for current smoking status are summarized in Table 4. Stronger associations with current smoking status were observed for friends smoking status (AOR = 3.07, 95% CI [2.99, 3.16]), receiving pocket money (AOR = 3.06, 95% CI [2.98, 3.14]), and perception that smoking increases body weight (AOR = 2.98, 95% CI [2.81, 3.16]).

Table 4. Associations of social, demographic and economic factors with current cigarette smoking among study participants in the Malawi GYTS 2005

Factor	Crude odds ratio OR (95%CI)	Adjusted odds ratio AOR (95%CI)
Age		
≤12	0.93 (0.90, 0.96)	1.03 (0.98, 1.07)
13	0.85 (0.82, 0.89)	0.92 (0.87, 0.97)
14	0.91 (0.88, 0.95)	0.80 (0.76, 0.84)
15+	1	1
Gender		
Male	1.31 (1.28, 1.33)	1.07 (1.04, 1.10)
Female	1	1
Parents smoked		
Yes	2.33 (2.28, 2.39)	1.70 (1.65, 1.75)
No	1	1
Friends smoked		
Yes	3.93 (3.84, 4.02)	3.07 (2.99, 3.16)
No	1	1
Received pocket money		
Yes	3.97 (3.87, 4.06)	3.06 (2.98, 3.14)
No	1	
Changes in body weight due to smoking		
Gain weight	2.94 (2.81, 3.07)	2.98 (2.81, 3.16)
Lose weight	0.49 (0.48, 0.51)	0.57 (0.55, 0.60)
Weight unchanged	1	1

AOR (95%CI) are adjusted for all the factors in the table.

All the factors in Table 5 were positively significantly associated with current smoking, except for the factor 'seeing advertisements in newspapers or magazines.' Students who had seen advertisements for cigarettes in newspapers or magazines were 4% (AOR = 0.96, 95% CI [0.93, 0.99]) less likely to have been current smokers.

Table 5. Associations of advertisement or promotion factors with current cigarette smoking among study participants in the Malawi GYTS 2005

Factor	Crude odds ratio OR (95%CI)	Adjusted odds ratio AOR (95%CI)
Seen actors smoking on TV, video, or movies		
Yes	2.11 (2.05, 2.18)	1.87 (1.80, 1.95)
No	0.80 (0.77, 0.83)	1.24 (1.18, 1.30)
Did not watch TV	1	1
Had something with a cigarette logo on it		
Yes	1.53 (1.50, 1.57)	1.31 (1.27, 1.35)
No	1	1
Saw cigarette brand names when watching sports events or other programs on TV		
Yes	1.76 (1.71, 1.81)	1.13 (1.09, 1.18)
No	0.85 (0.82, 0.88)	1.35 (1.30, 1.42)
Never watched TV	1	1
Heard cigarette brand names on radio		
Yes	1.39 (1.35, 1.43)	1.64 (1.56, 1.73)
No	0.63 (0.60, 0.66)	0.36 (0.33, 0.39)
Never listened to radio	1	1
Seen advertisements for cigarettes on billboards		
Yes	1.51 (1.48, 1.55)	1.49 (1.44, 1.55)
No	1	1
Seen advertisements for cigarettes in newspapers or magazines		
Yes	1.37 (1.34, 1.40)	0.96 (0.93, 0.99)
No	1	1
Seen advertisements for cigarettes at sports events, fairs, concert or community events		
Yes	2.31 (2.25, 2.38)	1.25 (1.20, 1.29)
No	0.53 (0.51, 0.55)	0.86 (0.82, 0.90)
Never attended public gatherings	1	1
Attended concert sponsored by a cigarette brand		
Yes	1.95 (1.91, 1.99)	1.29 (1.25, 1.33)
No	1	1
Cigarette representative ever offered a free cigarette		
Yes	2.08 (2.04, 2.13)	1.73 (1.68, 1.79)
No	1	1

AOR (95%CI) are adjusted for age and gender in addition to all the factors in the table.

Table 6. Associations of antismoking messages with current smoking status among study participants in the Malawi GYTS 2005

Factor	Crude odds ratio OR (95%CI)	Adjusted odds ratio AOR (95%CI)
Taught dangers of smoking		
Yes	0.77 (0.75, 0.79)	1.06 (1.02, 1.09)
No	1	1
Seen or heard antismoking media messages		
Yes	0.89 (0.86, 0.91)	0.89 (0.86, 0.93)
No	1	1
Seen antismoking messages at sports events, fairs, concert, community gathering or social gathering		
Yes	1.52 (1.47, 1.56)	1.60 (1.54, 1.66)
No	0.89 (0.85, 0.93)	1.06 (1.01, 1.12)
Never attended social gatherings	1	1
Taught effects of smoking like yellowing of teeth, causes wrinkles, or makes one smell badly		
Yes	0.76 (0.74, 0.78)	0.81 (0.79, 0.84)
No	1	1
Heard from youth groups discouraging young people from smoking		
Yes	0.64 (0.62, 0.65)	0.66 (0.64, 0.68)
No	1	1
Health professionals explained why smoking is dangerous to health		
Yes	1.07 (1.04, 1.09)	-
No	1	
Religious organizations discouraged young people from smoking		
Yes	0.88 (0.86, 0.90)	1.19 (1.15, 1.23)
No	1	1
Family members discussed harmful effects of smoking		
Yes	0.88 (0.86, 0.90)	0.94 (0.91, 0.97)
No	1	1
Thought cigarette smoking is harmful to health		
Yes	0.48 (0.47, 0.49)	0.44 (0.43, 0.45)
No	1	1

AOR (95%CI) are adjusted for age and gender in addition to all the factors in the table.

Respondents who had seen actors smoking on TV (AOR = 1.87, 95% CI [1.80, 1.95]), those who had heard of cigarette brand names on radio (AOR = 1.64, 95% CI [1.56, 1.73]), and those who were offered free cigarettes by a cigarette sales representative were more likely to smoke cigarettes than those who never watched TV, never listened to radio, and never offered free cigarettes from cigarette sales representatives.

We found that being taught dangers of smoking (AOR = 1.06, 95% CI [1.02, 1.09]), seeing antismoking messages at sports events, fairs, concerts, community gathering or social events (AOR = 1.60, 95% CI [1.54, 1.66]), and religious organizations discouraging young people from smoking (AOR=1.19, 95% CI [1.15, 1.23]) were positively associated with current cigarette smoking. The rest of the factors in Table 6 were negatively associated with current cigarette smoking. While explanation by health workers that smoking is dangerous was positively associated with current cigarette smoking in a bivariate analysis, this factor was not significantly associated with current cigarette smoking in a multivariate analysis. The largest magnitude of association was observed for the factor 'thinking that cigarette smoking is harmful to health.' Students who thought that cigarette smoking is harmful to health were 56% (AOR = 0.44, 95% CI [0.43, 0.45]) less likely to smoke than those who thought otherwise.

DISCUSSION

To our knowledge, the Malawi GYTS 2005 is the first ever nationally representative sample of in-school adolescents studied on tobacco use, including cigarette smoking. Previous surveys have been limited to specific geographic areas such Lilongwe and Blantyre (3, 4). The overall prevalence of current cigarette smoking was 2.5%, with 1.8% and 3.2% among females and males, respectively. The gender difference may be related to societal tolerance of smoking among males compared to females. Compared to the estimate obtained in the GYTS 2001 for Blantyre (3.0%) and Lilongwe (6.2%), the national prevalence is much lower. The reasons behind these differences are not known. However, we can suggest a few possibilities. Both studies in Blantyre and Lilongwe were conducted only in the urban areas of these districts. It is possible that smoking prevalence may be higher in urban commercial centres than the national estimates that also include rural areas. Secondly, it is possible that smoking prevalence has gone down. However, we do not have data for a national estimate for 2001 to verify if this assumption is correct. Nevertheless, between 2001 and 2005, there have been public health efforts, save for legislated changes, aimed to raise awareness among schoolchildren on the harmful effects of smoking.

In the developed world, adolescents may be motivated to initiate smoking in order to lose weight, which is perceived as a desirable outcome in these settings. Bean et al. (10) have reported that adolescent non-smokers believed that smoking would result in weight loss, while smokers believed that they would gain weight if they stopped smoking. However, Bentley et al. (11) reported that heavier built bodies were desirable among women in Malawi, in contrast to leaner bodies in the United States. Whether adolescents in Malawi hold different or similar views as their American counterparts deserve further study.

The low prevalence of smoking is also reflected in a low smoking prevalence among parents of the study participants. Slama (12) has reported smoking prevalence rates of 49% and 8% among men and women in low- and mid-income countries. Our estimates are much lower, especially for men (10.3% for Malawi versus 49% globally), but higher for Malawian women (10.1%) compared to the global estimates (8%). It is possible that the Malawi estimates may in fact be under-estimates as these (the estimates) were based on reports by smokers' children. Comparisons with data obtained when adults are surveyed need to be made with this caveat in mind.

Factors such as seeing actors smoking on television, having an item with a tobacco brand logo, seeing tobacco brands while watching games, hearing about tobacco brand names on radio, seeing tobacco advertisements in magazine and newspapers, and having seen adverts at sports or community events have been reported in previous studies to be associated with smoking among adolescents (9, 13, 14). Exposure to anti-tobacco initiatives such as being taught the dangers of smoking, having seen anti-smoking messages, having discussed smoking with family members and having heard anti-smoking messages on the media may have led to the majority (81.8%) believing that smoking is harmful to health. In general, being exposed to pro-tobacco media was associated with increased likelihood of being a smoker. This observation is in keeping with the Social Cognitive Theory (15, 16). The theory proposes that environment, people, and behaviour are constantly influencing each other in influencing behaviour. Of relevance to adolescent smoking is the recognition that the social environment that the adolescent is exposed to may influence when he or she initiates and/or maintains smoking.

We note some unexpected findings regarding smoking and explanatory variables. We found that adolescents who reported exposure to anti-tobacco advertisements were more likely to be current cigarette smokers. Study participants who reported being taught the dangers of smoking, having heard religious groups discouraging smoking, seeing anti-smoking messages at public events or social gathering, having had a health professional discuss smoking with them were more likely to be smokers. We are unable to obtain reasons for these paradoxical associations. However, potential explanations can be suggested. It is possible that adolescents who were smokers were more likely to have a discussion about smoking with a health professional as part of usual clinical care or due to illnesses associated with smoking (e.g., asthma or chronic cough). Schools with high smoking prevalence among students may also be more likely to have lessons aimed at discouraging students from smoking. Another alternative explanation is that the anti-tobacco messages were yet to be effective. Henriksen et al. (17) have reported that tobacco industry sponsored anti-tobacco messages may not result in decreasing tobacco use. These authors have reported that anti-tobacco messages from tobacco firms were more effective in building corporate image rather than preventing smoking. In Malawi, anti-tobacco message are likely to come from tobacco firms on radio advertisements aimed to promote smoking.

Malawi is the second leading grower of tobacco and no other country in the world is economically dependent on tobacco as Malawi (18-22). However, it appears that such a leading role in tobacco farming has not been translated into the country being a large cigarette consumer.

The limitations of the GYTS methodology has been reported elsewhere (6, 23). Firstly, data was collected from a self-completed questionnaire. For the main outcome of the current analysis, students were asked: During the past 30 days (one month), on how many days did you smoke cigarettes? Students may have intentionally miss-reported. It is also possible that some students may have genuinely forgotten whether they had smoked within the past 30 days. Another limitation is the GYTS definition of current smoking, defined as having smoked, even a single puff within the last 30 days. It should be clear that some students who may have smoked a single puff might have never smoked again. As to how many of such students there were in our sample is not known. Nevertheless, if the proportion of students who experimented with a single puff was high, our estimates lead us to exaggerate the public health importance of adolescent smoking in Malawi.

The GYTS methodology recruits study participants from schools. Our findings may not be applicable to out-of-school adolescents. Many secondary school-age adolescents are not enrolled in school. As school attendance is not compulsory and the out-of-school adolescent population is large, the overall prevalence of smoking among adolescents in the country may be assessed if both in-school and out of school adolescents are sampled. Furthermore, the GYTS methodology administers the questionnaire only to those students who are available in school on the day the survey is conducted, and as such, the findings may not be representative of all age-eligible students. However, the response rate was relatively high (84.3%) suggesting that most of the students who were eligible to participate did actually participate in the survey. In addition, the smoking status of the study participants was not validated by biomarkers such as salivary or urine cotinine. Even if these were used, they would have only been useful to determine the smoking status of students within the past few days. A student who had smoked for instance 29 days ago, may not exhibit biomarkers of smoking. Analysis of other bio-samples such as hair or finger nails for tobacco bi-products would also not distinguish between adolescents own smoking and environmental tobacco exposure.

In conclusion, we have estimated an overall prevalence of current cigarette smoking of 2.5% among in-school adolescents in Malawi, despite the country being the second leading grower of tobacco. This prevalence estimate is among the lowest in-school adolescents when compared to other estimates reported from similar settings.

ACKNOWLEDGMENTS

We thank all the study participants for their involvement in the study. We are also grateful to the Centers for Disease Control and Prevention (CDC) for making the data from the Malawi GYTS available to us for analysis. The CDC had no influence regarding the analysis that we conducted, nor the decision to have these findings published.

This chapter is a revised version of an original paper published in the Tanzania Journal of Health Research (Muula AS, Siziya S, Rudatsikira E. Prevalence and correlates of cigarette smoking among adolescents in Malawi: results from the Global Youth Tobacco Survey 2005. Tanzan J Health Res 2008; 10: 166-176) and the authors have obtained the permission from Tanzania Journal of Health Research to use this material.

REFERENCES

[1] Mathers CD, Loncar D. Projections of global mortality and burden of disease from 2002 to 2030. PLoS Med 2006; 3: e442.

[2] Pampel FC. Patterns of tobacco use in the early epidemic stages: Malawi and Zambia, 2000-2002. Am J Public Health 2005; 95: 1009-15.

[3] Muula AS, Mpabulungi L. Cigarette smoking prevalence among school-going adolescents in two African capital cities: Kampala Uganda and Lilongwe Malawi. Afr Health Sci 2007; 7: 45-9.

[4] Muula AS. Prevalence and determinants of cigarette smoking among adolescents in Blantyre City, Malawi. Tanzan Health Res Bull 2007; 9: 48-51.

[5] CDC. Global Youth Tobacco Survey Malawi. Centres for Disease Control and Prevention. URL: http://www.cdc.gov/tobacco/Global/GYTS/factsheets/afro/2005/malawi_factsheet.htm.

[6] Warren CW, Jones NR, Peruga A, Chauvin J, Baptiste JP, Costa de Silva V, el Awa F, Tsouros A, Rahman K, Fishburn B, Bettcher DW, Asma S, Centers for Disease Control and Prevention (CDC). Global youth tobacco surveillance, 2000-2007. MMWR Surveill Summ 2008; 57: 1-28.

[7] Warren CW, Riley L, Asma S, Eriksen MP, Green L, Blanton C, Loo C, Batchelor S, Yach D. Tobacco use by youth: a surveillance report from the Global Youth Tobacco Survey project. Bull World Health Organ 2000; 78: 868-76.

[8] Rudatsikira E, Dondog J, Siziya S, Muula AS. Prevalence and determinants of adolescent cigarette smoking in Mongolia. Singapore Med J 2008; 49: 57-62.

[9] Siziya S, Ntata PR, Rudatsikira E, Makupe CM, Umar E, Muula AS. Sex differences in prevalence rates and predictors of cigarette smoking among in-school adolescents in Kilimanjaro, Tanzania. Tanzan Health Res Bull 2007; 9: 190-195.

[10] Bean MK, Mitchell KS, Speizer IS, Wilson DB, Smith BN, Fries EA. Rural adolescent attitudes toward smoking and weight loss: relationship to smoking status. Nicotine Tob Res 2008; 10: 279-86.

[11] Bentley ME, Corneli AL, Piwoz E, Moses A, Nkhoma J, Tohill BC, Ahmed Y, Adair L, Jamieson DJ, van der Horst C. Perceptions of the role of maternal nutrition in HIV-positive breast-feeding women in Malawi. J Nutr 2005; 135: 945-9.

[12] Slama K. Global perspective on tobacco control. Part I. The global state of the tobacco epidemic. Int J Tuberc Lung Dis 2008; 12: 3-7.

[13] Laugesen M, Scragg R, Wellman RJ, DiFranza JR. R-rated film viewing and adolescent smoking. Prev Med 2007; 45: 454-9.

[14] Scragg R, Laugesen M. Influence of smoking by family and best friend on adolescent tobacco smoking: results from the 2002 New Zealand national survey of year 10 students. Aust NZ J Public Health 2007; 31: 217-23.

[15] Bandura A. Social cognitive theory: an agentive perspective. Annu Rev Psychol 2001; 52: 1-26.

[16] Glanz K, Rimer BK, Lewis FM. Health Behaviour and Health Education. Theory, Research and Practice. San Francisco, CA: Wiley, 2002.

[17] Henriksen L, Dauphinee AL, Wang Y, Fortmann SP. Industry sponsored anti-smoking ads and adolescent reactance: test of a boomerang effect. Tob Control 2006; 15: 13-8.

[18] Davies P. Malawi: addicted to the leaf. Tob Control 2003; 12: 91–3.

[19] Ota?ez MG, Mamudu H, Glantz SA. Global leaf companies control the tobacco market in Malawi. Tob Control 2007; 16: 261-9.

[20] Diao X, Robinson S, Thomas M, Wobst P. Assessing impacts of declines in the world price of tobacco on China, Malawi, Turkey, and Zimbabwe. Washington, DC: International Food Policy Research Institute, 2002. URL: http://www.ifpri.org/divs/tmd/dp/papers/tmdp91.pdf.

[21] FAO. Issues in the global tobacco economy: selected case studies. Rome: Food and Agriculture Organization of the United Nations, 2003. Accessed 2015 October 25: URL: http://www.ftp.fao.org/docrep/fao/006/y4997E/y4997e01.pdf.

[22] Jaffe S. Malawi's tobacco sector: standing on one strong leg is better than on none. Washington, DC: World Bank, 2003.

[23] Siziya S, Muula AS, Rudatsikira E. Correlates of current cigarette smoking among school-going adolescents in Punjab, India: results from the Global Youth Tobacco Survey 2003. BMC Int Health Hum Rights 2008; 8: 1.

In: Smoking and Adolescence ISBN: 978-1-63484-311-9
Editors: M. L. Mazabam, S. Siziya et al. © 2016 Nova Science Publishers, Inc.

Chapter 10

ADOLESCENTS AND CIGARETTE SMOKING IN SOMALILAND

Seter Siziya[1,*], BA(Ed), MSc, PhD, Emmanuel Rudatsikira[2], MD, MPH, DrPH, and Adamson S Muula[3], MBBS, MPH, PhD

[1]Department of Community Medicine, University of Zambia, Medical School, Lusaka, Zambia

[2]Departments of Epidemiology and Biostatistics and Global Health, Loma Linda University, School of Public Health, Loma Linda, California, USA

[3]Department of Community Health, University of Malawi, College of Medicine, Blantyre, Malawi

Tobacco is a leading cause of death globally. There are limited reports on current cigarette smoking prevalence and its associated-antismoking messages among adolescents in conflict zones of the world. We, therefore, conducted secondary analysis of data to estimate the prevalence of current cigarette smoking, and to determine associations of antismoking messages with smoking status. We used data from the Somaliland Global Youth Tobacco Survey (GYTS) of 2004 to estimate the prevalence of smoking. We also assessed whether being exposed to

---

* Correspondence: Professor Seter Siziya, Clinical Sciences Department, School of Medicine, Copperbelt University, Ndola Central Hospital, 6th Floor, P. O. Box 71191, Ndola, Zambia. E-mail: ssiziya@gmail.com.

anti-smoking media, education and having discussed with family members on the harmful effects of smoking were associated with smoking. Logistic regression analysis was used to assess these associations. Current smoking was defined as having reported smoking cigarettes, even a single puff, in the last 30 days preceding the survey (main outcome). Altogether 1563 adolescents participated in the survey. However, 1122 had data on the main outcome. Altogether, 15.8% of the respondents reported having smoked cigarettes (10.3% among males, and 11.1% among females). Factors that were associated with reported non-smoking were: discussing harmful effects of smoking cigarettes with their family members (OR = 0.61, 95% CI [0.52, 0.71]); being taught that smoking makes teeth yellow, causes wrinkles and smokers smell badly (OR = 0.62, 95% CI [0.52, 0.74]); being taught that people of the respondent's age do not smoke (OR = 0.81, 95% CI [0.69, 0.95]); and having reported that religious organizations discouraged young people smoking (OR = 0.70, 95% CI [0.60, 0.82]). However, exposure to a lot many antismoking messages at social gatherings was associated with smoking. Exposure to antismoking print media was not associated with smoking status. A combination of school and home based antismoking interventions may be effective in controlling adolescent smoking in Somaliland.

INTRODUCTION

Tobacco use is a leading cause of morbidity and mortality globally. Tobacco's contribution to ill health is projected to rise if current smoking trends are not reduced across the world (1). Although much of the long-term effects of smoking are observed in adulthood, the majority of smokers initiate the habit of smoking as adolescents.

There is a growing body of literature on adolescent tobacco use. Much of the research on the estimate of the prevalence and associated factors of adolescent smoking has been driven by the Global Youth Tobacco Survey (GYTS); an initiative spearheaded by the United States' Centers for Diseases Control and Prevention (CDC), the World Health Organization (WHO) and the Canadian Public Health Association (2), and a group of authors who have been conducting secondary analysis of GYTS data (3). Traditional reporting of results from the GYTS has concentrated on ages 13 to 15 years, and estimates of prevalence and the general socio-environment that may be associated with teenage smoking.

Odenwald et al. (4) have reported on the more than usual use of khat in Somalia as an indication of heightened prevalence of substance abuse in an environment of civil strife as is characteristic of most of Somalia. The prevalence of any tobacco use was 32.8% (26.8% among males, and 33.1% among females) and 15.8% currently smoked cigarettes (10.2% among males, and 11.1% among females) in the GYTS 2004 among adolescents 13 to 15 years of age (5).

While the prevalence of cigarette smoking in Somaliland has been reported, we are unaware of efforts to associate antismoking messages with current smoking status, and attempt to explain the prevalence of cigarette smoking within a conceptual or theoretical framework of health behaviors. We therefore carried out this study to estimate the prevalence of current cigarette smoking among all study participants in the Somaliland GYTS, identify positive antismoking messages, and explain their associations with current smoking status within theory-based outlook.

OUR STUDY

The Republic of Somaliland is what was previously known as the Somaliland Protectorate under the British rule from 1884 to 1969. The country attained independence in June 1960 around the same time that Italian Somalia also achieved independence from Italy. On July 1st 1960 Somaliland joined the former Italian Somalia to form the Somali Republic. A civil war was fought from 1980 onwards resulting in the eventual collapse of the Somali Republic. Somaliland shares borders with Republic of Djibouti to the west, Federal Republic of Ethiopia to the south and, the Red Sea to the North and Somalia to the east.

In this chapter we perform a secondary analysis of data from the Somaliland GYTS conducted in 2004. The Somaliland GYTS was a school-based survey of students in public primary classes 6 to 8, and Secondary 1. These classes were selected because they contained the majority of 13 to 15 years old adolescents in Somaliland. A two-stage cluster sample design was used to produce representative data for all of Somaliland. At the first stage, schools were selected with probability proportional to enrollment size. At the second stage, classes were randomly selected and all students in selected classes were eligible to participate. The overall response rate was 82.9%; the school response rate was 88%, the student response rate was 94.2%. Altogether 1563 students participated in the Somaliland GYTS.

A GYTS questionnaire was administered to students in their classrooms during one subject session. Only students who were present on the day a particular school was visited participated in the study. Students who were eligible but absent were not followed up. Questionnaires were self-completed on computer scan able survey sheets.

Students were asked among others the following questions: During the past 30 days (one month), on how many days did you smoke cigarettes? Has anyone in your family discussed the harmful effects of smoking with you? During the past 30 days (one month), how many antismoking media messages (e.g., television, radio, billboards, posters, newspapers, magazines, movies) have you seen or heard? When you go to sports events, fairs, concerts, community events, or social gatherings, how often do you see anti-smoking messages? During this school year, were you taught in any of your classes about the effects of smoking like it makes your teeth yellow, causes wrinkles, or makes you smell bad?; During the past year, did any health professionals explain to you why smoking is dangerous to your health? During the past year, did any religious organization discourage young people of your age from smoking? Responses to the questions were all pre-coded. A comprehensive description of the GYTS methodology has been reported elsewhere (6-8).

We obtained the data set from the CDC. Data were analyzed in SPSS 14.0 (Chicago, IL, United States of America). Current cigarette smoking was defined as having smoked a cigarette, even a single puff, within the last 30 days prior to the survey. A weighted analysis was conducted to obtain the prevalence of current cigarette smoking as well as other relevant characteristics. Associations between current smoking and categorical variables forming tables with two rows and two columns were assessed using the Yates corrected Chi-square test, and the Pearson Chi-square test was used for higher contingency tables. Age and gender adjusted odds ratios of current smoking and 95% CI were also obtained in a multivariate logistic regression analysis. A cut off point for statistical significance was set at the 5% level.

In order to understand and explain the results of the quantitative analysis in this study, three health behavior theories i.e., the Health Belief Model (HBM), the Knowledge, Attitude and Practice (KAP) model and the social cognitive theory (SCT) were used to explained the observed effect estimates with relation to explanatory variables (9-13). The SCT suggests that people's acquisition and maintenance of behavioral patterns is dependent on their own cognitive capacity, as well as on social-physical environment in which they are situated. The HBM on the other hand, promotes four constructs representing the perceived threat and net benefits: perceived susceptibility, perceived severity, perceived benefits, and perceived barriers. These concepts were proposed as accounting for people's "readiness to act." Other aspects of the model such as "cues to action," and efficacy, were added later to the model. Cues to action would activate readiness and stimulate overt behavior. In the KAP model, it is postulated that increased knowledge spurs people into changing their attitudes and eventually their behaviors. How knowledge specifically leads to behavioral change is not well explained.

FINDINGS

Altogether, 1,563 adolescents participated in the survey. For 1,285 study participants who reported their gender, 63.3% and 36.7% were males and females, respectively. However, 1,122 responded to the question on whether they smoked cigarettes in the previous 30 days. Altogether, 15.8% of the respondents reported having smoked cigarettes in the previous 30 days. There was no significant difference in the rate of reported smoking between gender (10.3% in males versus 11.1% in females).

Table 1. Characteristics of the study population stratified by gender in the Somaliland Global Youth Tobacco Survey 2004

Factor	Total n * (%)**	Males n * (%)**	Females n * (%)**	p value
Age				
≤ 11	347 (22.9)	211 (26.6)	66 (14.1)	<0.001
12	307 (20.2)	112 (13.8)	144 (31.2)	
13	129 (8.6)	55 (6.9)	31 (6.6)	
14	103 (6.9)	37 (4.7)	40 (8.9)	
15	142 (9.8)	69 (9.2)	41 (9.5)	
16	192 (13.2)	125 (16.5)	54 (12.1)	
17+	259 (18.2)	167 (22.4)	76 (17.7)	
Gender				
Male	813 (63.3)	-	-	-
Female	472 (36.7)	-	-	
Frequency of antismoking media messages seen or heard				
A lot	835 (59.6)	468 (61.1)	288 (64.9)	<0.001
A few	338 (25.1)	186 (25.8)	94 (21.7)	
None	210 (15.2)	100 (13.2)	59 (13.4)	

Table 1. (Continued)

Factor	Total	Males	Females	p value
	n * (%)**	n * (%)**	n * (%)**	
Family member discussed harmful effects of smoking				
Yes	1045 (76.4)	615 (81.7)	309 (70.6)	<0.001
No	327 (23.6)	140 (18.3)	130 (29.4)	
Frequency of antismoking messages seen at sports events, fairs, concerts, community events or social gathering				
A lot	490 (34.5)	266 (34.1)	163 (37.5)	<0.001
Some	281 (19.8)	158 (20.5)	68 (15.6)	
None	655 (35.8)	354 (45.3)	205 (46.8)	
Taught dangers of smoking				
Yes	713 (50.9)	404 (52.4)	249 (55.3)	0.008
No	660 (49.1)	351 (47.6)	193 (44.7)	
Taught that smoking makes teeth yellow, causes wrinkles and smokers smell badly				
Yes	738 (52.0)	478 (60.6)	179 (39.5)	<0.001
No	657 (48.0)	298 (39.4)	264 (60.6)	
Frequency of antismoking posters seen				
A lot	566 (40.5)	314 (41.7)	160 (36.4)	<0.001
Some	339 (24.2)	173 (23.0)	111 (25.3)	
None	490 (35.3)	266 (35.4)	166 (38.3)	
Frequency of antismoking messages seen on billboards				
A lot	641 (45.2)	389 (50.3)	167 (37.1)	<0.001
Some	352 (24.7)	166 (21.5)	133 (29.2)	
None	419 (30.1)	216 (28.2)	148 (33.7)	
Frequency of antismoking messages seen in newspapers or magazines				
A lot	516 (36.9)	270 (35.7)	179 (39.9)	<0.001
Some	500 (36.7)	282 (37.9)	147 (34.3)	
None	372 (26.4)	204 (26.4)	117 (25.9)	
Taught that most people of respondent's age do not smoke cigarettes				
Yes	630 (46.3)	367 (49.5)	178 (41.7)	<0.001
No	753 (53.7)	391 (50.5)	255 (58.3)	

Factor	Total	Males	Females	
	n * (%)**	n * (%)**	n * (%)**	p value
Health professional explained why smoking is dangerous to health				
Yes	602 (46.7)	352 (49.9)	177 (41.5)	<0.001
No	674 (53.3)	348 (50.1)	241 (58.5)	
Religious organization discouraged young people from smoking				
Yes	990 (73.9)	540 (74.7)	322 (74.9)	0.878
No	358 (26.1)	189 (25.3)	110 (25.1)	
Youth groups discouraged young people from smoking				
Yes	748 (58.9)	453 (62.2)	211 (53.6)	<0.001
No	513 (41.1)	272 (37.8)	177 (46.4)	
Current smoker				
Yes	183 (15.8)	65 (10.3)	37 (11.1)	0.248
No	939 (84.2)	554 (89.7)	283 (88.9)	

Numbers not adding up because of missing information.
*unweighted frequencies.
**weighted percentages.

Males tended to be older than females. Female respondents were more exposed than males to antismoking media messages; antismoking messages at sports events, fairs, concerts, community events or social gathering; teaching on the dangers of smoking; and antismoking messages in newspapers or magazines. No associations were observed between being exposed to religious organization that discouraged young people from smoking and gender. Further description of the study population is presented in Table 1.

Table 2 shows results of multivariate analysis after adjusting for age and gender. The following factors were not associated with reported smoking: being taught dangers of smoking, frequency of antismoking posters seen, frequency of antismoking messages seen in newspapers or magazines, youth groups discouraged young people from smoking, and health professionals explained why smoking is dangerous to health. Inconsistency results were obtained for the factor: frequency of antismoking messages seen on billboards. While there was no difference in the odds of reported smoking between those who had not seen messages on billboards and those who had seen a lot of messages, respondents who had seen a few messages were more likely to report smoking compared to those who had not seen any message.

Table 2. Results of antismoking messages and smoking status in multivariate analysis, adjusted for age and gender in the Somaliland GYTS 2004

Factor	Adjusted odds ratio (95% Confidential Interval)
Frequency of antismoking media messages seen or heard	
A lot	0.68 (0.55, 0.84)
A few	0.75 (0.58, 0.96)
None	1
Family member discussed harmful effects of smoking	
Yes	0.61 (0.52, 0.71)
No	1
Frequency of antismoking messages seen at sports events, fairs, concerts, community events or social gathering	
A lot	1.30 (1.06, 1.50)
Some	0.90 (0.72, 1.13)
None	1
Taught dangers of smoking	
Yes	0.90 (0.72, 1.13)
No	1
Taught that smoking makes teeth yellow, causes wrinkles and smokers smell badly	
Yes	0.62 (0.52, 0.74)
No	1
Frequency of antismoking posters seen	
A lot	0.93 (0.73, 1.18)
Some	1.06 (0.83, 1.36)
No	1
Frequency of antismoking messages seen on billboards	
A lot	0.87 (0.66, 1.14)
Some	2.34 (1.86, 2.94)
None	1

Factor	Adjusted odds ratio (95% Confidential Interval)
Frequency of antismoking messages seen in newspapers or magazines	
A lot	1.17 (0.92, 1.48)
Some	0.82 (0.67, 1.00)
None	1
Taught that most people of respondent's age do not smoke cigarettes	
Yes	0.81 (0.69, 0.95)
No	1
Health professional explained why smoking is dangerous to health	
Yes	0.97 (0.83, 1.14)
No	1
Religious organization discouraged young people from smoking	
Yes	0.70 (0.60, 0.82)
No	1
Youth groups discouraged young people from smoking	
Yes	0.89 (0.76, 1.04)
No	1

As shown in Table 2, respondents who discussed harmful effects of smoking cigarettes with their family members were 39% (OR = 0.61, 95% CI 0.52, 0.71) less likely to report smoking compared to those who did not discuss with their family members. Compared to respondents who had not seen antismoking media messages, those who had seen a few or too many messages were 25% (OR = 0.75, 95% CI 0.58, 0.96) and 32% (OR = 0.68, 95% CI 0.55, 0.84) less likely to report smoking, respectively. Respondents who had seen too many antismoking messages at social gatherings were 1.30 (95% CI 1.06, 1.60) times more likely to report smoking compared to those who had not seen the antismoking message at social gatherings. Meanwhile, respondents who were taught that smoking makes teeth yellow, causes wrinkles and smokers smell badly were 38% (OR = 0.62, 95% CI 0.52, 0.74) less likely to report smoking compared to those who were not taught. Compared to respondents who were not taught that most people of the respondent's age do not smoke, those who were taught were 19% (OR = 0.81, 95% CI 0.69, 0.95) less likely to report smoking. Finally, respondents who reported that religious organizations discouraged young people from smoking were 30% (OR = 0.70, 95% CI 0.60, 0.82) less likely to report smoking compared to those who did not report the same.

DISCUSSION

The prevalence of current smoking was 15.8% with no gender difference in reported smoking prevalence between males and females. The effect of gender on susceptibility to smoking is unclear. Some studies found that boys were at increased risk, some studies found that it is girls who were at increased risk, while others found no significant difference males and females (14-19).

In multivariate analysis, some knowledge or information related factors were associated with reported non-smoking while others were associated with reported smoking.

Factors associated with knowledge of the harmful effects of smoking (having discussed with family or taught in school about harms of smoking) were associated with reported non-smoking. According to the HBM, teaching adolescents on the dangers of smoking may be important to enhance their perception of the severity of the condition. Individuals who perceived smoking as harmful to health would be less likely to smoke. In addition, the KAP model's aim would be to improve the knowledge levels of the adolescents thereby leading to behavioral change. Previous reports on school based smoking intervention programs have shown mixed results (20-22). We again believe that the content and mode of delivery of these programs do matter as to their effectiveness.

It is interesting to note that exposure to anti-smoking messages through health workers, and print media (posters, billboards, newspapers, and magazines) was not associated with current reported smoking status. However, having been exposed to anti-smoking messages through sports or community events seem to have achieved a negative result of exposure to these messages being associated with reported smoking. This finding highlights the fact that the content and the delivery mode of anti-smoking messages may result in possibly unintended consequences.

Cohen et al. (23) in their review of 399 televised antismoking advertisements that were designed to discourage adult and teen smoking found that most advertisements had emphasized the consequences of smoking more than the viewer's self-efficacy to quit smoking. Within the HBM and KAP models, these advertisements may have improved knowledge of harmful effects of smoking (perceived severity) but were limited in promoting self-efficacy that may spur the smoker to quit. Furthermore, advertisements were more likely to use informational and humor appeals, rather than sadness, fear, or anger appeals. Biener et al. (24) have reported that anti-smoking advertisements featuring messages about serious health consequences that had been independently rated as high in negative emotion were more likely to be recalled and were perceived as more effective by youth survey respondents than ads featuring messages about normative behavior for teens or ads relying on humor. Advertising intensity, while contributing to recall, was negatively related to perceived effectiveness.

Flay and Sobel (25), and Rogers and Storey (26) have reported that mass media anti- smoking messages that promote inter-personal communication are more effective than those that do not. We found that adolescents who were exposed to interpersonal communication were less likely to report smoking than if they had not. We also believe that many of the billboards, posters, and newspaper anti-smoking messages may have possibly been a health warning on a pro-tobacco advert. Such advertisements, promoting glamour are less likely to result in reduced smoking among adolescents. Thrasher et al. (27) have reported that cigarette packages whose warning labels contain prominent graphic imagery are more likely than text-only warning labels to promote smoking-related knowledge and smoking cessation.

Mass media campaigns are performed to promote health knowledge, change attitudes and may change behavior (28-32). The KAP model, if effective, would be expected to lead to reduced smoking rates among adolescents. Staten and Ridner (33) have reported that inappropriate messaging may be less effective if no targeting is used.

We found that adolescents who reported that their religion discouraged smoking were less likely to report smoking. The lower rates of reported smoking could have been mediated through social norms within society where if society perceives a practice as unbecoming, adolescents are less likely to smoke. However, results on the positive role of religion are not consistent. Knowledge of pronouncement that smoking was sin was not associated with lower level of smoking in Egypt (34).

Adolescents who were taught that people of their age do not smoke may have reported less smoking as a result of improved efficacy that they are able not to smoke, as well as in conformity to normative beliefs (social cognitive theory).

This study has a number of limitations. Firstly, data were collected through self-reports. To the extent that study participants misreported, either intentionally or inadvertently, our results may be biased. The study also only recruited students. Adolescents who were out of school were, therefore, not represented. Furthermore reported current cigarette smoking was not verified by appropriate biomarkers such as cotinine level or exhaled carbon monoxide (35-37).

In conclusion, in a study of school-going adolescents in Somaliland, we found that adolescents who were exposed to anti-tobacco messages or discussions in school and at home were less likely to report smoking than those who were not exposed to such experiences. A combination of school and home based antismoking interventions may be effective in the control of adolescent smoking in Somaliland. Exposure to anti-smoking print messages was not associated with reported non-smoking in the current study, and we propose that studies be done on the effectiveness of antismoking messages (in terms of size, color and content) on adolescent smoking in Somaliland.

ACKNOWLEDGMENTS

We thank the Centers for Disease Control and Prevention, National Center for Chronic Disease Prevention and Health Promotion, Office on Smoking and Health for making available the data used in this study.

This paper is a revised version of an original publication in the Conflict and Health (Siziya S, Rudatsikira E, Muula AS. Antismoking messages and current cigarette smoking status in Somaliland: results from the Global Youth Tobacco Survey 2004) and the authors have obtained the permission from the Conflict and Health to use this material.

REFERENCES

[1] Ezzati M, Lopez AD, Rodgers A, Hoorn S Vander, Murray CJ. Comparative Risk Assessment Collaborating Group: Selected major risk factors and global and regional burden of disease. Lancet 2002;360:1347-60.

[2] Warren CW, Jones NR, Peruga A, Chauvin J, Baptiste JP, Costa de Silva V, et al. Global youth tobacco surveillance, 2000–2007. MMWR Surveill Summ 2008;57:1-28.

[3] Siziya S, Muula AS, Rudatsikira E. Correlates of current cigarette smoking among school-going adolescents in Punjab, India: results from the Global Youth Tobacco Survey 2003. BMC Int Health Hum Rights 2008;8:1.

[4] Odenwald M, Hinkel H, Schauer E, Neuner F, Schauer M, Elbert TR, et al. The consumption of khat and other drugs in Somali combatants: across-sectional study. PLoS Med 2007;4:e341.

[5] Global Youth Tobacco Survey (GYTS). Somalia – Somaliland. URL: http://www.cdc.gov/Tobacco/global/GYTS/factsheets/emro/2004/somalia_factsheet.htm.

[6] Kyrlesi A, Soteriades ES, Warren CW, Kremastinou J, Papastergiou P, Jones NR, et al. Tobacco use among students aged 13–15 years in Greece: the GYTS project. BMC Public Health 2007;7:3.

[7] Stojiljkovic D, Haralanova M, Nikogosian H, Petrea I, Chauvin J, Warren CW, et al. Prevalence of tobacco use among students aged 13–15 years in the South-eastern Europe health network. Am J Health Behav 2008;32:438-45.

[8] Warren CW, Riley L, Asma S, Eriksen MP, Green L, Blanton C, et al. Tobacco use by youth: a surveillance report from the Global Youth Tobacco Survey project. Bull World Health Organ 2000;78:868-76.

[9] Glanz K, Rimer BK, Lewis FM. Health behavior and health education: Theory, research and practice. San Fransisco, CA: Wiley, 2002.

[10] Bandura A. Self-efficacy: The exercise of control. New York: Freeman, 1997.

[11] Champion VL: Instrument development for health belief model constructs. ANS Adv Nurs Sci 1984;6:73-85.

[12] Becker MH, Radius SM, Rosenstock IM. Compliance with a medical regimen for asthma: a test of the health belief model. Public Health Rep 1978;93:268-77.

[13] Eisen M, Zellman GL, McAlister AL. Health belief model-social learning theory approach to adolescents' fertility control: findings from a controlled field trial. Health Educ Q 1992;19:A249-62.

[14] Feighery E, Borzekowski DL, Schooler C, Flora J. Seeing, wanting, owning: the relationship between receptivity to tobacco marketing and smoking susceptibility in young people. Tob Control 1998;7:123-8.

[15] Gritz ER, Prokhorov AV, Hudmon KS, Mullin Jones M, Rosenblum C, Chang CC, et al. Predictors of susceptibility to smoking and ever smoking: a longitudinal study in a triethnic sample of adolescents. Nicotine Tob Res 2003;5:493-506.

[16] Kaufman NJ, Castrucci BC, Mowery PD, Gerlach KK, Emont S, Orleans CT. Predictors of change on the smoking uptake continuum among adolescents. Arch Pediatr Adolesc Med 2002;156:581-7.

[17] Straub DM, Hills NK, Thompson PJ, Moscicki AB. Effects of proand anti-tobacco advertising on nonsmoking adolescents' intentions to smoke. J Adolesc Health 2003;32:36-43.

[18] Ertas N. Factors associated with stages of cigarette smoking among Turkish youth. Eur J Public Health 2007;17:155-61.

[19] Global Youth Tobacco Survey Collaborating Group. Differences in worldwide tobacco use by gender: findings from the Global Youth Tobacco Survey. J Sch Health 2003;73:207-15.

[20] Huang TT, Unger JB, Rohrbach LA. Exposure to, and perceived usefulness of, school-based tobacco prevention programs: associations with susceptibility to smoking among adolescents. J Adolesc Health 2000;27:248-54.
[21] Wiehe SE, Garrison MM, Christakis DA, Ebel BE, Rivara FP. A systematic review of school-based smoking prevention trials with long-term follow-up. J Adolesc Health 2005;36:162-9.
[22] Hwang MS, Yeagley KL, Petosa R. A meta-analysis of adolescent psychosocial smoking prevention programs published between 1978 and 1997 in the United States. Health Educ Behav 2004;31:702-19.
[23] Cohen EL, Shumate MD, Gold A. Original: anti-smoking media campaign messages: theory and practice. Health Commun 2007;22:91-102.
[24] Biener L, Ji M, Gilpin EA, Albers AB. The impact of emotional tone, message, and broadcast parameters in youth antismoking advertisements. J Health Commun 2004;9:259-74.
[25] Flay BR, Sobel JL. The role of mass media in preventing adolescent substance abuse. In: Glynn TJ, Leukefled CG, Ludford JP, eds. Preventing adolescent drug abuse: intervention strategies. Rockville, MD: National Institute on Drug Abuse, US Department of Health and Human Services; 1983:5-35.
[26] Rogers M, Storey JD. Communication campaigns. In: Berger CR, Chaffee SH, eds. Handbook of communication science. Newbury Park, CA: Sage, 1987:817-46.
[27] Thrasher JF, Hammond D, Fong GT, Arillo-Santillan M. Smokers' reactions to cigarette package warnings with graphic imagery and with only text: a comparison between Mexico and Canada. Salud Publica Mex 2007;49(Suppl 2):S233-40.
[28] Maibach E, Flora J, Nass C. Changes in self-efficacy and health behavior in response to a minimal contact community health campaign. Health Commun 1991;3:1-15.
[29] Cummings KM, Sciandra R, Markello S. Impact of a newspaper mediated quit smoking program. Am J Public Health 1987;77:1452-3.
[30] Farquhar JW, Maccoby N, Wood PD, Alexander JK, Breitrose H, Brown BW Jr, et al. Community education for cardiovascular health. Lancet 1977;1:1192-5.
[31] Farquhar JW, Fortmann SP, Flora JA, Taylor CB, Haskell WL, Williams PT, et al. Effects of communitywide education on cardiovascular disease risk factors: the Stanford Five-City Project. JAMA 1990;264:359-65.
[32] Ershoff DH, Quinn VP, Mullen PD, Lairson DR. Pregnancy and medical cost outcomes of a self-help prenatal smoking cessation program in a HMO. Public Health Rep 1990;105:340-7.
[33] Staten RR, Ridner SL. College students' perspective on smoking cessation: "If the message doesn't speak to me, I don't hear it." Issues Ment Health Nurs 2007; 28:101-15.
[34] Radwan GN, Israel E, El-Setouhy M, Abdel-Aziz F, Mikhail N, Mohamed MK. Impact of religious rulings (Fatwa) on smoking. J Egypt Soc Parasitol 2003;33(Suppl 3):1087-101.
[35] Hung J, Lin CH, Wang JD, Chann CC. Exhaled carbon monoxide level as an indicator of cigarette consumption in a workplace cessation program in Taiwan. J Formos Med Assoc 2006;105:210-3.

[36] Jenkins RA, Counts RW. Personal exposure to environmental tobacco smoke: salivary cotinine, airborne nicotine, and nonsmoker misclassification. J Expo Anal Environ Epidemiol 1999;9:352-63.

[37] Low EC, Ong MC, Tan M. Breath carbon monoxide as an indication of smoking habit in the military setting. Singapore Med J 2004;45:578-82.

In: Smoking and Adolescence ISBN: 978-1-63484-311-9
Editors: M. L. Mazabam, S. Siziya et al. © 2016 Nova Science Publishers, Inc.

Chapter 11

CIGARETTE SMOKING AMONG ADOLESCENTS IN VILLE DE SUID, COTE D'IVOIRE

Seter Siziya*[1], *BA(Ed), MSc, PhD,
Emmanuel Rudatsikira*[2], *MD, MPH, DrPH,
and Adamson S Muula*[3], *MBBS, MPH, PhD
[1]Department of Community Medicine, University of Zambia, Medical School, Lusaka, Zambia
[2]Departments of Epidemiology and Biostatistics and Global Health, Loma Linda University, School of Public Health, Loma Linda, California, USA
[3]Department of Community Health, University of Malawi, College of Medicine, Blantyre, Malawi

Tobacco use is a leading cause of global morbidity and mortality. Predictors of cigarette smoking among adolescents have not been well described in developing countries. The objective of the study was to assess predictors of current cigarette smoking among school-going adolescents in Ville de Suid, Cote d'Ivoire. Secondary analysis of data from a cross sectional study within the Global Youth Tobacco Survey was used. Questionnaires were completed using the GYTS format. Analysis was carried out to derive frequencies, odds ratios and 95% confidence intervals. A total of 2694, 1452 (53.9%) males and 1242 (46.1%) females completed the questionnaires. Overall, prevalence of current cigarette smoking was 15.3%. Significantly more males (23.0%) than females (6.2%) were current smokers ($p < 0.001$). Cigarette smoking was associated with having smoking friends, pro-tobacco advertisement, owning an item with a tobacco brand logo, pocket money and younger age. Parental smoking was associated with smoking among males but not among females. Perception that smoking was harmful to health was associated with less likelihood of being a smoker. Cigarette smoking is a significant public health problem in Cote D'Ivoire. Public health efforts aimed to prevent adolescents should incorporate knowledge on the associated factors related to smoking.

INTRODUCTION

Tobacco use is a leading cause of global morbidity and mortality (1, 2). In the developing world however where the bulk of morbidity and mortality is due to infectious diseases tobacco use has not received adequate research attention. There is also limited data on cigarette smoking among adolescents. However, there has been growing interest in adolescent tobacco smoking mostly arising from the Global Youth Tobacco Survey Project spearheaded by the Centres for Diseases and Control (CDC) and participating countries (3-5).

Cigarette smoking among adolescents is of public health interest for several reasons. Some adult cigarette smokers may have initiated smoking as adolescents. Cigarette smoking is also risk factor for asthma, eczema, suicidal behaviour and illicit drug use (6-8).

Adolescent cigarette smoking has not been well characterised in Cote d'Ivoire. We report on the prevalence of cigarette smoking and associated factors among 13 to 15 years olds in Ville de Suid, Cote d'Ivoire. This information will enable informed design, implementation and evaluation of public health interventions aimed to reduce cigarette smoking in Cote d'Ivoire. This information may also provide data that may be used in cross country comparisons of cigarette smoking among adolescent regionally and globally.

OUR STUDY

Data for our current study was obtained from the Cote D'Ivoire Global Youth Tobacco Survey conducted in 2003. This was a cross sectional designed study which recruited school-going 13 to 15 years olds using a two-stage probability sampling technique. In the first stage of sampling, primary sampling units were schools which were selected with a probability proportional to their enrolment size. In the second step, a systematic sample of classes in the selected schools was obtained. All students in the selected classes were eligible to participate. A self-completed questionnaire was used and included core GYTS questions as has been described elsewhere (3-5). Current cigarette smoking was defined as having smoked, even a single puff within the past 30 days preceding the survey.

For the purposes of our study we aimed to estimate the prevalence of current cigarette smoking and stratified by gender, assess whether a selected list of variables (based on the literature on adolescents tobacco use) were associated with current cigarette smoking. Weighted data analysis was performed using SPSS 11.5 (Chicago, Illinois, United States). A weighting factor was used to reflect the likelihood of sampling each student and to reduce bias by compensating for differing patterns of non response. The weight used for estimation is given by the following formula:

W = W1 * W2 * f1 * f2 *f3 *f4, where
W1 = the inverse of the probability of selecting the school
W2 = the inverse of the probability of selecting the classroom within the school
f1 = a school-level non response adjustment factor calculated by school size category (small, medium, large)
f2= a class-level non response adjustment factor calculated for each school
f3 = a student-level non response adjustment factor calculated by class
f4 = a post stratification adjustment factor calculated by grade

We obtained frequencies and their 95% confidence intervals as estimation of prevalence. We also conducted logistic regression analysis to estimate the association between current cigarette smoking and relevant predictor variables. We report unadjusted bivariate analysis between current cigarette smoking and a predictor variable. We also report adjusted odds ratios for the factors in model 1 as well as for age and education level. All significant factors at the 5% level were considered in a Backward logistic regression analysis for each gender. The level of statistical significance was set at the 5% level.

OUR FINDINGS

A total of 2694, of whom 1452 (53.9%) were males and 1242 (46.1%) females completed the questionnaires. Overall prevalence of current cigarette smoking was 15.3%. Significantly more males (23.0%) than females (6.2%) were current smokers ($p < 0.001$). The proceeding analyses were stratified by gender.

Demographic, social and economic factors

Associations between demographic, social and economic factors on one hand and current smoking status on the other are shown in Table 1. Among male respondents, compared with those of age less than 13 years, respondents of age 13 years, 14 years, 15 years and more than 15 years were 24% less likely, 17% less likely, 51% more likely and 56% more likely to have been current smokers, respectively (Table 1). In terms of the school grade, compared with respondents in Grade 4, those in Grades 6 and 5 were 19% less likely and 9% more likely to have been current smokers, respectively. Compared with respondents who did not get pocket money in a usual month, those who received less than 1500 C Francs, and 5000 or more C Francs were 46% more likely and 16% less likely to have been current smokers, respectively.

Among female respondents, compared with those of age less than 13 years, those of age 13 years, and 14 years were 35% more likely and 26% less likely to have been current smokers, respectively. Although the school grade was significantly associated with current smoking status in bivariate analysis, it was not the case when other factors were considered in the analysis. Compared with respondents who did not get pocket money in a usual month, those who received 5000 or more CFA were 59% more likely to have been current smokers.

Parents and best friends smoking status

Table 2 shows the associations between parents and best friends smoking status and current smoking status of respondents. Male respondents who had parents who smoked cigarettes were 18% more likely to have been current smokers than respondents who never had parents who smoked cigarettes.

Table 1. Associations between demographic, social and economic factors on one hand and current smoking status on the other

Factor	n^1 $(\%)^2$	Crude OR (95% CI)	Adjusted OR (95% CI)	n^1 $(\%)^2$	Crude OR (95% CI)	Adjusted OR (95% CI)
Age						
<13	187 (13.5)	1	1	190 (2.7)	1	1
13	217 (14.4)	0.67 (0.58, 0.76)	0.76 (0.65, 0.89)	218 (6.9)	1.24 (1.01, 1.52)	1.35 (1.07, 1.71)
14	269 (18.7)	0.91 (0.81, 1.03)	0.83 (0.73, 0.96)	290 (5.0)	0.88 (0.72, 1.08)	0.74 (0.58, 0.95)
15	304 (27.8)	1.53 (1.38, 1.69)	1.51 (1.00, 1.20)	252 (8.3)	1.50 (1.25, 1.80)	1.01 (0.80, 1.27)
15+	467 (30.5)	1.74 (1.59, 1.90)	1.56 (1.39, 1.76)	286 (7.4)	1.32 (1.10, 1.58)	1.21 (0.98, 1.49)
Grade						
4	476 (20.1)	1	1	430 (3.8)	1	-
5	411 (22.6)	0.99 (0.92, 1.07)	1.09 (1.00, 1.20)	387 (6.6)	1.14 (0.99, 1.31)	
6	565 (25.8)	1.18 (1.10, 1.27)	0.81 (0.74, 0.89)	425 (8.0)	1.39 (1.22, 1.58)	
Pocket money received in a usual month						
None	896 (18.6)	1	1	761 (4.1)	1	1
<1500	154 (34.1)	0.71 (0.63, 0.79)	1.46 (1.26, 1.68)	97 (7.3)	1.02 (0.79, 1.32)	0.88 (0.63, 1.23)
1500-4999	217 (24.5)	1.12 (1.01, 1.25)	0.95 (0.84, 1.08)	197 (8.2)	0.91 (0.75, 1.10)	1.04 (0.83, 1.31)
5000+	175 (31.6)	0.79 (0.71, 0.88)	0.84 (0.73, 0.97)	182 (12.5)	0.56 (0.48, 0.67)	1.59 (1.28, 1.98)

n^1 - unweighted number of respondents; $(\%)^2$ - weighted percentage.

Table 2. Associations between parents and best friends smoking status on one hand and current smoking status on the other

Factor	n[1] (%)[2]	Crude OR (95% CI)	Adjusted OR (95% CI)	n[1] (%)[2]	Crude OR (95% CI)	Adjusted OR (95% CI)
Parents smoking status						
Yes	278 (31.8)	1.36 (1.28, 1.44)	1.18 (1.10, 1.27)	206 (7.8)	1.21 (1.07, 1.36)	
No	1123 (20.2)	1	1	995 (5.5)	1	-
Number of best friends who smoked cigarettes						
None	923 (10.8)	1	1	973 (2.9)	1	1
1	155 (35.0)	1.37 (1.24, 1.52)	1.23 (1.09, 1.37)	90 (16.9)	1.81 (1.52, 2.14)	2.08 (1.71, 2.53)
2+	366 (48.3)	2.38 (2.20, 2.57)	2.24 (2.04, 2.45)	173 (19.0)	2.08 (1.81, 2.39)	1.78 (1.51, 2.11)

n[1] - unweighted number of respondents; (%)[2] - weighted percentage.

In relation to the number of best friends who smoked cigarettes, male respondents who had 1, 2 or more best friends who smoked cigarettes were 2.24 and 1.23 times more likely to have been current smokers, respectively, compared with respondents to never had best friends who smoked cigarettes.

No significant association was observed between the smoking status of parents and current smoking status of the female respondents. Females who had 1, 2 or more best friends who smoked cigarettes were 1.78 and 2.08 times more likely, respectively, to have been current smokers compared to respondents did not have best friends who were smokers.

Pro-tobacco advertisements and campaigns against smoking

Associations between advertisements for and campaigns against smoking on one hand and current smoking status of the respondents on the other are shown in Tables 3a-c. Among male respondents, those who had seen 2-3 anti-smoking messages during the previous 30 days to the survey were 21% more likely to have been current smokers compared to those who had not seen any anti-smoking message in either electronic or print media. Male respondents who had sometimes seen anti-smoking messages at social gatherings were 14% less likely to have been current smokers compared with those that had not seen these messages at social gatherings. Compared to male respondents who had not seen actors smoking when watching television, video or movies, those that had sometimes or a lot of times seen actors smoking were 20% more likely and 11% less likely, respectively, to have been current smokers.

Male respondents who had an item like a t-shirt, pen or backpack with a cigarette brand logo on it were 14% more likely to have been current smokers compared with those that did not have something with a cigarette brand on it. When compared with male respondents who did not see advertisements for cigarettes on billboards during the previous 30 days to the survey, those who saw a few of the advertisements on cigarettes were 16% more likely to have been current smokers. Furthermore, male respondents who had seen a few of the advertisements or promotions for cigarettes in newspapers or magazines were 14% more likely to have been current smokers compared with those that had not seen these advertisements in these print media. Lastly, compared with male respondents who had not seen advertisements for cigarettes at social events, those that had sometimes and a lot of times seen these advertisements were 16% and 25%, respectively, more likely to have been current smokers.

Table 3. Associations between advertisements for and campaigns against smoking on one hand and current smoking status

Factor	n[1] (%)[2]	Crude OR (95% CI)	Adjusted OR (95% CI)	n[1] (%)[2]	Crude OR (95% CI)	Adjusted OR (95% CI)
Number of anti-smoking media messages seen during the past 30 days						
None	578 (16.3)	1	1	634 (4.1)	1	1
1 per month	301 (27.2)	1.17 (1.06, 1.28)	1.11 (0.99, 1.24)	234 (9.9)	1.59 (1.35, 1.89)	1.56 (1.25, 1.94)
2-3 per month	213 (29.1)	1.28 (1.15, 1.41)	1.21 (1.07, 1.37)	145 (4.3)	0.65 (0.50, 0.84)	0.37 (0.25, 0.54)
At least 1 per week	349 (26.2)	1.11 (1.01, 1.21)	1.06 (0.95, 1.18)	224 (9.6)	1.55 (1.31, 1.85)	1.51 (1.21, 1.89)
Frequency of anti-smoking messages seen at social gatherings						
None	648 (18.8)	1	1	761 (5.2)	1	-
Sometimes	226 (23.8)	1.03 (0.94, 1.13)	0.86 (0.76, 0.97)	120 (9.5)	1.39 (1.16, 1.68)	
A lot	570 (27.6)	1.26 (1.17, 1.36)	1.01 (0.92, 1.11)	355 (6.8)	0.98 (0.85, 1.14)	
Frequency of actors seen smoking on TV, videos or movies						
None	159 (18.2)	1	1	171 (3.6)	1	1
Sometimes	342 (27.0)	1.29 (1.18, 1.42)	1.20 (1.08, 1.34)	263 (3.9)	0.80 (0.65, 0.99)	0.62 (0.49, 0.80)
A lot	945 (22.2)	1.00 (0.92, 1.08)	0.89 (0.81, 0.97)	806 (7.6)	1.64 (1.40, 1.93)	1.72 (1.42, 2.08)
Had something such as a t-shirt or pen with a cigarette brand logo on it						
Yes	267 (31.8)	1.33 (1.25, 1.41)	1.14 (1.06, 1.24)	192 (12.4)	1.62 (1.45, 1.80)	1.25 (1.09, 1.42)
No	1162 (20.9)	1	1	1042 (5.1)	1	1
Frequency of seeing cigarette brand names on TV during the past 30 days						
None	227 (16.6)	1	-	200 (3.0)	1	-
Sometimes	534 (25.0)	1.23 (1.13, 1.32)		455 (7.7)	1.52 (1.30, 1.78)	
A lot	685 (23.3)	1.12 (1.04, 1.20)		581 (6.0)	1.17 (1.00, 1.36)	

Factor	n[1] (%)[2]	Crude OR (95% CI)	Adjusted OR (95% CI)	n[1] (%)[2]	Crude OR (95% CI)	Adjusted OR (95% CI)
A few (1-10)	666 (26.4)	1.25 (1.17, 1.34)	1.16 (1.06, 1.27)	547 (7.2)	1.22 (1.07, 1.38)	1.05 (0.89, 1.24)
A lot (>10)	341 (26.8)	1.28 (1.18, 1.39)	1.08 (0.96, 1.20)	242 (6.9)	1.15 (0.98, 1.35)	1.47 (1.19, 1.82)
Frequency of advertisements for cigarettes seen in newspapers or magazines during the past 30 days						
None	687 (19.2)	1	1	617 (4.6)	1	1
A few (1-10)	539 (27.3)	1.24 (1.15, 1.34)	1.14 (1.04, 1.25)	457 (9.5)	1.94 (1.64, 2.29)	1.67 (1.37, 2.04)
A lot (>10)	195 (23.6)	1.02 (0.93, 1.13)	0.90 (0.79, 1.02)	145 (3.1)	0.58 (0.45, 0.77)	0.45 (0.33, 0.63)
Frequency of advertisements for cigarettes seen at social gatherings						
None	570 (15.5)	1	1	695 (4.4)	1	1
Sometimes	330 (27.8)	1.27 (1.18, 1.38)	1.16 (1.05, 1.28)	204 (10.1)	1.54 (1.33, 1.78)	1.29 (1.07, 1.55)
A lot	543 (28.0)	1.29 (1.20, 1.38)	1.25 (1.14, 1.36)	335 (6.9)	1.02 (0.88, 1.17)	0.85 (0.72, 1.01)

n[1] - unweighted number of respondents; (%)[2] - weighted percentage.

Table 4. Association between knowledge of cigarette smoking being harmful to health and current smoking status

Factor	n[1] (%)[2]	Crude OR (95% CI)	Adjusted OR (95% CI)	n[1] (%)[2]	Crude OR (95% CI)	Adjusted OR (95% CI)
Cigarette smoking is harmful to health						
Yes	1356 (22.2)	0.78 (0.70, 0.85)	-	1178 (6.0)	0.70 (0.59, 0.83)	0.68 (0.55, 0.85)
No	92 (32.2)	1		63 (11.4)	1	1

n[1] - unweighted number of respondents; (%)[2] - weighted percentage.

Compared with female respondents who had not seen anti-smoking messages in either electronic or print media during the previous 30 days to the survey, those that had seen the anti-smoking messages at least 1 per week, 2-3 per month and 1 per month were 51% more likely, 56% more likely and 63% less likely, respectively, to have been current smokers. When compared with female respondents who did not see actors smoking on television, video or movies, those that had sometimes and a lot of times seen actors smoking on screens were 72% more likely and 38% less likely, respectively, to have been current smokers. In the meantime female respondents, who had something like a t-shirt, pen or backpack with a cigarette brand logo on it were 25% more likely to have been current smokers compared with those that had no cigarette brand on such materials. Compared with female respondents who had not seen advertisements for cigarettes on billboards, those who had seen a lot of the advertisements were 47% more likely to have been current smokers. In relation to number of cigarettes seen in newspapers or magazines, female respondents who seen a lot and a few advertisements for cigarettes were 55% less likely and 67% more likely, respectively, to have been current smokers compared with those who had not seen the advertisement. Lastly, female respondents who had sometimes seen advertisements for cigarettes at social events were 29% more like to have been smokers compared with those that had not seen the advertisements at social events.

Perception of effects of smoking on health

Table 4 shows associations between knowledge of cigarette smoking being harmful to health and the respondents' current smoking status. No significant association was observed between knowledge of cigarette smoking being harmful to their health and current cigarette smoking among males. Female respondents who thought that cigarette smoking is harmful to their health were 32% less likely to have been current smokers compared with respondents who did not think that cigarette smoking is harmful to their health.

DISCUSSION

Overall prevalence of cigarette smoking in this group of school going adolescents in Cote d'Ivoire was 15.3% with prevalence among males higher than in females (23.0% versus 6.2%). This prevalence is lower than that estimated in Arua, Uganda by Mpabulungi and Muula (9) were current cigarette smoking was 21.9% overall, 17.9% in females and 38.7% in males. Our current cigarette smoking prevalence estimates for Cote D'Ivoire however are much higher than the 5.8% estimated for Kampala, Uganda in 2002 (10).

We also found that older adolescents and those in higher school grades were less likely to be smokers compared to young study participants. It is unclear to us why younger adolescents were more likely to be smokers than older study participants. It may be possible that initiation of cigarette smoking occurs at younger ages but many adolescents eventually quit as they grow. This could explain a higher prevalence of current smoking among young adolescents and lower among older.

Adolescents who reported having more pocket money cash were more likely to be smokers. Having some pocket money and having more pocket money have been reported to be associated with adolescent cigarette smoking in many studies (11-13). It is likely that having disposable cash could facilitate adoption of smoking habit.

We also found that having friends who were also smokers was associated with being a smoker. Interestingly, parental smoking was associated with being a current smoker among males but not in females. Having friends who are smokers or having parents who smoke have been reported before as important predictors of adolescent smoking (14, 15). Smoking friends could influence initiation of smoking habit or adolescents who are smokers preferentially choose other smokers as friends.

Owning an item with a tobacco brand logo and exposure to pro-tobacco advertisement was associated with being a smoker. Among male respondents, those who had seen 2-3 anti-smoking messages during the previous 30 days to the survey were 21% more likely to have been current smokers compared to those who had not seen any anti-smoking message in either electronic or print media. Perception that smoking was harmful to health was associated with less likelihood of being a smoker. Positive attitudes toward smoking as promoted by mass media has been reported to influence adolescent smoking (16, 17).

Our study had several limitations. Due to the cross sectional nature of the study design, we cannot ascribe causation among any of the factors that have been identified as associated with current cigarette smoking. As the study participants were only recruited from schools, it is difficult to generalise these findings to all adolescents in the study area, including those not currently in school at the time of the survey. As the data collection mechanism relied on self reports without verification of current smoking by biomarkers such as cotinine levels and exhaled carbon monoxide, misreporting, both deliberate and inadvertent could not be verified (18-21). However, the study followed standard GYTS methodology as has been executed elsewhere.

In conclusion, cigarette smoking in a major public health problem in Ville de Suid, Cote d'Ivoire. There is need for public health interventions to curb adolescent smoking. School-based intervention should be designed with due consideration to the socio-demographic and societal factors that are associated with adolescent smoking (22).

ACKNOWLEDGMENTS

The GYTS is a collaborative project of WHO/CDC/participating countries. Analyses of GYTS data are not necessarily endorsed by the WHO/CDC/participating countries. We are thankful to the study participants and research assistants.

This paper is a revised version of an original publication in the Mali Medical (Siziya S, Rudatsikira E, Muula AS. Factors associated with current cigarette smoking among adolescents in Ville de Suid, Cote d'Ivoire. Mali Medical 2007; 22:40-46) and the authors have obtained the permission from the Mali Medical to use this material.

REFERENCES

[1] Murray CJ, Lopez AD. Global mortality, disability, and the contribution of risk factors: Global Burden of Disease Study. Lancet 1997;349:1498-504.

[2] Murray CJ, Lopez AD. Mortality by cause for eight regions of the world: Global Burden of Diseases Study. Lancet 1997;349:1269-76.

[3] The Global Youth Tobacco Survey Collaborative Group. Tobacco use among youth: a cross country comparison. Tob Control 2002;11:252-70.

[4] Sinha DN, Reddy KS, Rahman K, Warren CW, Jones NR, Asma S. Linking Global Youth Tobacco Survey (GYTS) data to the WHO framework convention on tobacco control: the case for India. Indian J Public Health 2006;50:76-89.

[5] Global Tobacco Surveillance System Collaborative Group. Global Tobacco Surveillance System (GTSS): purpose, production, and potential. J Sch Health 2005;75:15-24.

[6] Gilliland FD, Islam T, Berhane K, Gauderman WJ, McConnell R, Avol E, Peter JM. Regular smoking and asthma incidence in adolescents. Am J Respir Crit Care Med 2006;174:1094-100.

[7] Singh AK, Maheshwari A, Sharma N, Anand K. Lifestyle associated risk factors in adolescents. Indian J Pediatr 2006;73:901-6.

[8] Sidhartha T, Jena S. Suicidal behaviors in adolescents. Indian Journal of Pediatrics 2006;73:783-88.
[9] Mpabulungi L and Muula AS. Tobacco use among high school students in a remote district of Arua, Uganda. Rural Remote Health 2006;6:609.
[10] Mpabulungi L and Muula AS. Tobacco use among high school students in Kampala, Uganda: a questionnaire study. Croat Med J 2004;45:80-3.
[11] Mohan S, Sankara Sarma P, Thankappan KR. Access to pocket money and low educational performance predict tobacco use among adolescent boys in Kerala, India. Prev Med 2005;41:685-92.
[12] Sinha DN, Gupta PC, Pednekar M. Tobacco use among students in Bihar (India). Indian J Public Health 2004;48:111-7.
[13] Al-Damegh SA, Saleh MA, Al-Alfifi MA, Al-Hoqail IA. Cigarette smoking behavior among male secondary school students in the central region of Saudi Arabia. Saudi Med J 2004;25:215-9.
[14] Sen U, Basu A. Factors influencing smoking behavior among adolescents. Asian Pac J Cancer 2000;1:305-9.
[15] Uncu Y, Irqil E, Karadaq M. Smoking predictors among primary school students in Turkey. ScientificWorldJournal 2006;6:1667-73.
[16] Aloise-Young PA, Slater MD, Cruickshank CC. Mediators and moderators of magazine advertisement effects on adolescent cigarette smoking. J Health Commun 2006;11:281-300.
[17] Feighery EC, Henricksen L, Wang Y, Schleicher NC, Fortman SP. An evaluation of four measures of adolescent's exposure to cigarette marketing in stores. Nicotine Tob Res 2006;8:751-9.
[18] Hung J, Lin CH, Wang JD, Chann CC. Exhaled carbon monoxide level as an indicator of cigarette consumption in a workplace cessation program in Taiwan. J Formos Med Assoc 2006;105:210-3.
[19] Jenkins RA, Counts RW. Personal exposure to environmental tobacco smoke: salivary cotinine, airborne nicotine, and nonsmoker misclassification. J Expo Anal Environ Epidemiol 1999;9:352-63.
[20] Low EC, Ong MC, Tan M. Breath carbon monoxide as an indication of smoking habit in the military setting. Singapore Med J 2004;45:578-82.
[21] Mulcahy M, Evans DS, Hammond SK, Repace JL, Byrne M. Secondhand smoke exposure and risk following the Irish smoking ban: an assessment of salivary cotinine concentrations in hotel workers and air nicotine levels in bars. Tob Control 2005;14:384-8.
[22] World Health Organization Information Series on School Health, Document Five. Tobacco use prevention: an important entry point for the development of health promoting school. Geneva: WHO, 1998.

In: Smoking and Adolescence ISBN: 978-1-63484-311-9
Editors: M. L. Mazabam, S. Siziya et al. © 2016 Nova Science Publishers, Inc.

Chapter 12

CIGARETTE SMOKING BEHAVIOR AMONG JORDANIAN ADOLESCENTS

Emmanuel Rudatsikira[1], MD, MPH, DrPH,
Imad Al Doghim[2], MSc,
Adamson S Muula[3], MBBS, MPH, PhD,
and Seter Siziya[4,*], BA(Ed), MSc, PhD

[1]Department of Global Health Epidemiology and Biostatistics, School of Public Health, Loma Linda University, Loma Linda, California, USA
[2]Jordanian Royal Medical Services, Amman, Jordan
[3]Department of Community Health, University of Malawi, College of Medicine, Blantyre, Malawi
[4]Department of Community Medicine, University of Zambia, School of Medicine, Lusaka Zambia

Adolescent cigarette smoking has received particular attention in the past two decades. Comparison of prevalence estimates trends is likely to inform public health intervention strategies. In this chapter we compare the prevalence of current cigarette smoking among school going adolescents in Jordan between 1999 and 2003. Cross sectional,

* Correspondence: Professor Seter Siziya, Clinical Sciences Department, School of Medicine, Copperbelt University, Ndola Central Hospital, 6th Floor, P. O. Box 71191, Ndola, Zambia. E-mail: ssiziya@gmail.com.

questionnaire-based studies were conducted among school going adolescents in the Jordanian Global Youth Tobacco Survey in 1999 and 2003. The overall prevalence of smoking in 1999 was 16.9% (95% CI [15.7%, 18.1%]) versus 15.5% (95% CI [14.5%, 16.5%]) in 2003. In terms of gender distribution 26.9% (95% CI [24.5%, 29.3%]) males were current smokers in 1999, while 20.0% (95% CI [18.4%, 21.6%]) were smokers in 2003. Altogether, 12.4% (95% CI [10.3%, 14.5%]) females were smokers in 1999 and 10.1% (95% CI [8.9%, 11.2%]) females were smokers in 2003. Thus comparing the 1999 estimates to the 2003 suggests that there has been an overall drop in prevalence of current smoking among school going adolescents in Jordan. Widespread antismoking public health interventions may have resulted in the observed reduction in current smoking prevalence in Jordan between 1999 and 2003. There is need to continue monitoring the trends in smoking among adolescents.

INTRODUCTION

Tobacco is the single most important preventable cause of cardiovascular morbidity and cancers in the world (1-4). Many adult smokers initiate the habit as adolescents. Adolescent smoking is a public health significance as smoking is a marker of many other harmful lifestyle (5-7).

Akpinar et al. (8) have reported prevalence of 26.6% among 13 year olds and 43.7% among 17 years old in Turkey. In Syria, prevalence of adult cigarette smoking was reported at 56.9% and 35.3% among adult males and women, respectively (9). The Centers for Disease Control and Prevention has reported that 21% and 2.1% of male and female adolescents in Kurdistan Region of Iraq were smokers in 2005 (10).

Much of the data on cigarette smoking in Jordan among young people have mostly come from studies in which study participants were university students or patients attending dental services (11, 12). While these studies could be representative of their respective source populations, they are unlikely to be representative of the adolescent general population.

Two waves of the Global Youth Tobacco Survey (GYTS) were done in Jordan (1999 and 2003) using the GYTS standard methodology (13, 14) to estimate the prevalence of tobacco use and associated factors among school-going adolescents. The GYTS Collaborating Group and Warren et al. have reported prevalence of current smoking among adolescents in 1999 in Jordan as 16.6% (15, 16). While cross national comparisons of the prevalence of adolescent cigarette smoking have been conducted before (14, 17, 18), there is little information about same country comparison over the years. The objective of this study was to compare the prevalence of cigarette smoking among school going adolescents in Jordan in 1999 and 2003. We also assessed whether there had been changes in the number of cigarette smoked per day by adolescents who were current cigarette smokers.

OUR STUDY

Our study was secondary analysis of the data obtained from the Jordania Global Youth Tobacco Survey. A comprehensive description of the GYTS methodology has been reported elsewhere (20, 21). In brief, the GYTS is a cross sectional school-based survey of students aimed at ages 13-15 years. Two-stage sample design strategy is used in which schools are selected proportional to their enrollment size. Within any selected school, random selection of classes is done. All students within the selected classes are eligible to participate regardless of their actual ages. A standardized questionnaire is self-completed anonymously by the students and it takes students between 30 to 40 minutes to complete. The questionnaire is aimed at collecting the following information among young people: cigarette smoking and other tobacco use; knowledge and attitudes of towards cigarette smoking; role of the media and advertising and their use of cigarettes; access to cigarettes; tobacco-related school curriculum; exposure to environmental tobacco smoke (ETS) and cessation of cigarette smoking. For the purpose of this study however, only data related to estimation of prevalence of current cigarette smoking, gender distribution of current smoking and number of cigarettes smoked per day will be reported.

Current smoking is defined as having ever smoked even one puff in the past 30 days. The question asked was: "During the past 30 days, have you smoked part or all of a cigarette?" The number of cigarette smoked was assessed by asking the question: "During the past 30 days (1 month), on the days you smoked, how many cigarettes did you smoke?"

A weighting factor was used in the analysis to obtain prevalence of the outcome to reflect the likelihood of sampling each student and to reduce bias by compensating for differing patterns of non response. The weight used for estimation is given by the following formula:

$$W = W1 * W2 * f1 * f2 * f3 * f4$$

where W1 = the inverse of the probability of selecting the school
W2 = the inverse of the probability of selecting the classroom within the school
f1 = a school-level non response adjustment factor calculated by school size category (small, medium, large)
f2 = a class-level non-response adjustment factor calculated for each school
F3 = a student-level non response adjustment factor calculated by class
f4 = a post stratification adjustment factor calculated by grade.

Permission to conduct the study was obtained from the relevant authorities within the Ministries of Health and Education. Participation by the eligible students was voluntary. Data collection was conducted in school by trained assistants and questionnaires were administered without the presence of their teachers.

Data were analyzed using SUDAAN 9.0 (Research Triangle Institute, Research Triangle Park, Durhanm, North Carolina USA). Proportions and 95% confidence intervals (CI) were obtained as estimates of prevalence. Chi-square tests were used to compare the proportions. An α value was set at 0.05 and asop value of <0.05 was considered statistically significant.

Since the age distribution of study participants between the two survey waves was different, the two study groups were not comparable in this regard. As prevalence of smoking in part is dependent on age, there was need to standardize the estimates before meaningful comparisons could be done. The following formula was used:

$$(\Sigma Pj^*Aj)/N^*100$$

where Pj = 1999 age specific prevalence of current smoking for age j
Aj = number of participants in age category j in 2003
N= total number of study participants in 2003

The 100 in the denominator is required when prevalence Pj is reported as percent, otherwise Pj as ranging from 0 to 1, the 100 in the denominator is not required.

FINDINGS

Altogether, 3,912 adolescents participated in the 1999 survey. Information of gender was available for 3,681 (94.1%). Of those who had data available, 1,682 (45.7%) were males and (54.3%) were females in 1999. In 2003, 6,313 students participated and information on gender was available for 5,838 (92.5%) participants. Of these, 2,874 (51.2%) were males and 2,964 (50.8%) were females. The median age in both 1999 and 2003 surveys was 14 years. However, the age distribution of study participants between the two survey years was different as shown in Table 1.

Table 1. Age distribution of study participants in 1999 and 2003

Age (years)	**Frequency (%)**	
	1999	**2003**
	Total = 3862	Total = 5984
11 or younger	353 (8.9)	403 (7.2)
12	472 (11.8)	295 (5.5)
13	1043 (25.0)	520 (9.2)
14	1059 (26.5)	1640 (26.5)
15	745 (22.1)	1523 (25.2)
16	141 (4.3)	1414 (23.4)
17 or older	49 (1.4)	189 (3.1)

The overall prevalence of smoking in 1999 was 16.9% (95% CI [15.7, 18.1]) versus 15.5% (95% CI [14.5, 16.5]) in 2003. In terms of gender distribution, 26.9% (95% CI [24.5, 29.3]) males were current smokers in 1999, while 20.0% (95% CI [18.4, 21.6]) were smokers in 2003. Altogether, 12.4% (95% CI [10.3, 14.5]) females were smokers in 1999 and 10.1% (95% CI [8.9, 11.2]) females were smokers in 2003.

We also aimed to compare the age-distributed current cigarette smoking prevalence between 1999 and 2003. The results are reported in Table 2. When the 1999 overall prevalence (18.7%) was standardized to the 2003 age distribution, the prevalence was 22.0% and was statistically significantly different from the 2003 estimate ($p < 0.01$).

We also aimed to assess whether there has been a change in the number of cigarette smoked on each smoking day by the adolescent smoker. There was a statistical difference in the number of cigarettes smoked per day between the

1999 and 2003 surveys as reported in Table 3. However, no general pattern was observed.

Table 2. Age-specific current cigarette smoking prevalence among adolescents in Jordan 1999 and 2003

Age (years)	Prevalence		p value
	1999	2003	
<12	19.3	20.8	0.08
12	19.6	34.1	<0.01
13	13.8	20.5	0.08
14	15.8	14.2	0.02
15	20.6	20.5	0.45
16	36.2	24.9	<0.01
17+	42.6	35.9	0.54

Table 3. Number of cigarette smoked per day among current adolescent cigarette smokers in Jordan 1999 and 2003

Number of cigarettes per day	Prevalence		p value
	1999	2003	
<1	46.6	28.3	<0.01
1	28.0	24.8	<0.10
2-5	13.9	22.4	<0.01
6-10	6.2	11.6	<0.01
11-20	3.7	6.4	<0.01
>20	1.7	6.6	<0.01

DISCUSSION

The prevalence of current cigarette smoking among school-going adolescents in Jordan was 16.9% in 1999 and 24.6% in 2003. Our 1999 current smoking prevalence estimate is different from the 16.6% reported by the Global Youth Tobacco Survey Collaborative Group (GYTSG) in 2002 using the same data (15). The reason for the difference was that the GYTSG calculated the prevalence figure as number of participants reporting current smoking divided by total number of study participants. In our estimate, the numerator was the same as in the GYTSG but the denominator was only those who completed the question on current smoking. In the 1999 survey, 172 (4.4%) did not answer the question: "During the past 30 days, have you smoked part or all of a cigarette?" Including these study participants within the denominator was similar to assuming that they were all non-smokers. We chose to use only complete case analysis, and so our estimate is slightly higher, although the difference with the GYTSG was not statistically significant. The prevalence of smoking in 1999 at 16.9% was only slightly higher than 15.5% estimated in 2003, p=0.40. However if the 1999 prevalence was age-standardized to the 2003 sample, the prevalence of cigarette smoking significantly rises to 22.0%. This suggests that the prevalence estimate in the earlier sample was statistically different from the 2003 sample, if the age distributional differences between the samples are considered.

The Centers for Disease Control and Prevention (CDC) has reported an overall current smoking prevalence among school going adolescents in the Eastern Mediterranean region as 15.3% (14). Our estimates are not far different from the 'average' prevalence for the region. This suggests that most countries in the region have relatively high prevalence of smoking.

The decrease in current smoking prevalence in Jordan could be explained, partly if not to a great extent by the public health interventions that the Kingdom of Jordan has taken over the past several years (22). In 1998, the Jordanian government put in place anti-smoking legislation to prohibit smoking in public places, it has banned the advertisement of cigarettes in the media, and a national committee has been established to draw-up strategies and programs to combat smoking. In 2001, the government used postage stamps to carry adolescent relevant antismoking messages. The committee on the prevention of smoking in Jordan has wide representation including Health Ministry, UNICEF, the Public Security Department, Jordan Bar Association, the National Anti-smoking Society and the Ministry of Awqaf and Islamic Affairs.

We also aimed to assess whether there was a change among current cigarette smokers with regard to number of cigarettes smoked per day. The proportion of smokers smoking less than a cigarette a day to 5 cigarette a day were higher in 1999 as compared to 2003. However the proportion having at least 6 cigarettes per day were significantly higher in 2003. This may suggest that although overall smoking prevalence in 2003 was lower than in 1999, the proportion of smokers taking higher numbers of cigarettes increased over the period. Consideration that there is an increasing dose-response association between the number of cigarettes and adverse health outcomes, a significant proportion of adolescents were exposing themselves to greater potential harm in 2003. It is also important to recognize that adolescents who smoke cigarettes may also be engaging in other unhealthy behaviours (23). A holistic approach to overall healthy living is therefore likely to be of greater public health significant than individual behavior approach.

This study has a number of limitations. The data used were obtained through self-completed questionnaire. There is a possibility that some study participants may have misreported their exposure status. However, Brener et al. (24) has assessed a method of data collection the GYTS in the United States and they have reported high reliability. While reliability of data collection instrument was acceptable in the United States, we are not aware as to whether the methodology also has high reliability in the Eastern Mediterranean region. We suggest that future studies asses such issues. Also by asking how many cigarettes the adolescent smoked on the days s/he smoked assumed that the adolescent would smoke a regular number of cigarettes each day. This may result in mis-classification due to recall problems. It is also not known whether all or some study participants responded thinking that the researchers were asking for the 'average' number of cigarettes per smoking day. Obviously some study participants may have smoked more on certain days and not much on others. Another limitation of the GYTS methodology is that self reported history of current smoking is not verified by biomarkers such as salivary or blood cotinine level or exhaled carbon monoxide (25-27). We suggest that the Global Youth Tobacco Survey Collaborating Group consider validating the questionnaire with biomarkers in future surveys. As the GYTS methodology only allows recruitment of students who are present in school on the day that the survey is administered, our findings may not be applicable to all students. Also the findings may not be applicable to out-of-school adolescents. In between the two initiatives, the Jordanian National Anti-Smoking Strategy was launched (28). It is expected that such initiatives will support the reduction in the prevalence of smoking among all age groups in Jordan.

In conclusion, we find that the overall prevalence of current cigarette smoking among adolescents who participated in the Jordanian Global Youth Tobacco survey in 1999 was much higher that obtained in 2003. We suggest that public health interventions aimed to prevent smoking in Jordan may have started bearing fruit.

ACKNOWLEDGMENTS

The GYTS is a collaborative project of WHO/CDC/participating countries. Analyses of GYTS data are not necessarily endorsed by the WHO/CDC/participating countries. We are grateful also to Drs Mohammed Shreim and Ayub Hiba for coordinating the Global Youth Tobacco Surveys in Jordan.

This paper is revised from an original publication in the New Iraqi Journal of Medicine (Rudatsikira E, Al-Doghim I, Muula AS, Siziya S. Comparison of 1999 and 2003 current cigarette smoking behavior among Jordanian adolescents: the global youth tobacco surveys. New Iraqi J Med 2007;3:13-21) and the authors have obtained the permission from New Iraqi Journal of Medicine to use this material.

REFERENCES

[1] Ansary-Moqhaddam A, Huxley R, Barzi F, Lawes C, Ohkubo T, Fang X, et al. The effect of modificable risk factors on pancreatic mortality in populations of the asia Pacific region. Cancer Epidemiol Biomarker Prev 2006;15:2425-40.

[2] Brand RM, Jones DD, Lynch HT, Brand RE Watson P, Ashwathnayaran R, Roy HK. Risk of colon cancer in hereditary non-polyposis colorectal cancer patients as predicated by fuzzy modeling: influence of smoking. World J Gastroenterol 2006;12:4485-91.

[3] Kaur J, Bains K. A study of the risk factor profile of cardiovascular diseases in rural Punjabi male patients. Indian J Public Health 2006;50:97-100.

[4] Toustad S, Andrew-Johnston J. Cardiovascular risks associated with smoking: a review for clinicians. Eur J Cardiovasc Prev Rehabil 2006;13:507-14.

[5] Rudatsikira E, Siziya S, Kazembe LN, Muula AS. Prevalence and associated factors of physical fighting among school-going adolescents in Namibia. Ann Gen Psychiatry 2007;6:18.

[6] Dierker LC, Sledjeski EM, Botello-Harbaum M, Ramirez RR, Chavez LM, Canino G. Association between psychiatric disorders and smoking stages within a representative clinic sample of Puerto Rican adolescents. Compr Psychiatry 2007;48:237-44.

[7] Haddad LG, Malak MZ. Smoking habits and attitudes towards smoking among university students on Jordan. Int J Nurs Stud 2002;39:793–802.

[8] Akpinar E, Yoldascan E, Saatci E. The smoking prevalence and the determinants of smoking behaviour among students in Cukurova University, Southern Turkey. West Indian Med J 2006;55:414-9.

[9] Ward KD, Eissenberg T. Rastam S, Asfar T, Mzayek F, Fouad MF, et al. The tobacco epidemic in Syria. Tob Control 2006;15(Suppl 1):24-9.

[10] Centers for Disease Control and Preventation (CDC). Tobacco use among students aged 13-15 years – Kurdistan Region, Iraq, 2005. MMWR 2006 26;55:556-9.

[11] Alomari Q, Barrieshi-Nusair K, Said K. Smoking prevalence and its effect on dental attitudes and behaviour among dental students. Med Princ Pract 2006;15:195-9.

[12] Kyrlesi A, Soteriades ES, Warren CW, Kremastinou J, Papastergiou P, Jones NR, et al. Tobacco use among students aged 13-15 years in Greece: the GYTS project. BMC Public Health 2007;7:3.

[13] Arora M, Reddy KS. Global Youth Tobacco Survey (GYTS) – Delhi. India Pediatr 2005;42:850-1.

[14] Centers for Disease Control and Prevention (CDC). Use of cigarettes and other tobacco products among students aged 13-15 years – worldwide, 1999-2005. MMWR 2006;55:553-6.

[15] Global Youth Tobacco Survey Collaborative Group. Tobacco use among youth: a cross country comparison. Tob Control 2002;11:252-70.

[16] Warren CW, Riley L, Asma S, Eriksen MP, Green L, Blanton C, et al. Tobacco use by youth: a surveillance report from the Global Youth Tobacco Survey project. Bull World Health Organ 2000;78:868-76.

[17] Global Youth Tobacco Survey Collaborating Group. Differences in worldwide tobacco use by gender: findings from the Global Youth Tobacco Survey. J Sch Health 2003;73:207-15.

[18] Muula AS, Mpabulungi L. Cigarette smoking prevalence among school-going adolescents in two African capital cities: Kampala Uganda and Lilongwe Malawi. Afr Health Sci 2007;7:45-9.

[19] Global Tobacco Surveillance System Collaborating Group. Global Tobacco Surveillance System (GTSS): purpose, production, and potential. J Sch Health 2005;75:15-24.

[20] Centers for Disease Control and Prevention (CDC). Use of cigarettes and other tobacco products among students aged 13-15 years—worldwide, 1999-2005. MMWR 2006;55:553 -6.

[21] Rudatsikira E, Abdo A, Muula AS. Prevalence and determinants of adolescent tobacco smoking in Addis Ababa, Ethiopia. BMC Public Health 2007;7:176.

[22] Kandela P. Jordan starts campaign to tackle high rates of smoking. Lancet 2000;355:1800.

[23] Miller JW, Naimi TS, Brewer RD, Jones SE. Binge drinking and associated health risk behaviours among high school students. Pediatrics 2007;119:76-85.

[24] Brener ND, Kann L, McMannus T, Kinchen SA, Sundberg EC, Ross JG. Reliability of the 1999 youth risk behaviors survey questionnaire. J Adolesc Health 2002;31:336-42.

[25] Hung J, Lin CH, Wang JD, Chann CC. Exhaled carbon monoxide level as an indicator of cigarette consumption in a workplace cessation program in Taiwan. J Formos Med Assoc 2006;105:210-3.

[26] Jenkins RA, Counts RW. Personal exposure to environmental tobacco smoke: salivary cotinine, airborne nicotine, and nonsmoker misclassification. J Expo Anal Environ Epidemiol 1999; 9:352-63.

[27] Low EC, Ong MC, Tan M. Breath carbon monoxide as an indication of smoking habit in the military setting. Singapore Med J 2001;45:578-82.
[28] National Anti-smoking strategy to be announced today. Jordan Times 2002 May 2. URL: http://www.jordanembassy.org/0530200206. htm.

In: Smoking and Adolescence ISBN: 978-1-63484-311-9
Editors: M. L. Mazabam, S. Siziya et al. © 2016 Nova Science Publishers, Inc.

Chapter 13

CIGARETTE SMOKING AMONG ADOLESCENTS IN THE KURDISTAN REGION OF IRAQ

Seter Siziya[1,*], BA(Ed), MSc, PhD, Adamson S Muula[2], MBBS, MPH, PhD, and Emmanuel Rudatsikira[3], MD, MPH, DrPH

[1]School of Medicine, University of Zambia, Lusaka, Zambia
[2]Department of Community Health, University of Malawi, Blantyre, Malawi
[3]Departments of Global Health, Biostatistics and Epidemiology, School of Public Health, Loma Linda University, California, USA

Many adult cigarette smokers initiated the habit as adolescents. Adolescent tobacco use may be a marker of other unhealthy behaviours. There are limited data on the prevalence and correlates of cigarette smoking among in-school adolescents in Iraq. We aimed to estimate the prevalence of, and assess the socio-demographic correlates of current cigarette smoking among in-school adolescents in Kurdistan region of Iraq. Secondary data analysis of the Global Youth Tobacco Survey, conducted in the region of Kurdistan, Iraq in 2006. Logistic regression

* Correspondence: Professor Seter Siziya, Clinical Sciences Department, School of Medicine, Copperbelt University, Ndola Central Hospital, 6th Floor, P. O. Box 71191, Ndola, Zambia. E-mail: ssiziya@gmail.com.

analysis was conducted to assess the association between current cigarette smoking and explanatory variables. One thousand nine hundred eighty-nine adolescents participated in the Kurdistan-Iraq Global Youth Tobacco Survey. Of these, 58.1% and 41.9% were boys and girls respectively. The overall prevalence of current cigarette smoking was 15.3%; 25.1% and 2.7% in boys and girls respectively. The factors associated with adolescent smoking were: parents' smoking, smoking in closest friends, male gender, having pocket money and perceptions that boys or girls who smoked were attractive. We suggest that public health interventions aimed to curb adolescent cigarette smoking should be designed, implemented and evaluated with due recognition to the factors that are associated with the habit.

INTRODUCTION

Tobacco use is a leading cause of morbidity and mortality from non-communicable diseases globally (1, 2). Barzani has reported that the top five causes of mortality and morbidity in Kurdistan-Iraq are cardiovascular disease, cancer, respiratory disease, and hypertension, many of these associated with smoking (3).

Over the past 10 years, there has been growing research interest to estimate the prevalence of tobacco use among adolescents. This effort has largely been driven by the Global Youth Tobacco Survey Collaborating Group as part of the Global Tobacco Surveillance System initiated by the World Health Organization (WHO), CDC, and the Canadian Public Health Association.

Adolescent cigarette smoking is of public health significance. Many adult smokers had initiated the habit as adolescents. Also smoking among adolescents has short to medium term health effects in the smokers as well as peers who may be exposed to environmental smoke. Smoking in adolescents may also be a marker of other harmful lifestyles such as engagement in illicit drug use, alcohol use, psychiatric illnesses and sexual intercourse (4-6).

The Centers for Disease Control and Prevention (CDC) has reported on the prevalence of tobacco use including cigarette smoking among in-school adolescents in Kurdistan, Iraq (7). This study reported on the analysis of the Kurdistan-Iraq Global Youth Tobacco Survey. The study reported that 11.9%) were current cigarette smokers. Boys were significantly more likely than girls (21.0% versus 2.1%) to smoke cigarettes currently. Current smoking was defined as having reported smoking cigarettes, even a single puff, within the last 30 days of the survey.

The CDC's paper reported on prevalence of tobacco use and other social characteristics among in-school. This paper restricted data analysis to 13 to 15 year olds and did not assess the socio-demographic correlates of being a current cigarette smoker. While estimates of prevalence of tobacco use will certainly quantify the burden of the problem, it is not possible to identify factors that are associated with cigarette smoking without a deliberate assessment of the potential correlated. We therefore carried out a secondary analysis of the Kurdistan-Iraq Global Youth Tobacco Survey to identify the factors that are associated with current cigarette smoking among in-school adolescents in this region of Iraq.

OUR STUDY

The Kurdistan-Iraq Global Youth Tobacco Survey was conducted in the region which covers the governorates of Irbil, as-Sulaymaniyah, and Dahuk. The Kurdistan region borders Iran to the east, Turkey to the north and Syria to the west. Its capital is the city of Erbil.

The GYTS is a cross-sectional survey which aims to collect data from 13 to 15 year old in-school adolescents. Although the GYTS aims to collect data from 13 to 15 year olds, all students in the selected classes are invited to participate. In the Kurdistan region of Iraq, this age range is covered by the first through fourth years of secondary education.

The GYTS uses a cross sectional two-stage sampling design. In the first stage of sampling, the sampling frame included all schools containing secondary school grades 1 to 4. The probability of a school being selected was proportional to the enrolment size of the school in the selected grades. In the second stage of sampling, classes within the selected schools were selected randomly. All students present in the classes that had been selected were eligible to participate in the survey. There was no age restriction once a class had been selected. A total of 1,989 students completed the GYTS (58.1% male and 41.9% female). The school response rate was 100% (25 schools), the student and overall response rates was 95.6%.

The data from the Kurdistan-Iraq GYTS (2006) were collected anonymously from the eligible students who were present on the day of the survey at their school. A self-completed, computer scannable questionnaire was used. Students were asked questions about their smoking practices, socio-demographic information and exposure to tobacco-related media.

For the purpose of the current analysis, we were interested in the prevalence and factors associated with current cigarette smoking. Current cigarette smoking (the main outcome) was defined as self-report of having smoked a cigarette, even a single puff, within the last 30 days. No biomarkers were used to verify the self-reports. We also assessed the distribution of social characteristics among the study population. These characteristics included: gender, age, amount of pocket money usually received each month, parental smoking, smoking among closest friends, exposure to tobacco-related media and perceptions towards smoking.

A weighting factor was used in the analysis to obtain prevalence estimates to reflect the likelihood of sampling each student and to reduce bias by compensating for differing patterns of non response.

We also conducted weighted backward logistic regression analysis using SPSS software version 14.0 (Chicago, Illinois, United States of America) to assess what relationship existed between a selected list of explanatory variables and the main outcome. The explanatory variables were identified from the literature as having been associated with adolescent smoking in other settings. These variables included: gender, age, parental smoking, smoking in friends, exposure to tobacco-related media, perceptions towards tobacco and the amount of pocket money at the disposal of the adolescent (8-12).

OUR FINDINGS

One thousand nine hundred eighty-nine adolescents participated in the Kurdistan-Iraq Global Youth Tobacco Survey. Of these, 58.1% and 41.9% were boys and girls, respectively. The overall prevalence of current cigarette smoking was 15.3%; 25.1% and 2.7% in boys and girls respectively. Further description of the study participants is shown in Table 1.

Socio-demographic factors associated with current cigarette smoking

Table 2 shows multivariate analysis to identify the association between current cigarette smoking and the selected variables. We found that adolescents >15 years were more likely to be smokers compared to younger study participants.

Overall, some pocket money, male gender and lower school grades were associated with smoking.

Table 1. Characteristics of study participants in the Iraqi Kurdistan Global Youth Tobacco Survey 2006

Factor	Total n (%)	Male n (%)	Female n (%)
Age (years)			
17+	342 (19.2)	251 (26.6)	89 (9.2)
16	332 (16.7)	159 (16.5)	169 (17.1)
15	372 (18.8)	187 (18.6)	183 (19.4)
14	296 (15.3)	128 (13.0)	164 (18.6)
13	289 (14.7)	125 (13.0)	160 (17.0)
12	211 (10.3)	65 (7.1)	139 (14.4)
<12	98 (5.1)	51 (5.3)	41 (4.3)
Sex			
Male	982 (58.1)		
Female	969 (41.9)		
Schooling grade			
Fourth	278 (13.2)	80 (12.3)	192 (14.2)
Third	422 (22.9)	244 (22.6)	171 (23.5)
Second	555 (28.6)	304 (28.8)	243 (28.6)
First	709 (35.3)	352 (36.4)	344 (33.7)
Pocket money received in a usual month (Iraqi Dinars)			
30000+	142 (7.7)	93 (9.8)	47 (5.0)
21000-29999	107 (5.6)	65 (6.7)	42 (4.4)
11000-20999	114 (6.1)	73 (7.4)	41 (4.4)
6000-10999	191 (9.7)	110 (11.2)	80 (8.0)
1000-5999	275 (14.5)	155 (16.2)	116 (12.4)
<1000	262 (13.4)	118 (12.2)	137 (14.6)
0	858 (43.0)	352 (36.6)	485 (51.2)
Current smoker			
Yes	255 (15.3)	225 (25.1)	27 (2.7)
No	1615 (84.7)	675 (74.9)	914 (97.3)

Table 2. Demographic and economic factors associated with current smoking among adolescents in Kurdistan, Iraq, 2006

Factor	OR (95% CI)*
Age (years)	
17+	1.93 (1.86, 2.00)
16	1.30 (1.25, 1.35)
15	1.07 (1.03, 1.11)
14	0.62 (0.59, 0.65)
13	0.49 (0.46, 0.51)
12	0.43 (0.41, 0.46)
<12	1
Sex	
Male	2.21 (2.15, 2.27)
Female	1
Schooling Grades	
Fourth	0.84 (0.81, 0.87)
Third	0.94 (0.92, 0.97)
Second	0.70 (0.67, 0.72)
First	1
Pocket money received in a usual month (Iraqi Dinars)	
30000+	0.69 (0.66, 0.73)
21000-29999	1.04 (0.99, 1.09)
11000-20999	2.45 (2.35, 2.56)
6000-10999	1.44 (1.38, 1.49)
1000-5999	1.21 (1.17, 1.26)
<1000	1.03 (0.99, 1.07)
0	1

Also as shown in Table 3, we found that having a parent who was smoker (father or mother), having most or all of one's closest friends as smokers, perception that 1) boys who smoke have more friends, or 2) that a boy or girl who smoke was more attractive, were associated with being a current smoker.

We also assessed whether exposure to various sorts of media was associated with being a current smoker. As shown in Table 4, the analysis produced mixed results. We found that being exposed to a lot of tobacco advertisements at sports events, concerts and fairs and having seen a lot of movie actors smoking in movies or videos were associated with being a cigarette smoker. However, exposure to tobacco advertisement from billboards and magazines were not associated with being a smoker. In fact, being exposed to a lot of billboard and magazine tobacco advertisements was found to be protective from being a smoker.

Table 3. Social factors associated with current smoking among adolescents in Kurdistan, Iraq, 2006

Factor	OR (95% CI)*
Parents smoke	
Father only	1.14 (1.10, 1.18)
Mother only	1.65 (1.55, 1.77)
None of them	1
Closest friends smoke	
All of them	3.83 (3.66, 4.00)
Most of them	2.37 (2.29, 2.45)
Some of them	0.64 (0.63, 0.66)
None of them	1
Boys who smoke have more or less friends	
More friends	1.32 (1.28, 1.35)
Less friends	0.88 (0.86, 0.90)
No difference from non-smokers	1
Girls who smoke have more or less friends	
More friends	0.60 (0.58, 0.62)
Less friends	0.82 (0.80, 0.85)
No difference from non-smokers	1
Smoking cigarettes makes boys to look more or less attractive	
More attractive	1.15 (1.12, 1.18)
Less attractive	0.69 (0.67, 0.71)
No difference from non-smokers	1
Smoking cigarettes makes girls to look more or less attractive	
More attractive	1.26 (1.22, 1.30)
Less attractive	1.09 (1.06, 1.12)
No difference from non-smokers	1

Table 4. Associations of factors related to advertisements for smoking with current smoking among adolescents in Kurdistan, Iraq, 2006

Factors	OR (95%CI)
Frequency of seeing actors smoke when watching television, videos or movies	
A lot	1.14 (1.11, 1.17)
Sometimes	1.01 (0.98, 1.04)
Never watched	1
Frequency of tobacco advertisements seen on Billboards	
A lot	0.80 (0.78, 0.83)
A few	1.30 (1.27, 1.34)
None	1
Frequency of advertisements or promotions for cigarettes seen in newspapers or magazines	
A lot	0.90 (0.87, 0.93)
A few	1.01 (0.99, 1.04)
None	1
Frequency of advertisements for cigarettes seen at sports events, fairs, concerts or community events	
A lot	1.61 (1.57, 1.66)
Sometimes	0.94 (0.91, 0.96)
Never	0.75 (0.73, 0.78)
Never attended	1

DISCUSSION

The prevalence of current cigarette smoking among the study participants in the Kurdistan-Iraq Global Youth Tobacco Survey was 15.3%, higher among boys compared to girls (25.1% versus 2.1%). This prevalence is much higher than the 10.4% reported by Kyrlesi among Greek adolescents 13 to 15 years (13). Our estimates are also slightly different from those reported by the Centers for Disease Control (7) because in this previous analysis, analysis was only limited to 13 to 15 year olds. This previous study also did not assess the association between any explanatory variables and self-reported history of smoking.

Current cigarette smoking among Ethiopian in-school adolescents was 4.5% among boys and 1.0% among females in 2003 (10). Our estimate of

Kurdistan-Iraq adolescents is however much lower than has been reported for 16 to 18 year old Israeli adolescents (overall prevalence 25.7%, 26.2% in males and 21.1% among females respectively) (14).

Maziak et al. (15) reported on prevalence of cigarette smoking among university students in Syria. In this study, where study participants were much older (mean age 21.8 years) that in the Iraq GYTS, 30.9% males and 7.4% females were smokers. In a sample of Turkish youths (mean age 17.6%), the percentage of current smokers reported by Aras et al. (16) in males was 30.4% compared to 17.4% among females. The estimates reported by Aras et al. are much higher than what we have reported in this study.

Our study found that current smoking prevalence was higher among boys compared to girls (25.1% versus 2.1%). The male predominance in cigarette smoking has been reported elsewhere (10, 13-17). However fewer studies have reported why the gender disparity occurs. Maziak et al. (18, 19) have explored the reasons why most women in Syria were non-smokers. The reasons included religious convictions, perceptions about smoking among husbands, family values and traditions and limited economic resources. Family and societal values and traditions in Iraqi Kurdistan are more tolerant of smoking among boys that they are for smoking among girls. In 2002, Maziak (20) estimated that prevalence of current tobacco smoking was 48% among adult males versus 9% among women. Barzani has also reported that cultural and religious taboos towards smoking among women could be an important factor in Kurdistan-Iraq (3).

While male predominance in smoking has been reported in many settings, this finding is not universal. Steele et al. (21) had reported that girls were more likely to be current and former smokers in Minnesota, United States.

We also found that adolescents who had friends or parents who were smokers were also more likely to be smokers themselves. Similar findings have been reported elsewhere (9, 11, 12, 22). Parental smoking could influence the availability and access to cigarette by the adolescent as well as affect tolerance to smoking by the parent. Adolescents who have parents who are less tolerant to smoking are less likely to smoke themselves.

In the case of having friends who smoke as a factor associated with smoking, Simmons-Morton (23) and Hoffman et al. (24) have reported that both selection of friends and socialization effects may play a role. In terms of selection and socialization of friends, adolescents who are already smokers may be more likely to choose other smokers. Peer influence may also affect initiation of smoking in adolescents who start off as non-smokers but have selected smoker as friends. Choosing a friend who is a smoker may also be a predictor of the adolescent's tolerance to smoking. Kim and Clark (25) have reported that adolescents who attended schools with higher student smoking rates; adolescents who had easier access to cigarettes at home; and adolescents who had more friends smoking were all more likely to be adverse transitioners from low and mild smoking to heavy smoking by young adulthood.

When we assessed whether exposure to tobacco related advertisements was associated with being a current smoker, we found inconsistent results; some analysis showed exposure positively associated while others negatively associated with smoking (see Table 4). The mixed findings in terms of exposure to pro-tobacco advertisements and adolescent smoking may have arisen due to unmeasured confounders. Due to the secondary data analysis nature of study, we were only able to work with the available variables. It is possible that other factors in the socio-cultural milieu of the study area may have resulted in pro-tobacco advertisements having the unintended effects. For example, if the wide availability of tobacco advertisements was influencing the provision of aggressive anti-tobacco interventions, even with adolescents having been exposed to these adverts, if the interventions were successful, more advertising may not reap the intended effect.

Although we found that being exposed to a lot of magazine and billboard tobacco advertisements was negatively associated with being a smoker, we would hesitate in recommending exposure to such media as a reasonable measure to curb adolescents. Our decision is based on the following. Firstly, there is ample previous evidence that positively link pro-tobacco advertisements and adolescent smoking. Secondly, our results may have come about due to failure to control for unmeasured confounders. It is possible that having access to magazines may be a marker of some other variable. Exposure to billboards may also be a marker of residence status and possibly other socioeconomic status. We would however suggest that this issue about the relationship between exposure to tobacco related media and current cigarette smoking status be examined further in this setting. It is not adequate to always conclude that since pro-tobacco media advertisements had been associated with adolescent smoking, then similar findings may also be obtained in all settings.

We found that in general, the higher the amount of pocket money reported by the study participant, the more likely he or she was a smoker. Having access to pocket money may facilitate how an adolescent may access cigarettes. Unger et al. have reported that having access to pocket money was associated with being a smoker among adolescents in the United States (26). These authors suggested that limiting the amount of pocket money could be an effective strategy aimed to prevent adolescents smoking. Scragg et al. (27) has also reported similar findings in New Zealand. We believe that having some disposable income was a factor in influencing adolescents' access cigarettes. However, our results did not show a strictly linear pattern.

Various initiatives aimed to prevent tobacco use among adolescents in the Kurdistan region of Iraq have been planned and established. Barzani (3) has reported that a tobacco-control has been recognized as a priority within the Ministry of Health. A unit on tobacco control has been established. Barzani also reports that Kurdistan the law bans smoking in all government buildings, although strict implementation of the law has not been possible.

As reported above, the Kurdistan Region has been an autonomous region of Iraq for over a decade. Although the region has, to a large extent been spared from the conflict in the rest of the country, there may still be factors that have affected the region stemming from the conflict in the rest of the country. These factors may or may not affect the prevalence of smoking in the region.

The government of the Regional Government of Kurdistan-Iraq has planned for anti-tobacco education campaigns to be conducted in schools throughout the Kurdistan region during the 2006–07 academic year. These will include displayed of antismoking posters and distribution of pamphlets. While Kurdistan law bans smoking in all government buildings, including schools and administrative office buildings of MOH and the Ministry of Education (MOE), strict adherence to these regulations has not been possible.

The findings in this chapter are subject to some limitations. Firstly, the sample that we participated in the survey was limited to adolescents enrolled in school and present on the day of the survey. As such our findings may not be representative to all adolescents in the Kurdistan region of Iraq. We however believe that the findings are likely to be representative of the school-going adolescents as overall response rate was high i.e., 95.6%.

Secondly, the data were based on self-reports of students, who might have underreported or over-reported their behavior or attitudes. Brener et al. (28) has reported high reliability of adolescent reports on their behaviours for responses to tobacco-related questions on United States surveys similar to the GYTS. It however remains to be determined whether the high reliability of findings from the United States is comparable to experiences in Iraq. The self reports on history of current smoking from study participants were not confirmed with relevant biomarkers.

We also examined the variables as operating at the individual level. However authors like Nichter (29) and Wilcox (30) have called for the examination of the interaction between individual-level variable and societal level variables' interactions.

Furthermore, our study was based on a secondary analysis of already existing data. We therefore did not have control of which variables to collect from the study participants. The literature on adolescent smoking has reported that other variables such sibling smoking status (31, 32), alcohol use (33, 34) and religiosity (35-37) may be important factors associated with adolescents. We suggest that future survey's collect such data.

While we have assessed the relationship between the amount of pocket money and being a smoker, we also realize that like in many developing and emerging markets countries, smuggling of tobacco products, including cigarettes, may be an important source of tobacco among adolescents (38-41). There may therefore be different prices that an adolescent smoker may pay to access cigarettes dependent on the availability of smuggled, likely cheaper sources.

We are also unaware how the overall current conflict situation in Iraq may or may not have influence on the prevalence and associated factors of smoking in Kurdistan region of Iraq. We do recognize though that unlike the other areas of the country, this region has to a large extent been administered as an autonomous region of Iraq and has not been active geographic area of the conflict.

In conclusion, we have estimated adolescent smoking prevalence as 15.3% with males having higher prevalence than females. Evidence-based public health intervention should make use of our knowledge of the factors that are associated with smoking in Iraqi-Kurdistan. We suggest that research be conducted to assess the effectiveness of the interventions that are being provided in the region to prevent adolescent smoking. Also future studies should consider measuring other variables such as alcohol use, sibling smoking status and religiosity to enable assessment of how these factors may be associated with smoking in Iraq.

ACKNOWLEDGMENTS

We thank the Centers for Disease Control and Prevention (CDC), Atlanta, Georgia, United States for making the data available for our analysis. We do also recognize that our study would not have been possible without the consent and cooperation of the adolescents who participated in the Iraqi Kurdistan Global Youth Tobacco Survey. We particularly thank Dilyara Dilyara Barzani,

MD, MPH, Senior Health Adviser Ministry of Health Kurdistan Regional Government who was coordinator of the GYTS in Kurdistan-Iraq and provided us with further insights during data analysis.

This paper is a revised version of an original publication in the Conflict and Health (Siziya S, Muula AS, Rudatsikira E. Correlates of current cigarette smoking among in-school adolescents in the Kurdistan region of Iraq. Confl Health 2007;1:13) and the authors have obtained the permission to use this material.

REFERENCES

[1] Lopez AD, Mathers CD. Measuring the global burden of disease and epidemiological transitions: 2002–2030. Ann Trop Med Parasitol 2006;100:481-99.

[2] Mathers CD, Loncar D. Projections of global mortality and burden of disease from 2002 to 2030. PLoS Med 2006;3:e442.

[3] Barzani D.. Iraq: an important start in the Kurdish region. Tob Control 2006;15:3-4.

[4] Rudatsikira E, Siziya S, Kazembe LN, Muula AS. Prevalence and associated factors of physical fighting among school-going adolescents in Namibia. Ann Gen Psychiatry 2007;6:18.

[5] Ando M, Asakura T, Ando S, Simons-Morton BG. Psychosocial factors associated with smoking and drinking among Japanese early adolescent boys and girls: Cross-sectional study. Biopsychosoc Med 2007;1:13.

[6] Brook JS, Balka EB, Ning Y, Brook DW. Trajectories of cigarette smoking among African Americans and Puerto Ricans from adolescence to young adulthood: associations with dependence on alcohol and illegal drugs. Am J Addict 2007;16:195-201.

[7] Centers for Disease Control and Prevention (CDC). Tobacco use among students aged 13–15 years – Kurdistan Region, Iraq, 2005. MMWR 2006;55:556-9.

[8] Kokkevi A, Richardson C, Florescu S, Kuzman M, Stergar E. Psychosocial correlates of substance use in adolescence: a cross-national study in six European countries. Drug Alcohol Depend 2007;86:67-74.

[9] Muula AS. Prevalence and determinants of cigarette smoking among adolescents in Blantyre City, Malawi. Tanzania Health Res Bull 2007;9:48-51.

[10] Rudatsikira E, Abdo A, Muula AS. Prevalence and determinants of adolescent tobacco smoking in Addis Ababa, Ethiopia. BMC Public Health 2007;7:176.

[11] Scragg R, Laugesen M. Influence of smoking by family and best friend on adolescent tobacco smoking: results from the 2002 New Zealand national survey of year 10 students. Aust NZ J Public Health 2007;31:217-23.

[12] Livaudais JC, Napoles-Springer A, Stewart S, Kaplan CP. Understanding Latino adolescent risk behaviors: parental and peer influences. Ethnicity Dis 2007;17:298-304.

[13] Kyrlesi A, Soteriades ES, Warren CW, Kremastinou J, Papastergiou P, Jones NR, et al. Tobacco use among students aged 13–15 years in Greece: the GYTS project. BMC Public Health 2007;7:3.
[14] Samuels N. Cigarette use among Israeli adolescents: why do they smoke? Harefuah 2007;146:184.
[15] Maziak W, Hammal F, Rastam S, Asfar T, Eissenberg T, Bachir ME, et al. Characteristics of cigarette smoking and quitting among university students in Syria. Prev Med 2004;39:330-6.
[16] Aras S, Semin S, Gunay T, Orcin E, Ozan S. Sexual attitudes and risk-taking behaviors of high school students in Turkey. J Sch Health 2007;77:359-66.
[17] Mpabulungi L, Muula AS. Tobacco use among high school students in a remote district of Arua, Uganda. Rural Remote Health 2006;6:609.
[18] Maziak W, Asfar T, Mock J. Why most women in Syria do not smoke: can the passive barrier of traditions be replaced with an information-based one? Public Health 2003;117:237-41.
[19] Maziak W, Asfar T, Mzayek F. Socio-demographic determinants of smoking among low-income women in Aleppo, Syria. Int J Tuberculosis Lung Dis 2001;5:307-12.
[20] Maziak W. Smoking in Syria: profile of a developing Arab country. Int J Tuberculosis Lung Dis 2002;6:183-91.
[21] Steele JR, Raymond RL, Ness KK, Alvi S, Kearney I. A comparative study of sociocultural factors and young adults' smoking in two Midwestern communities. Nicotine Tob Res 2007;9(Suppl 1):S73-82.
[22] Akpinar E, Yoldascan E, Saatci E. The smoking prevalence and the determinants of smoking behaviour among students in Cukurova University, Southern Turkey. West Indian Med J 2006;55:414-9.
[23] Simons-Morton B. Social influences on adolescent substance use. Am J Health Behav 2007;31:672-84.
[24] Hoffman BR, Monge PR, Chou CP, Valente TW. Perceived peer influence and peer selection on adolescent smoking. Addict Behav 2007;32:1546-54.
[25] Kim H, Clark PI. Cigarette smoking transition in females of low socioeconomic status: impact of state, school, and individual factors. J Epidemiol Commun Health 2006;60(Suppl 2):13-9.
[26] Unger JB, Sun P, Johnson CA. Socioeconomic correlates of smoking among an ethnically diverse sample of 8th grade adolescents in Southern California. Prev Med 2007;44:323-7.
[27] Scragg R, Laugesen M, Robinson E. Cigarette smoking, pocket money and socioeconomic status: results from a national survey of 4th form students in 2000. NZ Med J 2002;115:U108.
[28] Brener ND, Collins JL, Kann L, Warren CW, Williams BI. Reliability of the Youth Risk Behavior Survey Questionnaire. Am J Epidemiol 1995;141:575-80.
[29] Nichter M. Smoking: What does culture have to do with it? Addiction 2003;98(Suppl 1):139-145.
[30] Wilcox P. An ecological approach to understanding youth smoking trajectories: Problems and prospects. Addiction 2003;98(Suppl 1):57-77.

[31] Edelen MO, Tucker JS, Ellickson PL. A discrete time hazards model of smoking initiation among West Coast youth from age 5 to 23. Prev Med 2007;44:52-4.

[32] Epstein JA, Bang H, Botvin GJ: Which psychosocial factors moderate or directly affect substance use among inner-city adolescents? Addict Behav 2007;32:700-13.

[33] Bricker JB, Peterson AV, Robyn Andersen M, Leroux BG, Bharat-Rajan K, Sarason IG. Close friends,' parents,' and older siblings' smoking: reevaluating their influence on children's smoking. Nicotine Tob Res 2006;8:217-26.

[34] Fisher LB, Miles IW, Austin SB, Camargo CA Jr, Colditz GA. Predictors of initiation of alcohol use among US adolescents: Findings from a prospective cohort study. Arch Pediatr Adolesc Med 2007;161:959-66.

[35] Ando M, Asakura T, Ando S, Simons-Morton BG. Psychosocial factors associated with smoking and drinking among Japanese early adolescent boys and girls: Cross-sectional study. Biopsychosoc Med 2007;1:13.

[36] Griffin KW, Botvin GJ, Epstein JA, Doyle MM, Diaz T. Psychosocial and behavioral factors in early adolescence as predictors of heavy drinking among high school seniors. J Stud Alcohol 2000;61:603-6.

[37] Sinha JW, Cnaan RA, Gelles RJ. Adolescent risk behaviors and religion: findings from a national study. J Adolescence 2007;30:231-49.

[38] Timberlake DS, Rhee SH, Haberstick BC, Hopfer C, Ehringer M, Lessem JM, Smolen A, Hewitt JK. The moderating effects of religiosity on the genetic and environmental determinants of smoking initiation. Nicotine Tob Res 2006;8:123-33.

[39] Novotny TE. The "ultimate prize" for big tobacco: opening the Chinese cigarette market by cigarette smuggling. PLoS Med 2006;3:e279.

[40] Wen CP, Peterson RA, Cheng TY, Tsai SP, Eriksen MP, Chen T. Paradoxical increase in cigarette smuggling after the market opening in Taiwan. Tob Control 2006;15:160-5.

[41] Collin J, Legresley E, MacKenzie R, Lawrence S, Lee K. Complicity in contraband: British American Tobacco and cigarette smuggling in Asia. Tob Control 2004;13(Suppl 2):ii104-11.

In: Smoking and Adolescence ISBN: 978-1-63484-311-9
Editors: M. L. Mazabam, S. Siziya et al. © 2016 Nova Science Publishers, Inc.

Chapter 14

ADOLESCENT CIGARETTE SMOKING IN GREECE

George Rachiotis[1], MD, PhD, Adamson S Muula[2], MBBS, MPH, PhD, Emmanuel Rudatsikira[3], MD, MPH, DrPH, Seter Siziya[4], BA, Ed, MSc, PhD, Athina Kyrlesi[1], MD, PhD, Konstantinos Gourgoulianis[5], MD, PhD, and Christos Chadjichristodoulou[1,*], MD, PhD

[1]Department of Hygiene and Epidemiology, Medical Faculty, University of Thessaly, Larissa, Greece
[2]Department of Community Health, University of Malawi, College of Medicine, Blantyre, Malawi
[3]Departments of Epidemiology and Biostatistics and Global Health, Loma Linda University, School of Public Health, Loma Linda, California, USA
[4]Department of Community Medicine, University of Zambia, Lusaka, Zambia and [5]Department of Pulmonology, Medical Faculty, University of Thessaly, Larissa, Greece

---

[*] Correspondence: Christos Chadjichristodoulou, MD, PhD, Department of Hygiene and Epidemiology, Medical Faculty, University of Thessaly, 22 Papakyriazi Str, Larissa, Thessaly, 41222 Greece. E-mail: chatzi@med.uth.gr.

Data about the predictors of smoking among adolescents in Greece are sparse. We tried to identify factors associated with current cigarette smoking among in-school adolescents in Greece in the context of GYTS study. A secondary analysis of data from a questionnaire study using the Global Youth Tobacco Survey methodology was conducted to identify factors associated with smoking among adolescents in Greece. Data were collected in 2004–2005. The outcome variable was cigarette smoking within the past 30 days preceding the survey while independent variables included age, gender, parental educational status, parental smoking, perception of harmfulness of smoking, and the amount of pocket money at the adolescent's disposal. Altogether, 6141 adolescents (51.5% males and 48.5% females) participated in the study. In multivariate analysis, cigarette smoking was associated with male gender (OR = 1.62; 95% CI [1.08, 3.08]), parental smoking (OR = 2.59; 95% CI [1.45, 5.89]), and having pocket money ≥16 Euros (OR = 2.64; 95% CI [1.19, 5.98]). Male gender, parental smoking, and having pocket-money ≥ 16 Euros were independently associated with current smoking among Greek students. These findings could be taken into account in order to formulate a comprehensive anti-smoking strategy in Greece.

INTRODUCTION

Tobacco is a leading cause of illness in the developed world where non-communicable diseases contribute to the greatest burden of disease (1). Many adult smokers initiate the smoking habit during adolescence or as young adults (2). Much of the severe health consequences of smoking are in adulthood. However, there are also significant short and intermediate term effects of smoking that may be experienced such as asthma and chronic cough (3, 4). Information on adolescent smoking is valuable not just because smoking is independently associated with adverse health effects, but also through the clustering of other harmful lifestyles among adolescents who smoke (5). Arvanitidou et al. (6) have reported that the odds of alcohol use among adolescents in Greece who reported smoking habit were 5.2 compared to non-smokers.

Known risk factors associated with cigarette smoking among adolescents include age (7), gender (7, 8), having smoking friends and or smoking parents, the perception that smoking is or not harmful (9), and the amount of pocket money (10).

Greece is a leading tobacco-producer country within European Union. In addition, in Greece the prevalence of smoking is 37% and the annual per capita consumption of cigarettes was one of the highest in the European Union (11, 12).

Kyrlesi et al. (13) have reported on the prevalence of tobacco use among middle school adolescents in Greece using the same data from which our study is based. The study by Kyrlesi et al. only reported on prevalence of tobacco use, exposure to second hand smoke, tobacco related media and advertising, cessation experience and access of tobacco products (13). Factors associated with cigarette smoking were not explored. Using the same database, we explored the factors that may be associated with cigarette smoking among in-school adolescents in Greece. We believe while knowledge of prevalence of various behaviors is important, understanding the factors that may be associated with the behavior may better inform public health policy decision.

OUR STUDY

Our study involved the secondary analysis of the Global Youth Tobacco Survey (GYTS) conducted in Greece among middle-school students in Greece, 2004–2005. A comprehensive description of the data collection methodology was reported previously by Kyrlesi et al. (13). In brief, a two-stage cluster sampling design was instituted in which in the first phase all schools containing the middle-school grades in Greece were identified and 100 schools were selected (25 schools from each region). This was considered adequate to obtain a sample design that would produce representative estimates for each region. In the first stage of sampling, the probability of schools being selected was proportional to the number of students enrolled in the specified grades (grades 1–3 at all middle schools). In the second sampling stage, classes within the selected schools were randomly selected. All students in selected classes attending school on the day of the survey were eligible to participate. The Committee on Health Promotion of the Ministry of National Education and Religions approved the survey. Parents were notified by a letter in advance of the survey and students gave verbal consent to complete the questionnaire. Further description of the GYTS methodology has been described elsewhere (14).

The GYTS questionnaire included data demographic variables and experience with cigarette smoking. Self-completed questionnaires were used. A project coordinator supervised the data collection process and reported to supervisor on a daily basis. Completed questionnaires were sent to the Centers for Disease Control and Prevention for processing where they were transformed into electronic files. Statistical analyses

A weighting factor was used in the analysis to reflect the likelihood of sampling each student and to reduce bias by compensating for differing patterns of non-response. The weight used for estimation is given by the following formula:

W = W1 * W2 * f1 * f2 *f3 *f4,

where

W1 = the inverse of the probability of selecting the school

W2 = the inverse of the probability of selecting the classroom within the school

fl = a school-level non response adjustment factor calculated by school size category (small, medium, large)

f2 = a class-level non response adjustment factor calculated for each school

f3 = a student-level non response adjustment factor calculated by class

f4 = a post stratification adjustment factor calculated by grade.

We conducted logistic regression analysis using SUDAAN software version 9.0 (Research Triangle Institute, NC, USA) to estimate the association between relevant predictor variables and current cigarette. To assess current smoking status participants were asked "During the past 30 days, on how many days did you smoke cigarettes?" In the analysis current smokers were those who reported having smoked one or more days during the last 30 days preceding the survey. The study was based on adolescents who by some authors are defined as 12 to 18 years; however age of adolescence varies by culture and much younger and much older persons may be included in the definition. In the Greece GYTS, the data collection questionnaire asked the question: How old are you? The options available were: a) 11 years or young; b) 12 years: c) 13 years; d) 14 years; d) 15 years; e) 16 years and f) 17 years or older. We report unadjusted Odds Ratios for selected predictor variables while considering current cigarette smoking as dependent variable. We thereafter report results of adjusted odds ratios for the factors.

FINDINGS

From 7,126 eligible students, 6,378 actually took part (response rate 89%) of whom 50.4% were males. Overall, a third of fathers/step fathers (36.4%) and mothers/step mothers (37.0%) had attained university level of education. While 26.2% of the participants' fathers smoked, 11.9% of their mothers smoked. Among males at age groups 11–12 and 16–17 years old the prevalence of smoking was 9.4% and 48.2%, respectively. Most (91.7%) of the participants felt that cigarette smoking is harmful. Overall, 12.5% of the participants (13.3% of males and 11.8% of females) smoked cigarettes (see Table 1).

Table 1. Characteristics of the study population

Characteristics	Total	Males	Females
	n (%)	n (%)	n (%)
	6146 (100)	3096 (50.4)	3045 (49.6)
Age (years)			
11-12	627 (10.2)	357 (11.5)	270 (8.9)
13	1757 (28.6)	884 (28.6)	873 (28.6)
14	1910 (31.1)	911 (29.4)	999 (32.8)
15	1465 (23.9)	730 (23.6)	735 (24.1)
16-17	382 (6.2)	214 (6.9)	168 (5.6)
Education father/stepfather			
Elementary school or less	1296 (19.8)	663 (21.4)	477 (15.7)
Middle school	1025 (16.1)	493 (15.9)	502 (16.5)
High school	1803 (28.3)	834 (27.0)	934 (30.7)
University	2238 (36.4)	1106 (35.7)	1132 (37.1)
Education mother/stepmother			
Elementary school or less	950 (15.5)	521 (16.8)	429 (14.1)
Middle school	911 (14.8)	433 (14.0)	478 (15.7)
High school	2006 (32.7)	990 (32.0)	1016 (33.3)
University	2274 (37.0)	1152 (37.2)	1122 (36.9)
Visiting grand parents			
Every day	2266 (37.3)	1199 (39.1)	1067 (35.4)
2-5 times/week	2153 (35.4)	1080 (35.2)	1073 (35.7)
Once a month or less	429 (7.1)	202 (6.6)	227 (7.5)
Never	1231 (20.2)	585 (19.1)	646 (21.4)
Parental smoking			
None	1947 (32.1)	1020 (33.3)	927 (30.8)
Father only	1589 (26.2)	819 (26.8)	770 (25.6)
Mother only	724 (11.9)	347 (11.3)	377 (12.5)
Both parents	1813 (29.9)	873 (28.5)	940 (31.2)

Table 1. (Continued)

Characteristics	Total n (%)	Males n (%)	Females n (%)
Smoking status grand parents			
None	3146 (53.4)	1568 (52.8)	1578 (54.0)
One or more grand parents	2747 (46.6)	1404 (47.2)	1343 (46.0)
Accepting cigarette offered by one of best one's friends smoking			
Definitely not	4287 (70.7)	2166 (70.7)	2121 (70.7)
Probably not	873 (14.4)	441 (14.4)	432 (14.4)
Probably yes	697 (11.5)	342 (11.2)	355 (11.8)
Definitely yes	204 (3.4)	111 (3.6)	93 (3.1)
Perception cigarette smoking is harmful			
Definitely yes or probably yes	5573 (91.7)	2760 (90.1)	2813 (93.2)
Definitely not or probably not	507 (8.3)	303 (9.9)	204 (6.8)
Pocket money (Euro)			
<8	2267 (44.7)	1371 (45.6)	1296 (43.7)
8-15	1647 (27.6)	753 (25.1)	894 (30.1)
16-23	709 (11.9)	348 (11.6)	361 (12.2)
24-31	369 (6.2)	202 (6.7)	167 (5.6)
32+	581 (9.6)	332 (11.0)	249 (8.4)
Current cigarette smoking			
Yes	5174 (87.5)	2576 (86.7)	2597 (88.2)
No	741 (12.5)	394 (13.3)	347 (11.8)

Among females at these age groups the prevalence of smoking was 12.8% for age group 11–12 years, and 47.6% for age group 16–17 years. Factors associated with smoking in bivariate analysis are in Table 2. Males were more likely to smoke than females (OR = .26; 95% CI [1.05, 1.50]). Subjects aged 13–14 years were less likely to smoke than those who were 11–12 years old (OR = 0.30; 95% CI [0.22, 0.41] for 13 years old and OR = 0.50; 95% CI [0.81, 1.38] for 14 years old) while the oldest individuals (16–17 years old) were more than 5 times likely to smoke than those aged 11–12 years (OR = 5.27; 95% CI [2.96, 9.39]).

For both males and females respondents, having both parents smokers was associated with a more than two times the odds of smoking (OR = 2.72; 95% CI [1.98, 3.74) for males and OR = 2.13; 95% CI [1.54, 2.96] for females). Boys with only father smoking were more likely to smoke than those who had non-smoking fathers (OR = 1.87; 95% CI [1.34, 2.61]). Likewise, girls with only mother smoking were more likely to smoke than those with non-smoking mothers (OR = 1.67; 95% CI [1.07, 2.60]).

Table 2. Variables associated with current smoking (Bi-variate analysis)

Variables	Total Odds ratio (95% confidence interval)	Males Odds ratio (95% confidence interval)	Females Odds ratio (95% confidence interval)
Age (years)			
11-12	1.00	1.00	1.00
13	0.30 (0.22, 0.41)	0.56 (0.35, 0.89)	0.20 (0.11, 0.35)
14	0.50 (0.31, 0.79)	0.63 (0.40, 0.97)	0.47 (0.36, 0.63)
15	1.05 (0.81, 1.38)	1.65 (1.09, 2.51)	1.04 (0.66, 1.64)
16-17	5.27 (2.96, 9.39)	7.21 (4.42, 11.76)	4.89 ([3.48, 6.86)
Gender			
Females	1.00	1.00	-
Males	1.26 (1.05, 1.50)		-
Education father/ stepfather			
Elementary school or less	1.00	1.00	1.00
Middle school	0.81 (0.56, 1.17)	0.76 (0.58, 1.00)	0.85 (0.55, 1.33)
High school	0.53 (0.40, 0.69)	0.47 (0.33, 0.68)	0.60 (0.41, 0.90)
University	0.52 (0.42, 0.69)	0.54 (0.39, 0.75)	0.49 (0.32, 0.77)
Education mother/ stepmother			
Elementary school or less	1.00	1.00	1.00
Middle school	1.00 (0.74, 1.34)	0.95 (0.62, 1.46)	0.71 (0.47, 1.08)
High school	0.54 (0.41, 0.71)	0.48 (0.32, 0.71)	0.61 (0.41, 0.93)
University	0.53 (0.41, 0.71)	0.55 (0.38, 0.81)	0.61 (0.42, 0.89)
Parental smoking			
None	1.00	1.00	1.00
Father only	1.57 (1.22, 2.02)	1.87 (1.34, 2.61)	1.27 (0.82, 1.97)
Mother only	1.38 (1.00, 1.89)	1.11 (0.69, 1.81)	1.67 (1.07, 2.60)
Both parents	2.48 (1.99, 3.09)	2.72 (1.98, 3.74)	2.13 (1.54, 2.96)
Perception cigarette smoking is harmful			
Definitely not or probably not	1.00	1.00	1.00
Definitely yes or probably yes	1.20 (0.92, 1.56)	1.13 (0.88, 1.45)	1.23 (1.04, 1.47)

Table 2. (Continued)

Variables	Total Odds ratio (95% confidence interval)	Males Odds ratio (95% confidence interval)	Females Odds ratio (95% confidence interval)
Pocket money (Euro)			
<8	1.00	1.00	1.00
8-15	2.29 (1.53, 3.41)	2.06 (1.23, 3.45)	3.14 (1.50, 6.60)
16-23	3.39 (2.34, 4.91)	3.31 (2.03, 5.39)	4.91 (2.47, 9.75)
24-31	4.15 (2.78, 6.20)	4.03 (2.37, 6.85)	6.04 (2.92, 12.47)
32+	7.26 (4.73, 11.14)	6.78 (3.86, 11.91)	10.96 (5.09, 23.58)

Participants whose parents had attained high school level of education or higher were less likely to smoke than those whose parents had elementary education or less. Pocket money was associated with increased odds of smoking. Compared to boys who reported having eight Euro or less per week, those who had more 32 Euro or more were more than six times likely to smoke (OR = 6.78; 95% CI [3.86, 11.91]). For girls, those who had more than 32 Euro per week were more than 10 times likely to smoke than those who had seven Euro or less (OR = 10.96; 95% CI [5.09, 23.58]).

Variables associated with smoking in multivariate analysis are in Table 3. Males subjects were more likely to smoke than females (OR = 1.62; 95% CI [1.08, 3.08]). compared to teens who had non-smoking parents, those whose both parents or whose father only were smokers were more than twice likely to smoke (OR = 2.59; 95% CI [1.45, 5.89] and OR = 2.49; 95% CI [1.12, 6.08] respectively).

Participants who reported having more than 16 Euro per week or more were more likely to smoke than those who had seven Euro or less (OR = 2.64; 95% CI [1.19, 5.58] for 16–23 Euro per week, OR = 3.46; 95% CI [1.41, 7.79] for 24–31 Euro/week, and OR = 4.93; 95% CI [1.59, 14.21 for more than 32 Euro/week). There was a dose-response relationship between smoking and the amount of pocket money respondents spent per week (p-value for trend = 0.03).

Table 3. Variables associated with current smoking in Multivariate analysis among adolescents in Greece, 2005

Variable	Odd ratios with 95% CI[1]
Age (years)	
11-12	1.00
13	0.42 (0.23, 0.93)
14	0.37 (0.27, 0.87)
15	0.86 (0.39, 1.82)
16-17	1.75 (0.79, 4.08)
Gender	
Females	1.00
Males	1.62 (1.08, 3.08)
Education father/ stepfather	
Elementary school or less	1.00
Middle school	0.78 (0.37, 1.87)
High school	0.67 (0.33, 1.49)
University	0.89 (0.38, 1.74)
Education mother/ stepmother	
Elementary school or less	1.00
Middle school	0.71 (0.40, 1.89)
High school	1.02 (0.47, 2.32)
University	0.89 (0.34, 2.28)
Parental smoking	
None	1.00
Father only	2.49 (1.12, 6.08)
Mother only	2.38 (0.91, 5.36)
Both parents	2.59 (1.45, 5.89)
Pocket money (Euro)	
<8	1.00
8-15	2.22 (0.98, 5.43)
16-23	2.64 (1.19, 5.58)
24-31	3.46 (1.41, 7.79)
32+	4.93 (1.59, 14.21)

CI[1] confidence interval.

DISCUSSION

Using the GYTS, Kyrlesi et al. (13) reported that among 13 to 15 year olds, 16.2% were current users of all tobacco products, 1 in 4 had started smoking by 10 years, 94.1% reported environmental tobacco exposure at home, and

10.4% were current cigarette smokers among 13 to 15 year olds. However, the predictors of smoking or social correlates were not reported among school-going adolescents in Greece. Our study explored the association between a selected list of variables and current cigarette smoking.

In bivariate analysis, we found that older age, male gender, having smoking parents, lower parental education status, and high amount of pocket money at the adolescent's disposal were positively associated with being a current cigarette smoker. In multivariate analysis, male gender, smoking status of parents and pocket money were positively associated with being a current smoker. Previous studies elsewhere have reported the association between cigarette smoking and age, gender, parental smoking status, and pocket money (7-10).

Males were more likely to be smokers than females. Similar findings have been reported in other studies and may suggest societal tolerance of male smoking (9, 15, 16). However, Hublet et al. (8) have reported that female adolescents have higher prevalence of cigarette smoking than males in Sweden (13.7% vs. 5.5%), Norway (19.9% vs. 15.4%), Austria (24.7% vs. 19.5%), Belgium (19.0 vs. 16.8%) and Finland (18.0 vs. 16.4), which is an indication that gender difference in cigarette smoking may be context-specific. Furthermore, it's of considerable interest that in some countries (e.g., Greece, Japan, Malawi and Ethiopia) apparently smoking is more prevalent among adolescent boys than girls, in other countries (e.g., Sweden, Norway, Austria, Finland, New Zealand, Australia) smoking is more prevalent among adolescent girls. In particular, for Greece we speculate that the previous finding could be associated with the ongoing – and not yet completed –process of "westernization" of the Greek society.

Findings from this study indicate that subjects whose parents smoked were more likely to be smokers than those whose parents were not smokers; which is consistent with previous studies (9). This suggests the influence parents have on the lifestyle of their children.

In this study, participants who had more than 16 Euro per week as pocket money were more likely to smoke than those who had seven Euros or less per week. This finding may suggest that having disposable income may influence smoking practice and/or that those adolescents with no money or very little may be purchasing bare essentials. Mohan et al. (10) have also reported on a four times the risk of being a smoker among adolescents who received pocket money versus none in India. The public health significance of this finding is that parents and other guardians who provide adolescents with cash should take interest in how that money is used.

We also found that the higher the educational level of the father, the less likely that the teenager was a smoker. On the other hand, it did not appear that the educational status of the mother was associated with being a smoker or non-smoker. We suggest that it is possible that the educational status, and therefore the socio-economic status of the male parent could influence adolescent behavior more than that of the mother.

Our study has the following limitations. Firstly the data were collected through self-completion of the questionnaire. It is possible that recall bias could affect the accuracy of the reports as well as deliberate miss-reporting. As our assessment of current smoking status was not validated by biomarkers such as nicotine or cotinine levels or exhaled carbon monoxide, it is difficult to estimate the extent of any reporting biases that may have occurred (17, 18). However our study used a standardized questionnaire that enables within country and across country comparisons of smoking status. The prevalence estimates also obtained are likely to closely represent the smoking prevalence among school-going adolescents. It is not known how representative our sample was to out of school adolescents.

As it has been noted above (11), Greece recorded a high smoking prevalence (37–40% of total population are current smokers). It has been suggested that Greece probably presents a pattern of smoking epidemic similar to that observed in United States and Western Europe during the sixties when more than 40% of adult smoked and smoking rates were almost equal between socioeconomic groups (19, 20). In addition a study on the prevalence of current smoking among students (GYTS project) revealed that 16% of the adolescents aged 13–15 years were current smokers (13). The high prevalence of smoking among adults and adolescents reflects the state of antismoking and public health activities in Greece. Indeed, the first (and the only one till now) nationwide antismoking campaign has been implemented in 1978 (21).

We believe that there is an urgent need for designing and implementing a national programme against smoking in Greece. In the context of that programme special attention should be paying to the determinants of smoking among students.

In conclusion, among school-going adolescents in Greece, we found that cigarette smoking is strongly associated with the amount of pocket money as well as the smoking status of parents. These findings indicate the need to implement public health interventions paying attention to the determinants of smoking in this group.

ACKNOWLEDGMENTS

This study was supported by a grant from the Greek Ministry of Health and Social Solidarity.

This paper is a revised version of a paper originally published in the BMC Public Health (Rachiotis G, Muula AS, Rudatsikira E, Siziya S, Kyrlesi A, Gourgoulianis K, Chadjichristodoulou C. Factors associated with adolescent cigarette smoking in Greece: results from a cross sectional study. BMC Public Health 2008;8:313) and the authors have obtained the permission from the BMC Public Health to use this material.

REFERENCES

[1] Mathers CD, Loncar D. Projections of global mortality and burden of disease from 2002 to 2030. PLoS Med 2006;3:e442.

[2] MacKey J, Ericksen M. Tobacco atlas. World Health Organization (WHO), 2002.

[3] Eisner MD, Iribarren C. The influence of cigarette smoking on adult asthma outcomes. Nicotine Tob Res 2007;9:53-6.

[4] Jindal SK, Aggarwal AN, Chaudhry K, Chabra SK, D'Souza GA, Gupta D, et al. A multicentric study on epidemiology of chronic obstructive pulmonary disease and its relationship with tobacco smoking and environmental tobacco smoke exposure. Indian J Chest Dis Allied Sci 2006;48:23-9.

[5] Petridou E, Zavitsanos X, Desspris N, Grangakis C, Mandyla M, Doxiadis S, et al. Adolescents in high-risk trajectory: clustering of risky behaviour and the origins of socioeconomic health differentials. Prev Med 1997;26:215-9.

[6] Arvanitidou M, Tirodimos I, Kyriakidis I, Tsinaslanidou Z, Seretopoulos D. Decreasing prevalence of alcohol consumption among Greek adolescents. Am J Drug Alcohol Abuse 2007;33:411-417.

[7] Abdullah AS, Ho WW. What Chinese adolescents think about quitting smoking: a qualitative study. Subst Use Misuse 2006;41:1735-43.

[8] Hublet A, De Bacquer D, Valimaa R, Godeau E, Schmid H, Rahav G, et al. Smoking trends among adolescents from 1990 to 2002 in ten European countries and Canada. BMC Public Health 2006;6:280.

[9] Rudatsikira E, Abdo A, Muula AS. Prevalence and determinants of adolescent tobacco smoking in Addis Ababa, Ethiopia. BMC Public Health 2007;7:176.

[10] Mohan S, Sankara Sarma P, Thankappan KR. Access to pocket money and low educational performance predict tobacco use among adolescent boys in Kerala, India. Prev Med 2005;41:685-92.

[11] World Health Organization. Compating the tobacco epidemic. The World Health Report 1999. Geneva: WHO, 1999.

[12] House of Lords. Select Committee on European Communities. 30th report. Tobacco production in the European Community [http://www.parliament.uk].

[13] Kyrlesi A, Soteriades ES, Warren CW, Kremastinou J, Papastergiou P, Jones NR, et al. Tobacco use among students aged 13–15 years in Greece: the GYTS project. BMC Public Health 2007;7:3.
[14] Global Youth Tobacco Survey Collaborative Group. Tobacco Use among Youth: A cross-country comparison. Tob Control 2002;11:252-70.
[15] Muula AS. Prevalence and determinants of cigarette smoking among adolescents in Blantyre City, Malawi. Tanzan Health Res Bull 2007;9:48-51.
[16] Ando M, Asakura T, Ando S, Simons-Morton BG. Psychosocial factors associated with smoking and drinking among Japanese early adolescent boys and girls: cross-sectional study. Biopsychos Med 2007;1:13.
[17] Hung J, Lin CH, Wang JD, Chann CC. Exhaled carbon monoxide level as an indicator of cigarette consumption in a workplace cessation program in Taiwan. J Formos Med Assoc 2006;105:210-3.
[18] Low EC, Ong MC, Tan M. Breath carbon monoxide as an indication of smoking habit in the military setting. Singapore Med J 2004;45:578.
[19] Rachiotis G, Behrakis PK, Vasiliou M, Yfantopoulos J. Quality of life and smoking among industrial workers in Greece. Med Lav 2006;97:44-50.
[20] Rachiotis G, Papanayiotou G, Kambosi C, Behrakis P, Kremastinos D. Increased risk for Coronary Heart Disease in blue-collar workers in a military industry plan in Greece? Med Lav 2005;96:162-8.
[21] Doxiadis SA, Trichopoulos DV, Phylactou HD. Impact of a nationwide anti-smoking campaign. Lancet 1985;8457:712-3.

In: Smoking and Adolescence ISBN: 978-1-63484-311-9
Editors: M. L. Mazabam, S. Siziya et al. © 2016 Nova Science Publishers, Inc.

Chapter 15

CIGARETTE SMOKING AMONG ADOLESCENTS IN LITHUANIA

Bradley Jamison*[1], *MPH, PhD,
Adamson S Muula*[2], *MBBS, MPH, PhD,
Seter Siziya*[3,*], *BA(Ed), MSc, PhD,
Sara Graham*[1], *MSc, MPH, MD,
and Emmanuel Rudatsikira*[1], *MD, MPH, DrPH
[1]Department of Global Health, Loma Linda University, School of Public Health, Loma Linda, California, USA
[2]Department of Community Medicine and Public Health, University of Malawi, College of Medicine, Blantyre, Malawi
[3]Department of Community Medicine, University of Zambia, School of Medicine, Lusaka, Zambia

The majority of people who suffer morbidity due to smoking may have initiated smoking during adolescent period. In this chapter we look at the prevalence and associated factors for cigarette smoking among school-going adolescents in Lithuania. Data from the Global Youth Tobacco Survey (GYTS) 2005 were used to conduct this study. Data were analyzed using SUDAAN software 9.03. Comparisons for categorical

* Correspondence: Professor Seter Siziya, Clinical Sciences Department, School of Medicine, Copperbelt University, Ndola Central Hospital, 6th Floor, P. O. Box 71191, Ndola, Zambia. E-mail: ssiziya@gmail.com.

variables were done using the Pearson's Chi-square test. The cut off point for statistical significance was set at 5% level. Logistic regression analyses were conducted to determine factors associated with the outcome. Unadjusted odds ratios (OR) and adjusted odds ratios (AOR) together with their 95% confidence intervals (CI) are reported. Of the 1,822 respondents, 35.8% males and 27.1% females reported being current cigarette smokers ($p < 0.001$). Having friends who smoke cigarettes was associated with smoking after controlling for age, gender, parental smoking status, and perception of risks of smoking (AOR = 3.76; 95% CI [2.33, 6.90] for some friends using tobacco; and AOR = 17.18; 95% CI [10.46, 28.21] for most or all friends using tobacco). Male gender and having one or both parents who smoke cigarettes were associated with smoking (AOR = 1.31; 95% CI [1.03, 1.66]) and AOR = 1.76; 95% CI [1.37, 2.27]) respectively). There is a high prevalence of cigarette smoking among Lithuanian adolescents. Male adolescents and adolescents who have friends or parents who smoke should be the main target for tobacco control in Lithuania.

INTRODUCTION

Tobacco use is a leading cause of adult mortality across the world. It is estimated that tobacco-attributable deaths are projected to rise from 5.4 million in 2005 to 8.3 million in 2030. By 2015, tobacco use is projected to cause 50% more deaths than AIDS (1, 2).

Much of the morbidity and mortality associated with tobacco use, such as cancers, chronic lower respiratory obstructive conditions and cardiovascular morbidity and mortality are experienced after several decades of smoking (1-4). The majority of people who suffer morbidity later in life had initiated smoking as adolescents or young adults (5).

Studies conducted in Lithuania include that of Garmiene et al. (6) who reported a smoking prevalence of 1.2% among fifth grade adolescents of whom 6.5% girls and 23.0% boys had ever tried smoking. This report however was from one setting (Kaunas) and included only 369 school children. The results of the Lithuanian GYTS 2005 that have been published (7) were limited to the analysis of data for the age group 13 to 15 years; and only reported the prevalence of tobacco use. Factors associated with current smoking were not reported in this report. However, these factors have been reported elsewhere (8-10), but public health actions have to be at local, national and regional level. We thus aimed to determine the prevalence and associated factors for cigarette smoking among school-going adolescents in Lithuania.

OUR STUDY

Our study involved secondary analysis of existing data from the Lithuania Global Youth Tobacco Survey (GYTS) conducted in 2005. A comprehensive description of the methods and procedures is presented elsewhere (7-9). In brief, the Lithuanian GYTS conducted in 2005 was a cross sectional study, that was aimed to recruit school-going adolescents of ages 13 to 15 years using a two-stage probability sampling technique. In the first stage, primary sampling units were schools which were selected with a probability proportional to their enrolment size. In the second step, a systematic sample of classes in the selected schools was obtained. All students in the selected classes, irrespective of their actual ages (even when outside the 13 to 15 year age group) were eligible to participate. The school and class response rates were 100%. However, out of the total sample eligible for participation, 82.8% eventually participated, representing 17.2% of the eligible students who were either absent or refused to participate in the survey.

A questionnaire was used and included 'core GYTS' and other additional questions as has been described elsewhere regarding the GYTS methodology (7-9). Responses to questions were close ended with multiple-choice style format. The questionnaire included questions among others on tobacco use, knowledge and attitudes regarding tobacco, and pro- and anti-tobacco media and advertising exposure.

For purposes of analysis, current cigarette smoking was defined as per GYTS convention which is having smoked a cigarette, even a single puff, within the last 30 days (7). Using the socio-ecological model (SEM) of health behavior (11), we selected the variables to be analyzed. In brief the SEM recognizes that for a behavior such as adolescent smoking, various factors operating at the individual, interpersonal, organizational, structural level and policy levels interact. The questions and possible responses that were selected for analysis in this study are shown in Table 1.

Data were analyzed using SUDAAN software 9.03 (Research Triangle Institute, Research Triangle Park, North Carolina, United states of America). Comparisons for the categorical variables were statistically conducted using the Pearson's Chi-square test. The cut off point for statistical significance was set at the 5% level.

Table 1. Variables considered in the study

Question	Options provided	Re-coding for analysis
During the past 30 days (one month), on how many days did you smoke cigarettes?	0 day; 1 or 2 days; 3 to 5 days; 6 to 9 days; 10 to 19 days; 20 to 29 days; all 30 days	Any number of days except 0, were coded as current smoker= yes (1)
Do you think boys who smoke cigarettes have more or less friends?	More friends, less friends, no difference from non-smokers	Re-coded as binary variable, less friends and makes no difference combined and recoded = 0; more friends recoded =1
Do you think girls who smoke cigarettes have more or less friends?	More friends, less friends; No difference from non-smokers	Re-coded as binary variable, less friends and makes no difference combined and recoded = 0; more friends recoded =1
Do you think smoking cigarettes makes girls look more or less attractive	More attractive; Less attractive; Smoking doesn't make a difference	Less attractive and doesn't make a difference recoded= 0; more attractive coded=1
Do you think smoking cigarettes makes boys look more or less attractive	More attractive; Less attractive; Smoking doesn't make a difference	Less attractive and doesn't make a difference recoded= 0; more attractive coded=1
Do you think cigarette smoking is harmful to your health?	Definitely not Probably not Probably yes; Definitely yes	Definitely yes or probably yes coded=1; otherwise 0
Do any of your closest friends smoke cigarettes?	none of them, some of them, most of them, all of them	indicator variables created, with one of the categories as referent
During the past 30 days (one month), when you watched sports events or other programs on TV how often did you see cigarette brand names?	I never watch TV; a lot; sometimes, never.	Never and I never watch TV combined and coded=0; a lot or sometimes coded=1

Question	Options provided	Re-coding for analysis
During the past 30 days (one month), how many advertisements for cigarettes have you seen on billboards?	a lot, a few, none	None = 0; a lot or a few = 1
During the past 30 days (one month), how many advertisements or promotions for cigarettes have you seen in newspapers or magazines?	a lot, a few, none	Non e= 0; a lot or a few = 1
When you go to sports events, fairs, concerts, community events, or other events, how often do you see anti-smoking information?	a lot, a few, none	None = 0; a lot or a few = 1

In order to estimate the associations between the explanatory variables and the outcome variable, bivariate logistic regression analyses were conducted, and obtained unadjusted odds ratios (OR) and their 95% confidence intervals (CI); and finally, a multivariate logistic regression model was run to determine independent predictors for the outcome, and the results are presented as adjusted odds ratios (AOR) and their 95% CI.

These data were obtained on request from the Centers for Diseases Control and Prevention, Atlanta, Georgia. The study was approved by the Committee on Health Promotion of the Ministry of National Education and Religion (8). Parents were informed of the study through a letter, and students gave verbal consent to participate in the survey. To preserve individual confidentiality, the questionnaire was self-completed anonymously by the student.

FINDINGS

A total of 1,853 students participated in the survey. Of the 1,822 (98.3%) students who reported their sex, 948 (52.0%) were female. The median age was 14 (Q1 = 13, Q3 = 15) years. Altogether, 35.8% males and 27.1% females reported being current cigarette smokers ($p < 0.001$).

Table 2 indicates that participants were exposed to tobacco advertisements through TV (70.7%), billboards (100%), and newspapers or magazines

(63.4%). More than 1 in 2 respondents (54.1%) reported having seen cigarette advertisements at sports events in the past 30 days.

Table 2. Exposure to cigarette advertisements among adolescents in Lithuania

Characteristics	Number of participants	% of total (95% CI)	p value
See cigarette adverts when watching TV	1735	70.7 (68.5, 72.9)	
Males	826	73.0 (69.8, 76.0)	0.082
Females	909	68.7 (65.5, 71.7)	
Seen cigarette adverts on billboards in past 30 days	1428	100	
Males	657	100	-
Females	771	100	
Seen cigarette adverts in newspapers or magazines in past 30 days	1808	63.4 (61.2, 65.7)	
Males	862	60.4 (57.1, 63.7)	0.017
Females	946	66.2 (63.1, 69.2)	
Seen cigarette adverts at sports events in past 30 days	1800	54.1 (51.7, 56.4)	
Males	861	54.9 (51.4, 58.3)	0.358
Females	939	53.3 (50.0, 56.4)	

Table 3 indicates that the vast majority (92.0%) of the respondents felt that cigarette smoking is harmful. More than two-thirds (69.5%) of the respondents thought that males who smoked cigarettes had more friends while 37.1% thought so for females. There were 1.74 times more respondents who thought that male smokers were attractive compared to those who thought so for female smokers (12.2% and 7.0%, respectively).

Table 3. Attitudes towards cigarette smoking distributed by gender in Lithuania

Characteristics	Number of participants	% of total (95% CI)	p value
Felt that boys who smoke cigarette have more friends	832	69.5 (66.3, 72.5)	
Males	391	68.4 (66.3, 72.5)	0.657
Females	441	70.3 (66.0, 74.6)	
Felt like girls who smoke cigarettes have more friends	921	37.1 (34.0, 40.3)	
Males	467	37.8 (33.5, 42.4)	0.618
Females	454	36.3 (32.0, 40.9)	
Felt that boys who smoke cigarettes are attractive	1180	12.2 (10.4, 14.2)	
Males	518	16.1 (13.1, 19.7)	0.001
Females	662	9.1 (7.1, 11.6)	
Felt that girls who smoke cigarettes are attractive	1426	7.0 (5.8, 8.5)	
Males	646	10.3 (8.2, 13.0)	<0.001
Females	780	4.3 (3.0, 6.1)	
Felt that cigarettes smoking is harmful to health	1809	92.0 (90.6, 93.2)	
Males	864	89.6 (87.3, 91.6)	<0.001
Females	945	94.1 (92.3, 95.5)	

Table 4 shows that age, parental and best friend smoking status were significantly associated with current cigarette smoking in bivariate analyses. These factors remained significantly associated with the outcome in a multivariate analysis. Having friends who smoke cigarettes was very strongly associated with tobacco use after controlling for age, gender, parental smoking status, and perception of hazards caused by smoking. For those respondents who had most or all friends who smoked cigarettes, we found a more than a seventeen-fold increase in the odds of smoking compared to those who had no smoking friends (AOR = 17.18; 95% [10.46, 28.21]). Those who had some friends who smoked were more than three times likely to smoke than those who had no smoking friends (AOR = 3.76; 95% CI [2.33; 95% CI [2.33, 6.90]). Males were more likely to report cigarette smoking than females (AOR = 1.31; 95% CI [1.03, 1.66]).

Table 4. Factors associated with current cigarette smoking in Lithuania

Characteristic	Cigarette smokers n (%)	OR (95% CI)	AOR (95% CI)
Overall	533 (31.3)		
Age (years)			
<14	109 (18.8)	1	1
14	167 (27.5)	1.56 (1.18, 2.05)	1.16 (0.85, 1.58)
15	203 (44.1)	3.35 (2.53, 4.42)	2.22 (1.61, 3.06)
6+	54 (60.3)	6.04 (3.78, 9.64)	4.06 (2.37, 6.96)
Gender			
Female	237 (27.1)	1	1
Male	284 (35.8)	1.54 (1.25, 1.89)	1.31 (1.03, 1.66)
Parental smoking status			
None	156 (22.7)	1	1
One or both parents smoked	372 (37.4)	1.99 (1.60, 2.48)	1.76 (1.37, 2.27)
Best friends smoking status			
None	21 (6.7)	1	1
Some	212 (23.9)	4.35 (2.72, 6.95)	3.76 (2.33, 6.90)
Most or all	292 (61.0)	22.52 (13.94, 36.37)	17.18 (10.46, 28.21)
Perception that smoking is harmful to health			
No	45 (35.9)	1	1
Yes	484 (30.9)	0.81 (0.55, 1.18)	0.83 (0.52, 1.32)

DISCUSSION

We found a prevalence of current cigarette smoking of 35.8% and 27.1% among Lithuanian school-going adolescent males and females respectively. Although there is male predominance, the smoking prevalence among females is much higher than the average prevalence of cigarette smoking among female youth in Europe (12) but similar to what has been reported in Cyprus (13). Christophi et al. (13) have reported smoking prevalence of 36% among boys and 23% among girls in high schools in Cyprus. Among in-school adolescents in some European countries, Warren et al. (7) have reported prevalence of current cigarette smoking of 8.5% in Albania (2004), 26.5% in Belarus (2004), 10.4% in Greece (2005), 32.9% in Latvia (2007) and 24.1% in Croatia (2007).

The male predominance in cigarette smoking has been reported in Africa, India and Europe but is not universal (14). A comprehensive report of global adolescent smoking patterns by Warren et al. (7) has shown in general male predominance is high in Africa and Asia, while in the United States and parts of Europe, the gap between the sexes is limited. We do not know the reasons behind these patterns but we suggest that they may have to do with cultural acceptability of female smoking. If smoking among women is perceived in negative terms more than male smoking is in any particular society, we hypothesize that females in that society are less likely to smoke. The findings in the current study that about 2 in 3 adolescents reported that boys who smoke have more friends while only 1 in 3 thought that girls who smoke have more friends supports the assertion that male smokers are more accepted by society in Lithuania than female smokers.

We found that exposure to pro-tobacco advertisement exceeded half of the sample, and in some of the exposures approaching three-quarters. Data on adolescent smoking has shown that pro-teen advertisements are an important factor in influencing initiation and maintenance of adolescent smoking (4, 15). The findings that smoking in a parent, best friend and increasing age were positively associated with smoking have also been reported elsewhere (16-19).

This study has several inherent limitations. Firstly, the data were collected via a self-reported questionnaire. Like all questionnaires, the possibility of mis-reporting both intentional and unintentional threatens the validity and reliability of the findings. No biomarkers were assessed to confirm current cigarette smoking status. However, data from the United States using a similar questionnaire as the GYTS have reported high reliability among students in reporting personal health-compromising behaviors (20, 21). The extent as to whether similarly high reliability values could be obtained in settings outside of the United States is not known. Secondly, only students enrolled and available in schools during the administration of the questionnaire and completed it, were surveyed; leaving out 17.2% of adolescent students. To the extent that these students are not representative of all the adolescents in school, and of the overall adolescent population in the country (including out of school adolescents) our findings may not be generalized to the in-school adolescents, and to the adolescent population in Lithuania.

In conclusion, our study has found that the prevalence of cigarette smoking among adolescent students was 35.8% for males and 27.1% for females. Being male and having friends or parents who smoke were associated with cigarette smoking. Male adolescents and adolescents who have friends or parents who smoke should be the main target for tobacco control guided by the WHO Framework Convention on Tobacco Control that Lithuania ratified in 2004.

Acknowledgments

We gratefully acknowledge the wonderful efforts by the Lithuanian 2005 GYTS research team in successfully completing the collection of data. To the students we say thank you for your participation, and we hope that the results of this study will be used to improve your health and that of the other adolescents in Lithuania.

This paper is a revised version of an original publication in BMC Research Notes (Jamison B, Muula AS, Siziya S, Graham S, Rudatsikira E. Cigarette smoking among school-going adolescents in Lithuania: Results from the 2005 Global Youth Tobacco Survey. BMC Res Notes 2010;3:130) and the authors have obtained the permission from BMC Research Notes to use this material.

References

[1] Mathers CD, Loncar D. Projections of global mortality and burden of disease from 2002 to 2030. PLoS Med 2006;3:e442.

[2] Peto R, Lopez AD. Future worldwide health effects of current smoking patterns. In: Koop CE, Pearson CE, Schwarz MR, eds. Critical issues in global health. San Francisco, CA: Jossey-Bass, 2001.

[3] Ezzati M, Lopez AD: Estimates of global mortality attributable to smoking in 2000. Lancet 2003;362:847-52.

[4] Warren CD, Jones NR, Eriksen MP, Asma S, Global Tobacco Surveillance System (GTSS) collaborative group: Patterns of global tobacco use in young people and implications for future chronic disease burden in adults. Lancet 2006;367:749-53.

[5] Bourgkard E, Wild P, Massin N, Meyer JP, Otero Sierra C, Fontana JM, et al. Association of physical job demands, smoking and alcohol abuse with subsequent premature mortality: a 9-year follow-up population-based study. J Occup Health 2008;50:31-40.

[6] Garmiene A, Zemaitiene N, Zaborskis A. Family time, parental behavior model and the initiation of smoking and alcohol use by ten-year-old children: an epidemiological study in Kaunas, Lithuania. BMC Public Health 2006;6:287.

[7] Warren CW, Jones NR, Peruga A, Chauvin J, Baptiste JP, Costa de Silva V, et al. Global youth tobacco surveillance, 2000-2007. MMWR Surveill Summ 2008;57:1-28.

[8] Kyrlesi A, Soteriades ES, Warren CW, Kremastinou J, Papastergiou P, Jones NR, et al. Tobacco use among students aged 13-15 years in Greece: the GYTS project. BMC Public Health 2007;7:3.

[9] Rudatsikira E, Muula AS, Siziya S, Mataya RH. Correlates of cigarette smoking among school-going adolescents in Thailand: findings from the Thai Global Youth Tobacco Survey 2005. Int Arch Med 2008;1:8.

[10] Stigler MH, Perry CL, Arora M, Reddy KS. Why are urban Indian 6th graders using more tobacco than 8th graders? Findings from Project MYTRI. Tob Control 2006;15(Suppl 1):i54-60.

[11] Naylor PJ, Macdonald HM, Reed KE, McKay HA. Action schools! BC: a socioecological approach to modifying chronic disease risk factors in elementary school children. Prev Chronic Dis 2006;3:A60.

[12] Baska T, Warren CW, Baskova M, Jones NR. Prevalence of youth cigarette smoking and selected social factors in 25 European countries: findings from the Global Youth Tobacco Survey. Int J Public Health 2009;54:439-45.

[13] Christophi CA, Kolokotroni O, Alpert HR, Warren CW, Jones NR, Demokritou P, et al. Prevalence and social environment of cigarette smoking in Cyprus youth. BMC Public Health 2008;8:190.

[14] Global Youth Tobacco Survey Collaborating Group. Differences in worldwide tobacco use by gender: findings from the Global Youth Tobacco Survey. J Sch Health 2003;73:207-15.

[15] Centers for Disease Control and Prevention (CDC). Youth exposure to alcohol advertising in magazines--United States, 2001-2005. MMWR 2007;56:763-7.

[16] Braun S, Mejia R, Ling PM, Perez-Stable EJ. Tobacco industry targeting youth in Argentina. Tob Control 2008;17:111-7.

[17] Madan Kumar PD, Poorni S, Ramachandran S. Tobacco use among school children in Chennai city, India. Indian J Cancer 2006;43:127-31.

[18] Weiss JW, Cen S, Schuster DV, Unger JB, Johnson CA, Mouttapa M, et al. Longitudinal effects of pro-tobacco and anti-tobacco messages on adolescent smoking susceptibility. Nicotine Tob Res 2006;8:455-65.

[19] Dirocco DN, Shadel WG. Gender differences in adolescents' responses to themes of relaxation in cigarette advertising: Relationship to intentions to smoke. Addict Behav 2007;32:205-13.

[20] Brener ND, Collins JL, Kann L, Warren CW, Williams BI. Reliability of the Youth Risk Behavior Survey Questionnaire. Am J Epidemiol 1995;141:575-80.

[21] Martin Gl, Newman IM. Assessing the validity of self-reported adolescent cigarette smoking. J Drug Educ 1983;18:275-84.

In: Smoking and Adolescence ISBN: 978-1-63484-311-9
Editors: M. L. Mazabam, S. Siziya et al. © 2016 Nova Science Publishers, Inc.

Chapter 16

CIGARETTE SMOKING AMONG ADOLESCENTS IN PUNJAB, INDIA

Seter Siziya[1,*], BA(Ed), MSc, PhD, Adamson S Muula[2], MBBS, MPH, PhD, and Emmanuel Rudatsikira[3], MD, MPH, DrPH

[1]School of Medicine, University of Zambia, Lusaka, Zambia
[2]Department of Community Health, University of Malawi, Blantyre, Malawi
[3]Departments of Global Health, Biostatistics and Epidemiology, School of Public Health, Loma Linda University, California, USA

Smoking is a leading cause of morbidity and mortality globally. There is therefore need to identify relevant factors associated with smoking among adolescents in order to better tailor public health interventions aimed at preventing smoking. In this chapter we used data from the Global Youth Tobacco Survey (GYTS) conducted in 2003 in Punjab, India, on 2,014 adolescents of whom 58.9% were males. We conducted a weighted logistic regression analysis, adjusting for age and gender, to determine associations between predictor variables and current tobacco smoking status. A total of 2,014 adolescents participated in the survey in 2003, and of these 58.9% were males. Male respondents tended to be older than females (21.2% of males, and 13.1% of females were of age 16 years or

[*] Correspondence: Professor Seter Siziya, Clinical Sciences Department, School of Medicine, Copperbelt University, Ndola Central Hospital, 6th Floor, P. O. Box 71191, Ndola, Zambia. E-mail: ssiziya@gmail.com.

above). The percent of males and females in the other age groups were: 23.0% and 28.6% for <14 years, 27.3% and 31.0% for 14 years, and 28.4% and 27.0% for 15 years, respectively. The following factors were positively associated with smoking: adolescents who received pocket money; adolescents who had parents who smoked, chewed or applied tobacco; adolescents who said that boys or girls who smoke or chew tobacco have more friends; adolescents who said that smoking or chewing tobacco makes boys look less attractive; adolescents who said that there is no difference in weight between smokers and non-smokers; adolescents who said that smoking makes one gain weight; and adolescents who had most or all of their closest friends who smoked. The factors that were negatively associated with smoking were: adolescents who said that boys or girls who smoke or chew tobacco have less number of friends; adolescents who said that girls who smoke or chew tobacco are less attractive; and adolescents who had some of their closest friends who smoked. The observed associations between current smoking on one hand and peer smoking, and perception that boys who smoke are less attractive on the other, deserve further studies. The factors reported in the current study should be considered in the design of public health interventions aimed to reduce adolescent cigarette smoking.

Introduction

Tobacco smoking among adolescents is of public concern because of the immediate and long-term health sequelae such as asthma, chronic cough, cancers, chronic obstructive airways disease and cardiovascular diseases (1-3). In the past decade data on adolescent smoking behaviours have been accumulating, partly due to work done by the Global Youth Tobacco Survey (GYTS) collaborative group and its partners (4-7). The prevalence of smoking cigarettes among school going adolescents in India using the GYTS data of 2000 and 2001 have been reported to vary from one State/Union to another between 0.5% in Gao and 22.8% in Mizoram, with the North-Eastern States/Unions having higher rates than the South-Western States/Unions (4). Current cigarette smoking was defined as having ever smoked even one puff in the past 30 days preceding the study. Jindal et al. (8) have reported that the prevalence of having ever smoked in Northern India was lowest in Punjab (2.9% for boys and 1.5% for girls) and highest in Chandigarh (8.5% for boys and 9.8% for girls).

Knowledge of the prevalence of smoking among adolescent is important in estimating the burden of the problem and facilitates evaluation of public health interventions as change in prevalence over time can be assessed. However, prevalence alone without information on the predictors of smoking will fail to provide further indicators that may be useful in targeted-interventions given the scarcity of public health resources. It is therefore important also to identify socio-demographic factors that are associated with cigarette smoking.

There have been reports elsewhere that gender, having parents or friends who were smokers, body image consideration and feeling of acceptance among peers may be important factors associated with smoking among adolescents (9-12). We therefore designed the current study to assess whether these factors were also associated with current smoking among adolescents in the 2003 Punjabi GYTS.

OUR STUDY

The Punjabi GYTS conducted in 2003 was a cross sectional study, that was aimed to recruit school-going adolescents of ages 13 to 15 years using a two-stage probability sampling technique. In the first stage, primary sampling units were schools which were selected with a probability proportional to their enrolment size. In the second step, a systematic sample of classes in the selected schools was obtained. All students in the selected classes were eligible to participate. An 85-item questionnaire was used and included 'core GYTS' and other additional questions as has been described elsewhere regarding the GYTS methodology (4-6, 13).

Data analysis was performed using a Statistical Package for Social Sciences (SSPSS) 14.0 for windows (Chicago, Illinois, United States). For the estimation of prevalence or proportions, the GYTS data are weighted to adjust for design effect (selection of school and class levels), nonresponse (school, class and student levels), and post-stratification of the sample population relative to the grade and sex distribution in the total population. A similar method of analysis has been used previously (4) and is reported by the CDC in the GYTS Dataset Help File (14). Weights were applied to effectively resize the sample so that it is representative of the population from which it is sampled from. The weighting factor is given by the formula:

$$W = W1 * W2 * f1 * f2 * f3 * f4$$

where W1 = the inverse of the probability of selecting a school

W2 = the inverse of the probability of selecting a classroom within a school
f1 = a school-level non response adjustment factor calculated by school size category (small, medium, large)
f2 = a class-level non response adjustment factor calculated for each school
f3 = a student-level non response adjustment factor calculated by class
f4 = a post-stratification adjustment factor calculated by sex and grade

For the purposes of this assessment we aimed to assess whether parental or friends' smoking status, perceptions of body image and acceptance among peers were associated with current smoking status. We also assessed the association between adolescent perception that individuals who smoke have more friends and their smoking status.

FINDINGS

Characteristics of the study participants A total of 2,014 adolescents participated in the survey in 2003, and of these 58.9% were males. Male respondents tended to be older than females (21.2% of males, and 13.1% of females were of age 16 years or above) The percent of males and females in the other age groups were: 23.0% and 28.6% for <14 years, 27.3% and 31.0% for 14 years, and 28.4% and 27.0% for 15 years, respectively. About 0.4% of the respondents reported that both parents or guardians used tobacco in any form (e.g., chew, smoke), and 13.6% reported that only the father used tobacco, while only one adolescent reported that only the mother used tobacco.

Overall, 3.3% of all respondents were current cigarette smokers. Boys were 1.18 (95%CI 1.16, 1.20) times more likely to be smokers than girls. Compared to adolescents of age <14 years, those of ages 14, 15 and 16+ years were 30% less likely (OR = 0.70, 95%CI 0.68, 0.71), 25% less likely (OR = 0.75, 95%CI 0.73, 0.77), and 55% more likely (OR = 1.55, 95% CI 1.52, 1.59), respectively, to be smokers.

Table 1 shows factors that were associated with current cigarette smoking. The following factors were positively associated with smoking: Adolescents who received pocket money were more likely to be smokers compared to adolescents who did not receive pocket money (OR = 1.25; 95%CI 1.23, 1.26).

Table 1. Factors associated with current smoking status among school going adolescents in Punjab, India

Factor	*Adjusted Odds ratio (95% confidence interval)
Received pocket money in a usual month	
No	1
Yes	1.25 (1.23–1.26)
Parents use tobacco	
No	1
Yes	1.35 (1.32–1.37)
Felt boys who used tobacco had more friends	
No difference between smokers and nonsmokers	1
Have fewer friends	0.84 (0.81–0.86)
Have more friends	2.74 (2.67–2.82)
Felt girls who used tobacco had more friends	
No difference between smokers and nonsmokers	1
Have fewer friends	0.43 (0.42–0.44)
Have more friends	1.34 (1.31–1.38)
Perception on attractiveness of boys who smoked	
No difference between smokers and nonsmokers	1
Less attractive	1.15 (1.13–1.17)
Perception on attractiveness of girls who smoked	
No difference between smokers and nonsmokers	1
Less attractive	0.87 (0.86–0.89)
Perception that smoking makes one lose or gain weight	
Lose weight	1
No difference between smokers and nonsmokers	1.19 (1.16–1.22)
Gain weight	1.47 (1.44–1.51)
Closest friends smoke	
None of them smokes	1
Some of them	0.73 (0.72–0.75)
Most or all of them smoke	3.83 (3.72–3.95

*weighted analysis adjusted for age and gender.

Adolescents who had parents who smoked, chewed or applied tobacco were more likely to be smokers compared to adolescents who did not have parents who smoked or chewed tobacco (OR = 1.34; 95% CI 1.32, 1.37). Respondents who said that boys or girls who smoke or chew tobacco have more friends were more likely to be smokers compared to those who said that boys or girls who smoke or chew tobacco are not different from non-smokers in the number of friends they have (OR = 2.74; 95% CI 2.67, 2.82, and OR = 1.34; 95% CI 1.31, 1.38, respectively). Adolescents who said that there is no difference in weight whether one smokes or not, and those who said that smokers gain weight were 1.19 (95% CI 1.16, 1.23) and 1.47 (95% CI 1.44, 1.51), respectively, times more likely to be smokers compared with those who said that smoking makes one lose weight. Adolescents who said that boys who smoke or chew tobacco are less attractive were 15% (OR = 1.15; 95% CI 1.13, 1.17) more likely to smoke cigarettes compared to those who said that there was no difference, or they were more attractive than non-smokers. Lastly, adolescents who had most or all of their closest friends who smoked were 3.83 (95% CI 3.72, 3.95) times more likely to smoke compared with adolescents who had none of their closest friends who smoked cigarettes.

The following factors were negatively associated with smoking cigarettes: Adolescents who said that boys or girls who smoke or chew tobacco have less number of friends were 16% (OR = 0.84, 95% CI 0.81, 0.86) and 57% (OR = 0.43; 95% CI 0.42, 0.44), respectively, less likely to be smokers when compared with those that said that there was no difference in the number of friends one had between smokers and non-smokers. We also found that adolescents who said that girls who smoke or chew tobacco are less attractive were 13% (OR = 0.87; 95% CI 0.86, 0.89) less likely to be smokers compared to those who said that there was no difference in attractiveness between smokers and non-smokers, or smokers were more attractive than non-smokers. Finally, adolescents who had some of their closest friends who smoked were 27% (OR = 0.73, 95% CI 0.72, 0.75) less likely to be smokers compared to adolescents who had none of their closest friends who smoked.

DISCUSSION

Overall the prevalence of smoking was 3.3%, with more males than females being smokers. Higher prevalence of smoking among males compared to females have been reported in some settings (15), but not demonstrated in other settings (16). This suggests that the socio-cultural factors that impact on smoking may be different from one setting to the other.

The finding that receiving pocket money was associated with smoking in the current study has also been reported by Siziya et al. (17) in Kafue, Zambia, and by Mohan et al. (18) in Kerala, India. As we have argued before (17), having disposable cash may influence adolescents to spend the money on buying cigarettes.

In the current study, adolescents who perceived that girls who smoke are less attractive were less likely to be smokers compared to those who thought smoking made no difference, or made an individual look more attractive. This result contradicts that reported by Croghan et al. (19), who conducted a study among college students in the United States and found that perceived lower body image satisfaction and low self-esteem were associated with smoking. However, our other finding that adolescents who felt that boys who smoke are less attractive were more likely to smoke compared to those who felt that there was no difference between boys who smoked and non-smokers, or those who felt that boys who smoked were more attractive, supports the finding of Croghan et al. (19). The observed contradictions in the results may be a reflection of how body image is perceived differently between males and females in different societies.

We also assessed whether adolescents' perception of body weight was associated with current smoking. The hypothesis was that adolescents who thought that smoking would make one lose weight were more likely to be smokers as has been demonstrated in Western populations and Japan (20-23). We, however, found that adolescents who believed that smoking makes one gain weight were more likely to be smokers. This finding is different from what has been reported in Western countries where adolescent smokers generally believe smoking makes one lose weight and hence more attractive. There could be a difference in the definition of attractiveness in Punjab which is different from the predominant Western belief. In Malawi for instance, Bentley et al. (24) have reported that study participants indicated a large body silhouette as desirable compared to a smaller build. This is a setting where human immunodeficiency virus (HIV) and malnutrition are leading health problems and thinness is associated with disease and or poverty.

Compared with respondents who said that there is no difference between smokers and non-smokers in terms of the number of friends they have, respondents who felt that boys or girls who smoke have more friends were more likely to smoke, and those who said that boys or girls who smoke have less number of friends were less likely to smoke cigarettes. Although we obtained these consistency results, we are unable to suggest any causality between current smoking and perception of having more friends if one was a smoker. This observed association deserves further study.

Our study also found that adolescents who had parents, and most or all of their closest friends who were smokers were more likely to be smokers themselves. This finding has also been reported elsewhere (17, 25, 26). Although parental smoking may influence adolescents to start smoking, we cannot conclude the same for peer smoking. It may be that adolescents who smoke choose other adolescents who smoke to be their closest friends (27).

Our study had several limitations. Our study was based on self report and therefore subject to respondent recall and deliberate misreporting. The study also recruited only school-going adolescents who may not have been representative of the out of school adolescents. The findings of the study may also be limited by not controlling for unmeasured confounders and effect measure modifiers (28). For example, Bergen et al. (29) have reported that perceived academic performance was associated with tobacco use among adolescents. We did not account for perceived academic performance. Finally, data on current smoking were only collected through interviews and not verified by biomarkers such as cotinine assessment or exhaled carbon monoxide (30-33). However, the study used validated standard GYTS methodology, and weighted analysis that adjusted for design effects and non-responses, to ensure valid comparisons of our findings to other studies using the same methodology. Brener et al. (34) has also reported that adolescents in the United States reported reliably on health risk behaviours. The extent to which the reliability obtained by Brener et al. (34), can be extrapolated to the Punjab adolescent group is not known. In conclusion, the observed associations between current smoking on one hand and peer smoking, and perception that boys who smoke are less attractive on the other deserve further studies. The rest of the factors reported in the current study should be considered in the design of public health interventions aimed to reduce adolescent cigarette smoking.

ACKNOWLEDGMENTS

The GYTS is a collaborative project of the World Health Organisation (WHO), the Centers for Disease Control and Prevention (CDC), United States and participating countries. Analyses of GYTS data are not necessarily endorsed by the WHO/CDC/participating countries. We are thankful to the study participants and research assistants. We also thank Jagadish Mahanta, Silvano Gallus and Andrew Roddam for reviewing the manuscripts.

This paper is a revised version of a paper published in the BMC International Health and Human Rights (Siziya S, Muula AS, Rudatsikira E. Correlates of current cigarette smoking among school-going adolescents in Punjab, India: results from the Global Youth Tobacco Survey 2003. BMC Int Health Hum Rights 2008;8:1) and the authors have obtained the permission from BMC International Health and Human Rights to use this material.

REFERENCES

[1] Gilliland FD, Islam T, Berhane K, Gauderman WJ, McConnell R, Avol E, et al. Regular smoking and asthma incidence in adolescents. Am J Respir Crit Care Med 2006;174:1094-100.

[2] Jindal SK. Emergence of chronic obstructive pulmonary disease as an epidemic in India. Indian J Med Res 2006;12:619-23.

[3] Singh AK, Maheshwari A, Sharma N, Anand K. Lifestyle associated risk factors in adolescents. Indian J Pediatr 2006;73:901-6.

[4] The Global Youth Tobacco Survey Collaborative Group. Tobacco use among youth: a cross country comparison. Tob Control 2002;11:252-70.

[5] Sinha DN, Reddy KS, Rahman K, Warren CW, Jones NR, Asma S. Linking Global Youth Tobacco Survey (GYTS) data to the WHO framework convention on tobacco control: the case for India. Indian J Public Health 2006;50:76-89.

[6] Arora M, Reddy KS. Global Youth Tobacco Survey (GYTS)- Dehli. Indian Pediatr 2005;42:850-851.

[7] Global Tobacco Surveillance System Collaborative Group. Global Tobacco Surveillance System (GTSS): purpose, production, and potential. J Sch Health 2005;75:15-24.

[8] Jindal SK, Aggarwal AN, Gupta D, Kashyap S, Chaudhary D. Prevalence of tobacco use among school going adolescents in North Indian States. Indian J Chest Dis Allied Sci 2005;47:161-6.

[9] Ariza-Cardenal C, Nebot-Adell M. Factors associated with smoking progression among Spanish adolescents. Health Educ Res 2002;17(6):750-6.

[10] Uncu Y, Irqil E, Karadaq M. Smoking predictors among primary school students in Turkey. ScientificWorldJournal 2006;6:1667-73.

[11] Hublet A, De Bacquer D, Valimaa R, Godeau E, Schmid H, Rahav G, Maes L. Smoking trends among adolescents from 1990 to 2002 in ten European countries and Canada. BMC Public Health 2006;6:280.

[12] McKee SA, Nhean S, Hinson RE, Mase E. Smoking for weight control: effect of priming for body image in females restrained eaters. Addict Behav 2006;31:2319-23.

[13] Warren CW, Riley L, Asma S, Eriksen MP, Green L, Blanton C, et al. Tobacco use by youth: a surveillance report from the Global Youth Tobacco Survey project. Bull World Health Organ 2000;78:868-70.

[14] Centers for Disease Control and Prevention: GYTS Dataset Helpfile. CDC, Atlanta, Georgia, undated document.

[15] Menezes AM, Goncalves H, Anselmi L, Hallal PC, Araujo CL. Smoking in early adolescence: evidence from the 1993 Pelotas (Brazil) Birth Cohort Study. J Adolesc Health 2006;39:669-77.

[16] Global Youth Tobacco Survey Collaborating Group. Differences in worldwide tobacco use by gender: findings from the Global Youth Tobacco Survey. J Sch Health 2003;73:207-15.

[17] Siziya S, Rudatsikira E, Muula AS. Cigarettes smoking among school-going adolescents in Kafue, Zambia. Malawi Med J 2007;19:75-8.

[18] Mohan S, Sankara-Sarma P, Thankappan KR. Access to pocket money and low educational performance predict tobacco use among adolescent boys in Kerala, India. Prev Med 2005;41:685-92.
[19] Croghan IT, Bronars C, Patten CA, Schroeder DR, Nirelli LM, Thomas JL, et al. Is smoking related to body image satisfaction, stress, and self-esteem in young adults? Am J Health Behav 2006;30:322-333.
[20] Hayashi F, Takimoto H, Yoshita K, Yoshiike N. Perceived body size and desire for thinness of young Japanese women: a population- based study. Br J Nutr 2006;96:1154-62.
[21] Takimoto H, Yoshiike N, Kaneda F, Yoshita K. Thinness among young Japanese women. Am J Public Health 2004;94:1592-5.
[22] Carroll SL, Lee RE, Kaur H, Harries KJ, Strother ML, Huang TT. Smoking, weight loss intention and obesity-promoting behaviors in college students. J Am Coll Nutr 2006;25:348-53.
[23] van Berg P, Neumark-Sztainer D, Hannan PJ, Haines J. Is dieting advice from magazines helpful or harmful? Five-year associations with weight control behaviors and psychological outcomes in adolescents. Pediatrics 2007;119:e30-37.
[24] Bentley ME, Cornelli AL, Piwoz E, Moses A, Nkhoma J, Tohill BC, et al. Perceptions of the role of maternal nutrition in HIV-positive breast feeding women in Malawi. J Nutr 2005;135:945-9.
[25] Brook JS, Pahl K, Ning Y. Peer and parental influences on longitudinal trajectories of smoking among African-Americans and Puerto Ricans. Nicotine Tob Res 2006;8:639-51.
[26] Kalesan B, Stine J, Alberg AJ. The joint influence of parental modeling and positive parental concern on cigarette smoking in middle and high school students. J Sch Health 2006;76:402-7.
[27] de Vries H, Candel M, Engels R, Mercken L. Challenges to the peer influencer paradigm: results from 12–13 year olds from six European countries from the European Smoking Prevention Framework Approach. Tob Control 2006;15:83-9.
[28] Kalilani L, Atashili J. Measuring additive interaction using odds ratios. Epidemiol Perspec Innov 2006;3:5.
[29] Bergen HA, Martin G, Roeger L, Allison S. Perceived academic performance and alcohol, tobacco and marijuana use: longitudinal relationships in young community adolescents. Addict Behav 2005;30:1563-73.
[30] Thaqi A, Franke K, Merkel G, Wichmann HE, Heinrich J. Biomarkers of exposure to passive smoking of children: frequency and determinants. Indoor Air 2005;15:302-10.
[31] George L, Granath J, Cnattingius S. Self-reported nicotine exposure and plasma levels of cotinine in early and late pregnancy. Acta Obstet Gynecol Scand 2006;85:1331-7.
[32] Godtfredsen NS, Prescott E, Vestbo J, Osler M. Smoking reduction and biomarkers in two longitudinal studies. Addiction 2006;101:1516-22.

[33] Oruc EE, Kocyi-Kaymankcioglu B, Yilmaz-Demircan F, Gurbuz Y, Kalaca S, Kuckguzel SG, et al. An high performance liquid chromatographic method for the quantification of cotinine in the urine of pre-school children. Pharmazie 2006;61:823-7.
[34] Brener ND, Colins JL, Kann L, Warren CW, Williams BT. Reliability of the Youth Risk Behavior Survey Questionnaire. Am J Epidemiol 1995;141:575-80.

In: Smoking and Adolescence ISBN: 978-1-63484-311-9
Editors: M. L. Mazabam, S. Siziya et al. © 2016 Nova Science Publishers, Inc.

Chapter 17

CIGARETTE SMOKING AMONG ADOLESCENTS IN THAILAND

Emmanuel Rudatsikira*[1], *MD, MPH, DrPH,
Adamson S Muula*[2,*], *MBBS, MPH, PhD,
Seter Siziya*[3], *BA, Ed, MSc, PhD,
and Ronald H Mataya*[4], *MD

[1]Departments of Biostatistics and Epidemiology and Global Health, Loma Linda University, School of Public Health, Loma Linda, California, USA
[2]Department of Community Health, University of Malawi, College of Medicine, Blantyre, Malawi
[3]Department of Community Medicine, University of Zambia, School of Medicine, Lusaka, Zambia
[4]Department of Global Health, School of Public Health, Loma Linda University, California, USA

Many studies examining the social correlates of tobacco use among adolescents fail to recognise theories of health behaviour and health promotion in their analysis. Using the Socio-Ecological Model (SEM) we assessed the demographic and social factors associated with current

* Correspondence: Professor Adamson S Muula, 2Department of Community Medicine and Public Health, College of Medicine, University of Malawi, Blantyre, Malawi. E-mail: amuula@medcol.mw.

cigarette smoking among adolescents in Thailand. A secondary analysis of cross-sectional data from the Thai Global Youth Tobacco Survey (Thai GYTS) 2005 was analysed to obtain prevalence of selected attributes and assess factors associated with current cigarette smoking. Current cigarette smoking was defined as having smoked a cigarette, even a single puff, in the last 30 days. Logistic regression was conducted to estimate the level of association between the explanatory variables and current smoking. Of the 18,368 respondents, 22.0% males and 5.2% females reported being current smokers ($p < 0.001$). In multivariate logistic regression analysis, current smoking was negatively associated with the perception that smoking is harmful to health (OR = 0.47; 95% CI [0.33, 0.66]) and positively associated with male gender (OR = 3.46; 95% CI [2.72, 4.86]) and having smoking parents (OR = 1.62; 95% CI [1.25, 2.11]) and friends (OR = 5.07; 95% CI [3.54, 7.25]) for some friends smokers and OR = 26.71; 95% CI [18.26, 39.06] for most or all friends smokers. Compared to subjects 11 = 12 year olds, those who were older were less likely to report smoking (OR = 0.49; 95% CI [0.36, 0.66] for 13 years olds, OR = 0.56; 95% CI [0.40, 0.79] for 14 years olds, OR = 0.59; 95% CI [0.41, 0.86] for 15 years olds). Current cigarette smoking was associated with male gender, smoking parents or closest peers. Perception that smoking was harmful to health was associated with less likelihood of being a current smoker.

INTRODUCTION

Tobacco is the leading cause of morbidity and mortality globally (1-3). In Thailand current adult daily and occasional tobacco smoking prevalence was reported at 37.2% for males, 2.1% for females and19.5% overall (4). Tobacco farming is an important economic activity in the country. In 1995, 0.21% of Thailand's land was used for tobacco farming (5). In 1998, 0.181 billion cigarette sticks were exported while 1.7 billion sticks were imported by the country (5). The Thai tobacco industry is largely dominated by the state-owned Thai Tobacco Monopoly (TTM). The tobacco industry contributed 3.5%-4.5% of the total government revenue in the country between 2000 and 2005 (6).

Although the country derives significant financial resources from tobacco, it has two specific laws regarding tobacco use control since 1992 i.e., the Tobacco Products Control Act of 1992 and Non-smokers' Health Protection Act of 1992; the Tobacco Products Control Act of 1992 includes total advertising ban (7, 8).

Tobacco use is an important public health concern. Previous research has linked substance use, such as tobacco use, to other health-related risky behaviours, mental health problems, suicide, motor vehicle accidents, violent crime, dental problems and other major health problems, including cancer and heart disease (9-13). Research on the sequence of drug use suggests that cigarettes and alcohol may serve as "gateway" drugs to illicit drugs (10). As the adolescent and young adult years represent a critical period for the initiation of substance use this period also avails itself as critical in the institution of interventions to prevent substance use. Such public health interventions should, as far as is practicable, be based on an understanding of the many factors that shape use during the adolescent and young adult years.

Attempts to understand adolescent health behaviours have not always been linked to theories of health behaviours. We hypothesized that adolescents' cigarette use may be explainable through the Social ecological model (SEM) of health behaviour (14-17). The SEM has been applied to a broad range of health behaviours and among different subject populations. The model suggests that various factors including individual-level factors and the socio-cultural environment that an individual is exposed to contribute or interact to produce specific behaviors such as cigarette smoking. With regard to adolescent smoking, we hypothesized that adolescents who perceived that smoking was harmful to their health would be less likely to be current smokers. Belief that smoking is harmful, which may be influenced by education or thorough observation within one's society, as well as an individual's age. One's sex (which may influence gender) and smoking among peers and parents may also be perceived as operating within the SEM. If society is more permissive toward smoking by one gender, such gender may be more likely to smoke. Furthermore, adolescents who have their peers or parents who also smoke may be living in environments that are more tolerant towards smoking. We also aimed to assess other socio-demographic characteristics that could be associated with being a current cigarette smoker.

OUR STUDY

The current study was based on secondary analysis of data from the 2005 Thai Global Youth Tobacco Survey. Comprehensive descriptions of the Global Youth Tobacco Survey (GYTS) purpose and methodology have been described in the literature elsewhere (18-20). In brief, the GYTS uses a standard survey questionnaire with core questions and country-specific questions. The core questions are the same in all the countries where the survey is administered. The survey recruits in-school adolescents in classes with the majority of its students are between 13–15 years. A two-stage clustered sampling survey approach is used in which the primary sampling units are schools with students in the eligible age group (13 to 15 years). At the second stage of sampling, eligible classes (classes with the majority of students 13 to 15 years) within the selected schools are randomly selected. All students within the selected classes are eligible to participate in the study, regardless of their actual ages. However, students are free not to participate when identified as eligible for participation.

The GYTS data in this report include surveys completed in the following 5 regions in Thailand: Bangkok; Central-Western; North Eastern; Northern, and Southern. The school response rate was 100% while the student response rate was 99%.

Study participants self-complete questionnaires which had standard "core questions" and a few other country-specific questions (18-20). Questionnaires which were administered and anonymously self-completed within class time. Time taken to complete questionnaire was estimated at about 40 minutes. Some of the questions asked aimed to collect information on the following variables: age, history of having ever smoked, current smoking status, parental smoking, having friends who smoked, perception that smoking is harmful to health, exposure to tobacco advertisements and approval of smoking among boys and girls. These explanatory variables have been previously reported as being associated with smoking among adolescents in other settings (21-25).

Completed questionnaires were scanned by computer and data file generated in Access. Data were analyzed by SUDAAN software 9.0 (Research Triangle Institute, Research Triangle Park, North Carolina, United States). We generated frequencies and 95% confidence intervals of relevant variables such as demographics, approval of smoking among boys and girls and exposure to tobacco advertisements. To assess the associations between a selected list of variables identified from the literature as possibly associated with current cigarette smoking, logistic regression analysis was conducted both at bivariate and multivariate level. These explanatory variables were: gender; age; peer smoking; and parental smoking. Based on the SEM, we hypothesised that adolescents who believe that smoking was harmful to one's health, age, gender, peer and parental smoking would be associated with being a current cigarette smoker. Current smoking was defined as having ever smoked, even a single puff in the past 30 days preceding the survey.

The bivariate logistic regression analysis was conducted to obtained unadjusted odds ratios with current smoking status (Yes or Not) as the outcome of interest and each of the following variables as explanatory or predictor variables (age, gender, peer smoking, parental smoking, perception that smoking is harmful). Separate multivariable models were also conducted with the same outcome variable but each of the explanatory variables as the main exposure of interest with the rest of the variables being controlled for.

FINDINGS

A total of 18,368 students participated in the study of whom 9,851 (51.4%) were males and 9,312 (48.6%) were females. The median age was 14 years. Prevalence of current and ever cigarette smoking Of the 18,368 participants, 22.0%; 95% CI [19.8, 24.4] males and 5.2%; 95% CI [4.3, 6.2] females reported being current smokers ($p < 0.001$). An estimated 42.9%; 95% CI [40.7, 45.3] males and 18.4%; 95% CI [15.9, 21.1] females had ever smoked a cigarette ($p < 0.001$).

Prevalence to cigarette advertisements and attitudes towards smoking

Tables 1 and 2 show the prevalence of various exposures to pro-tobacco advertisements and perceptions towards smoking among the study sample. More than a third of the sample had seen tobacco advertisements on television in past 30 days, had an item with tobacco brand logo and had seen tobacco advertisements on the internet. Furthermore smokers were perceived favourably (see Table 1).

Factors associated with current cigarette smoking

Table 3 reports the results of both bivariate and multivariable logistic regression analysis. In bivariate analysis, the Table indicates that older students were less likely to report current smoking than those who were 11–12 years old (OR = 0.42; 95% CI [0.32, 0.56] for 13 years, OR = 0.63; 95% CI [0.44, 0.90] for 14 years olds, and OR = 0.54; 95% CI [0.38, 0.77] for 15 year-olds).

Table 1. Exposure to tobacco advertisement among adolescents in Thailand

Characteristic	Number of participants	% of total (95% CI)
Seen cigarette brand name on TV in past 30 days	13,037	33.8 (30.9, 36.4)
Males	6,899	39.3 (36.9, 41.6)
Females	6,138	27.3 (24.0, 30.8)
Has item with cigarette brand logo	18,428	40.8 (37.5, 45.2)
Males	9,440	43.7 (41.8, 45.7)
Females	8,988	37.7 (35.9, 40.2)
Seen tobacco adverts on the internet in past 30 days	18,588	45.5 (41.9, 48.8)
Males	9,536	48.4 (45.4, 51.4)
Females	9,049	41.2 (38.6, 44.7)

Table 2. Attitudes towards tobacco smoking distributed by gender in Thailand

Characteristic	Number of participants/ Total for category	% of total and 95% CI
Felt that boys who smoke have more friends	12,408	58.3 (55.8, 60.8)
Males	6,510	60.7 (58.2, 63.2)
Females	5,898	56.2 (52.2, 60.2)
Felt like girls who smoke had more friends	14,031	20.0 (19.4, 22.8)
Males	7,336	22.5 (20.9, 24.2)
Females	6,695	19.7 (17.1, 22.7)
Felt that boys who smoke are more attractive	14,720	16.5 (15.3, 17.8)
Males	7,310	21.4 (19.3, 23.7)
Females	7,410	12.5 (11.4, 13.7)
Felt that girls who smoke are more attractive	15,411	7.8 (6.7, 8.9)
Males	7,710	10.7 (9.6, 12.0)
Females	7,701	5.3 (3.8, 7.3)
Felt that smoking is harmful to health	18,871	86.7 (85.6, 88.1)
Males	9,695	82.3 (80.2, 84.2)
Females	9,176	90.8 (89.1, 92.3)

Males were more than five times likely to report smoking than females (OR = 5.17; 95% CI [4.08, 6.54]). Study participants with one or both parents smokers were 1.98 times likely to report smoking compared to those whose parents were non-smokers (OR = 1.98; 95% CI [1.56, 2.53]). Adolescents with most or all friends who smoked were more than twenty times likely to report smoking compared to those who had non-smoking friends (OR = 27.45; 95% CI [18.40, 40.96]). Participants who perceived that smoking was harmful were less likely to report smoking (OR = 0.34; 0.25, 0.47]).

Table 3. Factors associated with current smoking in Thailand in bivariate and multivariate logistic regression analysis

Characteristic	Current smoking (%, n)	Unadjusted Odds ratio (95% CI[1])	Adjusted OR (95% CI)
Age (years)			
11–12	20.0 (2144)	1	1
13	9.6 (4154)	0.42 (0.32, 0.56)	0.49 (0.36, 0.66)
14	13.6 (5226)	0.63 (0.44, 0.90)	0.56 (0.40, 0.79)
15	12.0 (3806)	0.54 (0.38, 0.77)	0.59 (0.41, 0.86)
16–17	15.8 (1214)	0.75 (0.50, 1.13)	0.75 (0.47, 1.20)
Gender			
Female	5.2 (9089)	1.00	1
Male	22.0 (9279)	5.17 [4.08, 6.54]	3.64 (2.72, 4.86)
Parental smoking status			
None	9.6 (9648)	1.00	1
One or both parents Smokers	17.3 (8805)	1.98 [1.56, 2.53]	1.62 (1.25, 2.11)
Best friends smokers			
None	4.0 (9445)	1.00	1
Some	15.7 (7664)	4.44 [3.12, 6.32]	5.07 (3.54, 7.25)
Most or all	53.5 (1627)	27.45 [18.40, 40.96]	26.71 (18.26, 39.06)
Perception that smoking is harmful			
No	27.7 (2362)	1.00	1
Yes	11.5 (16309)	0.34 [0.25, 0.47]	0.47 (0.33, 0.66)

CI[1] Confidence Interval.

In the multivariate analysis, the findings were not different from the bivariate analysis. Current smoking was negatively associated with increasing age and positively associated with male gender, and having friends and/or parents who smoked. The perception that smoking is harmful was negatively associated with smoking in multivariate analysis.

Table 2 indicates that participants were exposed to tobacco adverts through television (35.1%) and internet (45.5%). Four in ten respondents

(40.8%) reported having an item with cigarette brand on it. Compared to females, males had higher rates of those who reported having an item with cigarettes logo ($p < 0.001$) and those who were exposed to adverts on the internet and television ($p < 0.001$).

Table 3 indicates that most respondents (86.7%) felt that smoking is harmful. 58.3% thought that male smokers had more friends while 20.0% thought so for females. There were twice as many respondents who thought that male smokers were attractive compared to those who thought so for females (16.5% and 7.8%).

DISCUSSION

The current study reports results from a secondary analysis of the Global Youth Tobacco Survey-2005 for Thailand. Among the studied sample, 22% of males and 5.2% females reported being current cigarette smokers. Many adolescents had been exposed to tobacco advertisements and many perceived smokers favourably.

Males were at least five times more likely to be current smokers compared to females. This finding is similar to what Rudatsikira et al. (26) reported for the Mongolia GYTS. In that study, current cigarette smoking was 5.4 percent among males versus 4.4 percent among females. In logistic regression analysis the following results were obtained: older adolescents were less likely to be current smokers when compared to 11 to 12 year olds; having one or both parents being smokers or having friends who were smokers was associated with being a smoker in the study participants; and adolescents who believed that smoking was harmful to one's health were less likely to be smokers.

It is of interest that younger adolescents reported being current smokers compared to their older colleagues. However the significance of such finding deserves further study. One explanation is that younger adolescents are more likely to experiment and as the adolescent grows older, he or she is less likely to smoke. An alternative explanation is that older adolescents may be smoking equally or more than younger adolescents, but they are less likely to report. This could be solved by collecting biomarkers in future GYTS rounds in order to validate these self-reports on smoking.

Our findings also showed that males were more than 5 times likely to be smokers than females. This is an almost constant finding in GYTS reports and other studies where males are in general, more likely to report being smokers than females (27-30). In many studies that have reported harmful health behaviours such alcohol misuse, illicit drug use, truancy and violence, males far outnumber females. In case of substance use males report greater use than females for just about every measure (27, 28). There are some exceptions though where the gender disparity does not exist. Ng et al. (31), reported that smoking was perceived as evidence of masculinity among Indonesians. Based on the social ecological model we had hypothesized that age, normative beliefs about smoking, sex, parental and peer smoking would be associated with smoking. In both bivariate and multivariable analysis, adolescents who perceived that smoking was harmful to health were in fact less likely to be smokers. This probably suggests that adolescent education on the dangers of smoking may result in prevent them from taking up smoking. Of course, a much less likely reason for the finding would be that current smokers were more likely to downplay the hazards of smoking.

Having friends who are smokers was associated with being a current smoker among the study participants. Due to the cross sectional nature of the data collection in the GYTS, it is not possible to ascribe causation or the sequence of events in an adolescents' smoking trajectory. It is plausible to consider that adolescents who befriend smokers are more likely to be influenced into smoking. It is equally plausible that smoking adolescents are more likely to choose other smokers as their friends (32, 33).

Exposure to pro-tobacco advertisements has been reported to be associated with smoking among adolescents in diverse settings. As shown in Table 2, about a quarter of both males and females reported having seen a tobacco brand name on television in the past 30 days, and nearly 50% reported having seen tobacco advertisements on the internet. About 40% reported owning an item with a cigarette brand logo.

Over half of the study participants felt that boys who smoke had more friends than non-smokers while just about one-fifth thought that female smokers had more friends. Similarly, a higher proportion of the study participants reported that boys who smoke were more attractive (16.5%) while a smaller proportion (7.8%) felt that girls who smoke are more attractive. The majority of the study participants felt that smoking was harmful to one's health.

Thailand ratified the WHO Framework Convention on Tobacco Control (WHO FCTC) on November 8, 2004. Thailand has implemented tobacco price-based measures to control tobacco use. The retail price of domestic cigarette brands includes excise and value-added taxes and an additional import tariff is imposed on imported cigarette brands (6). In 1994, the country increased the level of excise tax (6) and in the subsequent decade this tax policy is credited to have resulted in raising US$1 billion as well as helping to reduce the cigarette smoking prevalence in virtually all age groups.

The Tobacco Products Control Law also prohibited tobacco companies from advertising through sponsorship of events (5). However, as can be seen in Table 2, about a third of the study participants had seen a tobacco advertisement on TV and about 40% own an item with a tobacco brand logo. This observation may imply that enforcement of the law regarding tobacco control is less than being fully effective.

The limitations of the Global Youth Tobacco Survey methodology have been described elsewhere (21, 29, 30, 34). In brief however, the following are known major limitations. Firstly data are only collected from school-going adolescents. To the extent that a significant proportion of the adolescent population is not in school, the estimates obtained from using these data may be biased. Also, data are only collected from the eligible students that are present in school on the day that the survey is administered in a particular school. No follow-up is made in respect of students who may be absent. However, in a majority of cases, the number of absent, but eligible students is minimal. However as some of the absent students may in fact be truant, and truant students may have different smoking practices than their non-truant peers, the estimates obtained from the GYTS may be slightly be biased. Furthermore, data are collected through self-reporting by the study participants.

There may be intentional as well as unintentional misreporting on any of the questions. However this is minimized by the fact that the survey is self-administered (as compared to interviewer administered) and study participants complete the surveys anonymously. The GYTS does not verify current cigarette smoking status through collection of biological specimens and assessing tobacco by-products such as cotinine and exhaled carbon monoxide (35-38). However, the fact that the GYTS uses a standard methodology of data collection makes comparisons in prevalence and other estimates among different settings possible.

We can also not claim to have controlled for all important confounders or described all important determinants. A recent study by Primack (39) has shown that exposure to films and music are associated with smoking, but only the relationship between music exposure and smoking persisted after rigorous covariate control. Exposure to books was however associated with lower odds of smoking.

In conclusion, we have estimated the prevalence of current cigarette smoking among in-school adolescents in Thailand based on data from the Thai

Global Youth Tobacco Survey 2005. Being male, having smoking friends or parents and perception that smoking is harmful to one's health was associated with being a current cigarette smoker.

Acknowledgments

The GYTS is a collaborative project of WHO/CDC/participating countries. Analyses of GYTS data are not necessarily endorsed by WHO/CDC/ participating countries.

This paper is a revised version of and earlier publication in the International Archives of Medicine (Rudatsikira E, Muula AS, Siziya S, Mataya RH. Correlates of cigarette smoking among school-going adolescents in Thailand: findings from the Thai global youth tobacco survey 2005. Int Arch Med 2008;1:8) and the authors have obtained the permission from International Archives of Medicine to use this material.

References

[1] Lopez AD, Mathers CD, Ezzati M, Jamison DT, Murray CJL. Global and regional burden of disease and risk factors, 2001: Systematic analysis of population health data. Lancet 2006;367:1747-57.

[2] Ezzati M, Lopez AD. Smoking and oral tobacco use. In: Ezzati M, Lopez AD, Rodgers A, Murray CJL, eds. Comparative quantification of health risks: Global and regional burden of disease attributable to selected major risk factors. Geneva: WHO, 2004:959-1108.

[3] Mathers D, Loncar D. Projections of global mortality and burden of disease from 2002 to 2030. Plos Med 2006;3:e442.

[4] National Statistical Office. The cigarette smoking and alcoholic drinking behavior survey. Bangkok: Thai Ministry of Information and Communication Technology, 2004.

[5] Shafey O, Dolwick S, Guindon GE, eds. Tobacco control country profiles. Atlanta, GA: American Cancer Society, 2003.

[6] [6]Sarntisart I. An economic analysis of tobacco control in Thailand. In Paper prepared for the World Health Organization Regional Office for South-East Asia. Presented at a meeting on the Economics of Tobacco Control in the South-East Asia Region, in Jakarta, Indonesia Washington, DC: World Bank, 2003.

[7] MacKenzie R, Collin J, Sriwongcharoen K, Muggli ME. If we can just 'stall' new unfriendly legislations, the scoreboard is already in our favour": transnational tobacco companies and ingredients disclosure in Thailand. Tob Control 2004;13(Suppl 2):ii79-87.

[8] Chantornvong S, McCargo D. Political economy of tobacco control in Thailand. Tob Control 2001;10:48-54.

[9] Tullis LM, Dupont R, Frost-Pineda K, Gold MS. Marijuana and tobacco: a major connection. J Addict Dis 2003;22:51-62.

[10] Hornik R. Alcohol, tobacco, and marijuana use among youth. Same-time and lagged and simultaneous change associations in a nationally representative sample of 9- to 18-year-olds. In: Romer D, ed. Reducing adolescent risk: Toward an integrated approach. Thousand Oaks, CA: Sage, 2003:335-343.

[11] US Department of Health and Human Services. Preventing tobacco use among young people: A report of the Surgeon General. Rockville, MD: DHHS, 1994.

[12] US Department of Health and Human Services. Centers for Disease Control and Prevention, National Center for Chronic Disease Prevention and Health Promotion, Office on Smoking and Health: Reducing tobacco use: A report of the Surgeon General. Atlanta, GA: DHHS, 2000.

[13] US Department of Health and Human Services. A comprehensive plan for preventing and reducing underage drinking, 2006. URL: http:// www.stopalcoholabuse.gov/media/underagedrinking/pdf.

[14] Fisher EB. The importance of context in understanding behavior and promoting health. Ann Behav Med 2008;35:3-18.

[15] Glanz K, Rimer BK, Lewis FM. Health behavior and health education: Theory, research and practice. San Francisco, CA: Wiley, 2002.

[16] Laver SM, Borne B van der, Kok G. Using theory to design an intervention for HIV/AIDS prevention in farm workers in rural Zimbabwe. Int Q Community Health Educ 2006;25(1-2):135-48.

[17] Adams MA, Hovell MF, Irvin V, Sallis JF, Coleman KJ, Liles S. Promoting stair use by modeling: an experimental application of the Behavioral Ecological Model. Am J Health Promot 2006;21:101-9.

[18] Warren CW, Riley L, Asma S, Eriksen MP, Green L, Blanton C, et al. Tobacco use by youth: a surveillance report from the Global Youth Tobacco Survey project. Bull World Health Organ 2000;78:868-76.

[19] Global Tobacco Surveillance System Collaborating Group. Global Tobacco Surveillance System (GTSS): purpose, production, and potential. J Sch Health 2005;75:15-24.

[20] Global Youth Tobacco Survey Collaborative Group. Tobacco use among youth: a cross country comparison. Tob Control 2002;11:252-70.

[21] Siziya S, Muula AS, Rudatsikira E. Correlates of current cigarette smoking among in-school adolescents in the Kurdistan region of Iraq. Confl Health 2007;1:13.

[22] Pinto Dda S, Ribeiro SA. Variables related to smoking initiation among students in public and private high schools in the city of Belem, Brazil. J Bras Pneumol 2007;33:558-64.

[23] Siziya S, Rudatsikira E, Muula AS, Ntata PR. Predictors of cigarette smoking among adolescents in rural Zambia: results from a cross sectional study from Chongwe district. Rural Remote Health 2007;7:728.

[24] Sen U, Basu A. Factors influencing smoking behavior among adolescents. Asian Pac J Cancer 2000;1:305-309.

[25] Babu DS, Chuttani CS, Murty NS Some epidemiological factors related to smoking among secondary school children of Delhi urban area. Int J Epidemiol 1978;7:183-4.

[26] Rudatsikira E, Dondog J, Siziya S, Muula AS. Prevalence and determinants of adolescent cigarette smoking in Mongolia. Singapore Med J 2008;49:57-62.

[27] Ruangkanchanasetr S, Plitponkarnpim A, Hetrakul P, Kongsakon R. Youth risk behavior survey: Bangkok, Thailand. J Adolesc Health 2005;36:227-35.

[28] Department of Health and Human Services. Results from the 2005 National Survey on Drug Use and Health: National findings, 2006. URL: http://www.drugabusestatistics.samhsa.gov/nsduh.htm

[29] Kyrlesi A, Soteriades ES, Warren CW, Kremastinou J, Papastergiou P, Jones NR, et al. Tobacco use among students aged 13–15 years in Greece: the GYTS project. BMC Public Health 2007;7:3.

[30] Rudatsikira E, Abdo A, Muula AS. Prevalence and determinants of adolescent tobacco smoking in Addis Ababa, Ethiopia. BMC Public Health 2007;7:176.

[31] Ng N, Weinehall L, Ohman A. 'If I don't smoke, I'm not a real man' Indonesian teenage boys' views about smoking. Health Educ Res 2007;22:794-804.

[32] Chassin L, Presson CC, Sherman SJ. Cognitive and social influence factors in adolescent smoking cessation. Addict Behav 1984;9:383-90.

[33] Wang MQ, Eddy JM, Fitzhugh EC. Smoking acquisition: peer influence and self-election. Psychol Rep 2000;86:1241-6.

[34] Centers for Disease Control and Prevention. Use of cigarettes and other tobacco products among students aged 13–15 years worldwide, 1999–2005. MMWR 2006;55:553-6.

[35] Anuntaseree W, Mo-Suwan L, Ovatlarnporn C, Tantana C, Ma-A-Lee A. Exposure to environmental tobacco smoke among infants in Southern Thailand: A study of urinary cotinine. Bull Environ Contam Toxicol 2008;80:34-7.

[36] Hung J, Lin CH, Wang JD, Chann CC. Exhaled carbon monoxide level as an indicator of cigarette consumption in a workplace cessation program in Taiwan. J Formos Med Assoc 2006;105:210-3.

[37] Jenkins RA, Counts RW. Personal exposure to environmental tobacco smoke: salivary cotinine, airborne nicotine, and non-smoker misclassification. J Expo Anal Environ Epidemiol 1999;9:352-63.

[38] Low EC, Ong MC, Tan M. Breath carbon monoxide as an indication of smoking habit in the military setting. Singapore Med J 2004;45:578-82.

[39] Primack BA, Dalton MA, Carroll MV, Agarwal AA, Fine MJ. Content analysis of tobacco, alcohol, and other drugs in popular music. Arch Pediatr Adolesc Med 2008;162:169-75.

In: Smoking and Adolescence ISBN: 978-1-63484-311-9
Editors: M. L. Mazabam, S. Siziya et al. © 2016 Nova Science Publishers, Inc.

Chapter 18

ADOLESCENT CIGARETTE SMOKING IN MONGOLIA

Emmanuel Rudatsikira*[1], *MD, MPH, DrPH,
Jargalsaikhan Dondog*[2], *MD, PhD,
Seter Siziya*[3,*], *BA(Ed), MSc, PhD,
and Adamson S Muula*[4,5], *MBBS, MPH, PhD

[1]Departments of Global Health, Epidemiology and Biostatistics, School of Public Health, Loma Linda University, Loma Linda, California, USA
[2]Health Promotion Department, Directorate of Medical Services, Mongolia and Department of General Practice, Medical University of Mongolia, Mongolia
[3]Department of Community Medicine, University of Zambia School of Medicine, Ndola, Zambia
[4]Department of Community Health, University of Malawi, College of Medicine, Blantyre, Malawi
[5]Department of Epidemiology, School of Public Health, University of North Carolina at Chapel Hill, North Carolina, USA

[*] Correspondence: Professor Seter Siziya, Clinical Sciences Department, School of Medicine, Copperbelt University, Ndola Central Hospital, 6th Floor, POBox 71191, Ndola, Zambia. E-mail: ssiziya@gmail.com.

Cigarette smoking is the single most important risk factor for non-communicable chronic medical conditions. Estimating the prevalence of cigarette smoking and its determinants will aid in the design, implementation and evaluation of public health interventions. In this chapter we estimate the prevalence and determinants of smoking among school-going adolescents in Mongolia. A cross-sectional study using standardised methodology was conducted among school-going adolescents in 2003 in Mongolia. Altogether 4,105 adolescents (mean age 14.1 years, standard deviation 0.8 year) participated in the study. Approximately 55% were females, 30.4% of the study population was 15 years old, 63.5% had never smoked and 93.2% perceived tobacco as 52% had friends, who were smokers. The prevalence of current cigarette smoking was 9.2%; 15.4% among males versus 4.4% among females. Cigarette smoking was associated with the male gender, parental and peer influence and having spending power. The perception that smoking was harmful to health was associated with lower odds of smoking. Cigarette smoking is prevalent among school-going adolescents in Mongolia. There is a need to implement public health interventions, with special attention to the determinants of smoking in this age group.

INTRODUCTION

Cigarette smoking is the major single known cause of non-communicable diseases, such as cancer and cardiovascular diseases (1-4). It is recognised that as the life expectancy of societies improve, the prominence of non-communicable chronic diseases, many of which are associated with cigarette smoking, will gain greater prominence (5-7). About 25% of all adolescents who experiment with cigarette smoking become regular smokers, and among the smokers, about one-third will die from a smoking-related health disease (8). Baigalmaa et al. (9) reported that Mongolia is among the top ten countries with the highest overall adult smoking prevalence. Reliable data on the prevalence and determinants of cigarette smoking among adolescents in the country are lacking. Globally, however, there has been growing interest in the prevalence of adolescent cigarette smoking. Tobacco firms preferentially target young people in their marketing efforts (10, 11). Public health interventions that aim to prevent and/or control tobacco use among adolescents are generally lacking in many countries, where adolescent tobacco use is of public health concern (12). We report on a study conducted in 2003 aimed to assess the prevalence and determinants of cigarette smoking among school-going adolescents in Mongolia.

OUR STUDY

A cross-sectional study utilising a multi-stage sample design was conducted in 2003. In the first stage, schools were selected from a list of schools in the country. The probability of a school being selected was proportional to enrollment size. The second stage involved randomly selecting classes in the eligible schools. In this phase, only classes within a selected school which had the majority of students within the 13–15 years age range, were eligible to be randomly chosen. All the students within the selected classes were eligible for participation, regardless of their actual ages. Altogether, 4,517 students were eligible to participate. However, only 4,183 (92.6%) eventually participated.

A modified Global Youth Tobacco Survey (GYTS) questionnaire was self-completed anonymously by the students. Students usually take between 30 and 45 minutes to complete the questionnaire (13-15). All questions were presented as multiple choice options and were completed at a single sitting. The GYTS core questionnaire aimed to collect the following information: experience of cigarette smoking; knowledge and attitudes of young people towards cigarette smoking; gender; age at initiation of smoking; amount of pocket money received each day and amount of money spent on cigarettes; and parental smoking and having friends who were smokers. For the purpose of this study, however, only data related to estimation of the prevalence of smoking, associated factors and amount of pocket money received per day are reported.

Data were analysed using SUDAAN version 9.0 (Research Triangle Institute, Research Triangle Park, Durham, NC, USA). A weighting factor was used to account for non-response and probability of being selected into the study. Proportions and 95% confidence intervals were obtained as estimates of prevalence. Bivariate logistic regression analysis was done to determine associations between current smoking status and other relevant variables according to the literature. Multivariable logistic regression analysis was also done to assess the association of each of the individual variables while adjusting for the other variables.

Permission to conduct the study was obtained from the Ministry of Education. All eligible students were also informed that participation was voluntary. Data collection was facilitated in schools by trained assistants without the presence of a teacher. In order to estimate how much disposable cash a study participant had, there was a question on how much pocket money a study participant received each day.

Table 1. Selected variables on smoking and demographics

Variables	Total % (95% CI[1])	Males % (95% CI)	Females % (95% CI)
No. of participants	4105	1850	2255
Age (years)			
All	100.0	45.1 (43.6, 46.6)	54.9 (53.4, 56.5)
11-12	6.1 (5.5, 6.9)	6.7 (5.6, 7.9)	5.7 (4.8, 6.7)
13	25.1 (23.8, 26.4)	23.8 (22.0, 25.8)	26.1 (24.3, 27.9)
14	29.3 (27.9, 30.7)	28.4 (26.4, 30.5)	30.0 (28.1, 31.9)
15	30.4 (29.1, 31.9)	31.9 (29.8, 34.0)	29.3 (27.4, 31.1)
16-17	9.1 (8.3, 10.0)	9.2 (8.0, 10.6)	9.0 (7.9, 10.3)
Smoker (current or previous)			
Yes	59.9 (58.3, 61.3)	45.4 (43.1, 47.7)	71.6 (69.7, 73.5)
Age started smoking (years)			
Never smoked	63.5 (62.0, 65.0)	49.4 (47.1, 51.8)	74.9 (73.1, 76.9)
11	7.2 (6.4, 8.0)	11.4 (10.0, 12.9)	3.6 (2.9, 4.4)
12-13	5.6 (4.8, 6.2)	8.9 (7.6, 10.3)	2.7 (2.1, 3.5)
14+	23.9 (22.7, 25.3)	30.4 (28.8, 32.6)	18.8 (17.3, 20.5)
Current smoking	9.2 (8.4, 10.2)	15.2 (13.6, 16.9)	4.4 (3.6, 5.4)
Parental smoking			
None	41.8 (40.3, 43.3)	42.4 (40.1, 44.7)	41.2 (39.2, 43.3)
Both parents	7.0 (6.3, 7.9)	6.8 (5.7, 8.1)	7.4 (6.4, 8.6)
Father only	47.9 (46.3, 49.4)	47.9 (45.6, 50.2)	47.9 (45.8, 50.0)
Mother only	3.3 (2.8, 3.9)	2.9 (2.3, 3.8)	3.5 (2.8, 4.3)
Friends smoking			
None	47.7 (46.2, 49.2)	37.0 (34.8, 39.2)	56.5 (54.4, 58.5)
Some	43.1 (41.6, 44.6)	50.8 (48.5, 53.1)	36.8 (34.8, 38.7)
Most	6.8 (6.1, 7.6)	8.2 (7.0, 9.6)	5.7 (4.8, 6.8)
All	2.4 (2.00, 2.9)	4.1 (3.2, 5.1)	1.1 (0.7, 1.6)
Exposed to ETS[2]	74.5 (73.2, 75.5)	76.0 (74.0, 77.9)	73.3 (71.4, 75.1)
Smoking is harmful			
Taught about dangers of smoking	54.5 (53.0, 56.1)	55.6 (53.2, 58.0)	53.6 (51.5, 55.7)
Definitely/probably not	7.5 (6.8, 8.4)	9.5 (8.2, 10.9)	5.9 (5.0, 7.0)
Probably yes	5.6 (4.9, 6.3)	6.1 (5.1, 7.3)	5.9 (5.0, 7.0)
Definitely yes	86.9 (85.8, 87.9)	84.4 (82.6, 86.0)	89.0 (87.6, 90.2)

CI[1] Confidence interval.

ETS[2] Environmental tobacco smoke.

Study participants were required to select the most appropriate option of the given reasonable ranges of money in Mongolian currency (1,200 tögrög [T] is equivalent to US$ 1). Current smoking was defined as having smoked even one puff in the past 30 days. Having ever smoked was defined as having smoked even a single puff in one's lifetime.

FINDINGS

Selected characteristics of the study population of 4,105 adolescent Mongolians (mean age 14.1 years, standard deviation [SD] 0.8 year) are presented in Table 1. Most of the sample were females (54.9%), 15 years old (30.4%), had never smoked (63.5%), had been taught about the dangers of smoking (54.5%), perceived smoking as definitely harmful (86.9%), had parents and friends who were smokers (58.2% and 52.3%, respectively), and were exposed to environmental tobacco smoke (74.5%) (see Table 1). Those who were 15 years or older had increased odds of smoking, compared to those aged 11–12 years (OR = 2.66; 95% CI [1.51, 4.68]) and even more so for those aged 16–17 years (OR = 4.03; 95% CI [2.20, 7.37]) (see Table 2).

The perception of cigarette smoking as harmful was associated with smoking among females. Those who perceived cigarette smoking as definitely not harmful or probably not harmful were six times more likely to smoke than females who perceived cigarette-smoking as definitely harmful (OR = 6.82; 95% CI [3.90, 11.92]).

There was a dose-response relationship between the amount of pocket money and smoking ($p < 0.001$). Those who had US$ 10 or more had a greater than six-time increase in the odds of smoking compared to those who had no pocket money (OR = 6.78; 95% CI [4.60, 10.01]). Further associations are presented in Table 2.

The results from multivariate analysis are presented in Table 3. The association between smoking and pocket money remained significant after adjusting for age, gender, parents' and friends' smoking status, and perception of cigarette smoking being harmful. Those who reported having less than US$ 10 had a greater than four times likelihood in the odds of smoking, compared to those who had no pocket money (OR = 4.33; 95% CI [2.73, 6.88]), while those who had US$ 5–9 had more than double the odds of smoking (OR = 2.50; 95% CI [1.66, 3.77]). Other variables associated with smoking in multivariate analysis included age, gender, friends who are smokers, and perception of cigarette smoking as harmful (see Table 3).

Table 2. Variables associated with current smoking in bivariate analyses

	Total	**Males**	**Females**
Variables	OR[1] (95% CI[2])	OR (95% CI)	OR (95% CI)
Age (years)			
11-12	1.00	1.00	1.00
13	0.87 (0.47, 1.61)	1.54 (0.67, 3.55)	0.46 (0.14, 1.52)
14	1.34 (0.75, 2.40)	2.29 (1.02, 5.15)	0.76 (0.25, 2.32)
15	2.66 (1.51, 4.68)	3.83 (1.73, 8.48)	2.23 (0.78, 6.33)
16-17	4.03 (2.20, 7.37)	6.17 (2.66, 14.30)	3.05 (1.00, 9.29)
Gender			
Females	1.00	-	-
Males	3.84 (3.01, 4.91)	-	-
Parental smoking			
None	1.00	1.00	1.00
Father only	1.15 (0.90, 1.46)	1.12 (0.84, 1.49)	1.17 (0.72, 1.90)
Mother only	1.80 (1.04, 3.09)	1.78 (0.88, 3.61)	2.62 (1.05, 6.52)
Both parents	1.81 (1.22, 2.68)	1.41 (0.84, 2.38)	3.10 (1.62, 5.92)
Friends smoking			
None	1.00	1.00	1.00
Some	6.91 (4.73, 10.09)	4.78 (3.06, 7.49)	8.12 (3.93, 16.7)
Most	38.10 (24.88, 58.34)	28.67 (16.88, 48.70)	50.7 (23.41, 109.88)
All	43.07 (25.23, 73.54)	25.07 (13.16, 47.73)	78.09 (27.37, 223.08)
Perception that smoking is harmful			
Definitely yes	1.00	1.00	1.00
Probably yes	1.80 (1.27, 2.56)	1.25 (0.82, 1.91)	2.51 (1.25, 5.04)
Definitely or probably no	2.70 (1.87, 3.90)	1.47 (0.89, 2.42)	6.82 (3.90, 11.92)
Pocket money (US$)			
0	1.00	1.00	1.00
<1	2.55 (1.77, 3.68)	2.46 (1.64, 3.69)	2.30 (1.11, 4.73)
1-4	2.77 (1.98, 3.88)	2.71 (1.75, 4.20)	3.33 (1.76, 6.31)
5-9	3.65 (2.48, 5.38)	3.13 (1.96, 4.99)	4.35 (2.08, 9.08)
10+	6.78 (4.60, 10.01)	7.68 (4.76, 12.40)	5.38 (2.51, 11.55)

OR[1] Odds ratio.

CI[2] Confidence interval.

Table 3. Variables associated with current smoking in multivariate analysis

Variables	Odd ratios (95% Confidence Interval)
Pocket money (US$)	
0	1.00
<1	2.31 (1.60, 3.34)
1-4	2.47 (1.59, 3.84)
5-9	2.50 (1.66, 3.77)
10+	4.33 (2.73, 6.88)
Age (years)	
11-12	1.00
13	1.47 (0.65, 3.29)
14	1.84 (0.85, 4.00)
15	2.90 (1.36, 6.20)
16-17	3.91 (1.74, 8.81)
Gender	
Female	1.00
Male	3.22 (2.45, 4.24)
Parental smoking	
None	1.00
Father only	1.10 (0.84, 1.44)
Mother only	1.43 (0.71, 2.89)
Both parents	1.52 (0.95, 2.43)
Friends smoking	
None	1.00
Some	4.49 (3.06, 6.60)
Most	24.25 (15.66, 37.54)
All	25.52 (13.72, 47.48)
Cigarette smoking is harmful	
Definitely yes	1.00
Probably yes	1.65 (1.03, 2.64)
Definitely or probably no	2.29 (1.46, 3.59)

DISCUSSION

The prevalence of current cigarette smoking among school-going adolescents in Mongolia was 9.2%. Males had a higher prevalence than females (15.4% vs. 4.4%). The overall prevalence of cigarette smoking is slightly lower than the 10.4% found in the GYTS in Greece in 2005, but the difference between males and females in Greece was small, with percentages of 11.3% versus 9.0%. (16) In Iraqi's Kurdistani region, however, cigarette smoking prevalence among the males in 2005 was 21%, while the female prevalence was 11.9% (17). In 2003 in the Philippines, the overall prevalence was 15.0%, with 21.8% for males and 8.8% for females (18). In Jakarta (Indonesia), Guangdong (China) and Nepal, male predominance in cigarette smoking has been reported, while in Delhi and Goa (India), and in the Czech Republic, no gender differences have been observed (19). In Colombia and Chile, more female than male adolescents have been reported to be cigarette smokers (19). In these settings, the same GYTS core questions were used. It is therefore clear that the gender difference in cigarette smoking has determinants that differ from setting to setting. Parna et al. (20) reported the prevalence of smoking among girls in Russian schools in Tallinn (34.6%), in Helsinki (39.5%), and in Moscow (32.1%). These reports have a higher prevalence than our results. In China, Johnston et al. have reported on current cigarette smoking at 9.3% among the eighth graders and 23% among 12th graders (21). All these studies have reported prevalence among adolescents of similar age range to those in our study, i.e., 13–15 years.

Although the magnitude of association between bivariate and multivariable analyses changed to varying degrees, overall, the direction of association was maintained. Parental smoking and peer smoking were both positively associated with cigarette smoking. A study of 2,763 high school students by Zhang et al. in the Henan Province, China, reported that peer and mother's smoking were positively associated with smoking in the study participants. If smoking was discouraged at school, this was associated with low smoking propensity by study participants (22). It is not possible however, from our study, to determine the direction of association between having a friend who smokes and one's smoking, i.e., whether friends influence one to initiate smoking or smokers are likely to choose other smokers as friends, as this was a cross-sectional study. However, as the literature has reported the importance of peer influence in initiating behaviour, it is reasonable to suggest that peer influence could be important also in the initiation of smoking among our study participants (23, 24). A smoker who has a friend who also smokes may reinforce each other in the maintenance of the habit.

Previous studies elsewhere have reported the association between age, gender, peer influence and cigarette smoking (23). It is also interesting that we identified a dose-response association between the amount of pocket money received and smoking. This finding may suggest that having a disposable income may influence smoking practice and conversely, those adolescents with very little or no pocket money may be only be able to afford bare essentials. Mohan et al. (25) have also reported that in India, adolescents who received pocket money have four times the risk of being a smoker versus those who do not. The public health significance of this finding is that parents and other guardians who provide adolescents with cash should take an interest in how the money is used. We found that adolescents who believed that smoking was harmful to health were less likely to be current smokers, compared to those who disbelieved. Rodriquez et al. have also reported that adolescents who had positive attitudes towards smoking were more likely to be smokers (26).

Our study has the following limitations. As the data were collected through self-completion of the questionnaire, it is possible to have deliberate misreporting. There may also be recall bias as study participants may fail to recall whether or not they smoked within the past 30 days prior to the day of completion of questionnaire. As our assessment of current smoking status was not validated by biomarkers, such as nicotine or cotinine levels or exhaled carbon monoxide, it is difficult to estimate the extent of any reporting biases that may have occurred (27-30). However, our study used a standardised questionnaire that enables within country and across country comparisons of smoking status. The prevalence estimates also obtained are likely to closely represent the smoking prevalence among school-going adolescents. It is not known how representative our sample was of the adolescent population in Mongolia. However, as the gross primary and secondary school enrolment ratios for Mongolia range between 84% and 97%, it implies that the majority of adolescents are in school (31). The Human Development Report states that 97.8% of persons aged 15 years and older are literate in Mongolia (32). The limitation of the gross enrolment ratio is that it measures the estimated number of students in a class expressed as a proportion of the total expected number of students at a particular age or ages. In a situation where class repletion is high, gross enrolment ratio could be high, despite having a significant proportion of adolescents out of school.

In conclusion, among school-going adolescents in Mongolia, we found that cigarette smoking is prevalent and strongly associated with the amount of pocket money, as well as the smoking status of friends and parents. These findings indicate the need to implement public health interventions, with special attention to the determinants of smoking in this group.

ACKNOWLEDGMENTS

The Global Youth Tobacco Survey (GYTS) is a collaborative project of World Health Organisation (WHO), the Centers for Disease Control and Prevention (CDC), and participating countries. Analyses of GYTS data are not necessarily endorsed by the WHO/CDC/participating countries. We are thankful to the study participants and research assistants.

This paper is a revised version of the original publication in the Singapore Medical Journal (Rudatsikira E, Dondog J, Siziya S, Muula AS. Prevalence and determinants of adolescent cigarette smoking in Mongolia. Singapore Med J 2008;49:57-62) and the authors have obtained the permission from the Singapore Medical Journal to use this material.

REFERENCES

[1] Brand RM, Jones DD, Lynch HT, Brand RE, Watsn P, Ashwathnayaran R, et al. Risk of colon cancer in hereditary non-polyposis colorectal cancer patients as predicted by fuzzy modeling: influence of smoking. World J Gastroenterol 2006;12(28):4485-91.

[2] Kaur J, Bains K. A study of the risk factor profile of cardiovascular diseases in rural Punjabi male patients. Indian J Public Health 2006;50:97-100.

[3] Tonstad S, Andrew-Johnston J. Cardiovascular risks associated with smoking: a review for clinicians. Eur J Cardiovasc Prev Rehabil 2006;13:507-14.

[4] Pesut D, Basara HZ. Cigarette smoking and lung cancer trends in Serbia - a ten-year analysis. Med Pregl 2006;59:225-9.

[5] Murray CJ, Lopez AD. Global mortality, disability, and the contribution of risk factors: Global Burden of Disease Study. Lancet 1997;349:1436-42.

[6] Murray CJ, Lopez AD. Mortality by cause for eight regions of the world: Global Burden of Diseases Study. Lancet 1997;349:1269-76.

[7] Mathers CD, Loncar D. Projections of Global Mortality and burden of disease from 2002 to 2030. PLoS Med 2006;3:e442.

[8] Global Youth Tabacco Survey Collaborative Group. Tobacco use among youth: A cross country comparison. Tob Control 2002;11:252-70.

[9] Baigalmaa D, Nishimura A, Ito K. Smoking cessation rate 12 months after a group counseling program in Mongolia. Asian Pac J Cancer Prev 2006;7:399-402.

[10] Aloise-Young PA, Slater MD, Cruickshank CC. Mediators and moderators of magazine advertisement effects on adolescent cigarette smoking. J Health Commun 2006;11:281-300.

[11] Feighery EC, Henricksen L, Wang Y, Schleicher NC, Fortmann SP. An evaluation of four measures of adolescents' exposure to cigarette marketing in stores. Nicotine Tob Res 2006;8:751-9.

[12] Abdullah AS, Husten CG. Promotion of smoking cessation in developing countries: a framework for urgent public health interventions. Thorax 2004;59:623-30.
[13] Warren CW, Riley L, Asma S, Eriksen MP, Green L, Blanton C, et al. Tobacco use by youth: a surveillance report from the Global Youth Tobacco Survey project. Bull World Health Organ 2000;78(7):868-76.
[14] Global Tobacco Surveillance System Collaborating Group. Global Tobacco Surveillance System (GTSS): purpose, production, and potential. J Sch Health 2005;75:15-24.
[15] Global Youth Tobacco Survey Collaborative Group. Tobacco use among youth: A cross country comparison. Tob Control 2002;11:252-70.
[16] Kyrlesi A, Soteriades ES, Warren CW, et al. Tobacco use among students aged 13-15 years in Greece: the GYTS Project. BMC Public Health 2007;7:3.
[17] Centers for Diseases Control and Prevention (CDC). Tobacco use among students aged 13-15 years-Kurdistan region, Iraq 2005. MMWR 2006;55:556-9.
[18] Centers for Diseases Control and Prevention (CDC). Tobacco use among students aged 13-15 years--Phillipines, 2000 and 2003. MMWR 2005;54:94-7.
[19] Global Youth Tobacco Survey Collaborating Group. Differences in worldwide tobacco use by gender: findings from the Global Youth Tobacco Survey. J Sch Health 2003;73:207-15.
[20] Pärna K, Rahu K, Fischer K, Mussalo-Rauhamaa H, Zhuravleva I, Umbleja T, et al. Smoking and associated factors among adolescents in Tallinn, Helsinki and Moscow: a multilevel analysis. Scand J Public Health 2003;31(5):350-8.
[21] Johnston L, O'Malley PM, Bachman JG. Monitoring the future. National survey results on drug use, 1975–2004: Vol. 1. Secondary school students. Rockville, MD: National Institute Drug Abuse, 05-5727, 2005.
[22] Zhang L, Wang WF, Zhou G. A cross-sectional study of smoking risk factors in junior high school students in Henan, China. Southeast Asian J Trop Med Public Health 2005;36:1580-4.
[23] Abdullah AS. Ho WW. What Chinese adolescents think about quitting smoking: a qualitative study. Subst Use Misuse 2006;41:1735-43.
[24] Hoffman BR, Sussman S, Unger JB, Valente TW. Peer influences on adolescent cigarette smoking: a theoretical review of the literature. Subst Use Misuse 2006;41:103-55.
[25] Mohan S, Sankara Sarma P, Thankappan KR. Access to pocket money and low educational performance predict tobacco use among adolescent boys in Kerala, India. Prev Med 2005;41:685-92.
[26] Rodriguez D, Romer D, Audrain-McGovern J. Beliefs about the risks of smoking mediate the relationship between exposure to smoking and smoking. Psychosom Med 2007;69:106-13.
[27] Hung J, Lin CH, Wang JD, Chan CC. Exhaled carbon monoxide level as an indicator of cigarette consumption in a workplace cessation program in Taiwan. J Formos Med Assoc 2006;105:210-3.
[28] Jenkins RA, Counts RW. Personal exposure to environmental tobacco smoke: salivary cotinine, airborne nicotine, and non smoker misclassification. J Expo Anal Environ Epidemiol 1999;9:352-63.

[29] Low EC, Ong MC, Tan M. Breath carbon monoxide as an indication of smoking habit in the military setting. Singapore Med J 2004;45:578- 82.
[30] Mulcahy M, Evans DS, Hammond SK, Repace JL, Byrne M. Secondhand smoke exposure and risk following the Irish smoking ban: an assessment of salivary cotinine concentrations in hotel workers and air nicotine levels in bars. Tob Control 2005;14:384-8.
[31] Unicef. The State of the World's Children 2007. URL: www.unicef.org/ infobycountry/mongolia_statistics.html.
[32] United Nations Development Report. Human Development Report. Fact sheet for Mongolia. URL: hdr.undp.org/hdr2006/statistics/countries/country_fact_sheets/cty_f s_M NG.html.

In: Smoking and Adolescence ISBN: 978-1-63484-311-9
Editors: M. L. Mazabam, S. Siziya et al. © 2016 Nova Science Publishers, Inc.

Chapter 19

PREVALENCE AND CORRELATES OF CURRENT CIGARETTE SMOKING AMONG ADOLESCENTS IN EAST TIMOR-LESTE

Seter Siziya[1*], BA(Ed), MSc, PhD, Adamson S Muula[2], MBBS, MPH, PhD, and Emmanuel Rudatsikira[3], MD, MPH, DrPH

[1]Department of Community Medicine, University of Zambia, School of Medicine, Lusaka, Zambia
[2]Department of Community Health, University of Malawi, College of Medicine, Blantyre, Malawi
[3]Departments of Epidemiology and Biostatistics and Global Health, Loma Linda University, School of Public Health, Loma Linda, California, USA

In this chapter we determine the prevalence and correlates for current cigarette smoking by using secondary data of the East Timor-Leste Global Youth Tobacco Survey conducted in 2006 in the study. Public and private schools registered with the Ministry of Education were included in the study. A two-stage cluster sample of 1790 students in Grades 7 to 9 was used to select the participants. Schools were selected with probability proportional to enrolment size, and classes were randomly selected in

* Correspondence: Professor Seter Siziya, Clinical Sciences Department, School of Medicine, Copperbelt University, Ndola Central Hospital, 6th Floor, POBox 71191, Ndola, Zambia. E-mail: ssiziya@gmail.com.

each school. All students in selected classes were eligible to participate in the survey. The school and student response rates were 96.0% and 84.5%, respectively. Out of 1790 adolescents, 52.1% were of ages less than 15 years, 51.8% were males, 42.8% reported having some pocket money in a month, and 72.7% had at least a parent who was a smoker. Prevalence of current cigarette smoking was 40.3%. Current smokers also reported having bought cigarettes from peddlers (32.4%), someone bought for them (16.7%), got from someone older (13.7%), borrowed (13.3%), and stole (3.4%). Males were more likely to be smokers than females (59.0% versus 19.3%). Factors positively associated with current smoking were: parental smoking; closest friend smoking; amount of pocket money; and exposure to anti-tobacco messages. East Timor has one of the highest prevalence of cigarette smoking among adolescents. The fact that exposure to anti-tobacco messages was associated with being a smoker may be evidence suggesting that anti-tobacco messages, especially from tobacco-related industry, may have unintended consequences.

INTRODUCTION

Tobacco use is the single most important preventable cause of morbidity and mortality from non-communicable diseases (1). There has been growing interest in adolescent tobacco smoking in the past decade (2). Adolescent tobacco use is of public health concern because it may lead to long-term smoking behavior into adulthood. Adolescent smokers may also suffer from immediate or medium term effects such as incident asthma (3). Smoking among adolescents may also be a marker of many other lifestyle and health concerns (4, 5). Francis et al. (6) have reported that adolescents who smoke are at higher risk of psychopathology compared to adolescents who are non-smokers. This clustering of unhealthy lifestyles has also been observed among adults (7).

The Global Youth Tobacco Survey has reported on the prevalence of cigarette smoking among 13 to 15 year old in-school adolescents in East Timor-Leste (8). In this age group, prevalence of current cigarette smoking was 32.4%. We are however unaware of any published reports on social correlates of cigarette smoking among adolescents in this setting. Using data from the Global Youth Tobacco Survey, we therefore conducted analysis to identify the factors that are associated with cigarette smoking among in-school adolescents.

Our study

Our study involved secondary analysis of data from the East Timor Global Youth Tobacco Survey (GYTS) conducted in 2006. The survey was school based and recruited students in Grades 7 to 9. The school population was all junior high school (both public and private schools) that were registered with the Ministry of Education, East Timor. Total number of schools was 127 schools, and total number of student was around 41,000 students.

Study administration and sampling followed the GYTS process as has been described elsewhere (2). In brief however, a two-stage cluster sample design was used to produce representative data for all of East Timor. At the first stage of sampling, schools were selected with probability proportional to enrolment size. At the second stage of sampling, classes were randomly selected and all students in selected classes were eligible to participate. The school response rate was 96.0%, while the student response rate was 84.5%, and the overall response rate was 81.1%. A total of 1,790 students participated in the survey.

East Timor shares a border with Indonesia and lies 800 km to the northwest of Australia. East Timor is a former Portuguese colony that was annexed by Indonesia in 1975. In 1999, following a referendum on independence from Indonesia, violent civil conflict led to the destruction of much of East Timor's infrastructure. The country has an estimated population of about 1 million inhabitants.

A self-completed questionnaire with core and country-specific questions as outlined in the GYTS methodology (2) was used to collect data. Completion of question occurred within one class period and coordinators supervised the process. Study participants were informed that they were free not to answer any of the questions they felt uncomfortable with.

Data analysis was performed using SPSS version 14.0 software (Chicago, Illinois, United States of America). Current cigarette smoking (the main outcome) was defined as having smoked a cigarette, even a single puff, in the last 30 days preceding the survey. The predictor variables were obtained from the literature as factors that have been previously reported as being associated with adolescent smoking in other settings. These factors include: smoking in close friends (9); gender (10); having pocket money or allowance (11); parental smoking (12) and exposure to tobacco related messages or advertisements (13).

A weighting factor was used in the analysis to reflect the likelihood of sampling each student and to reduce bias by compensating for differing patterns of non-response. We obtained frequencies as estimates of prevalence. We conducted a Backward logistic regression analysis to estimate the association between relevant predictor variables and current cigarette smoking.

FINDINGS

A total of 1,790 in-school adolescents participated in the East Timor Global Youth Tobacco Survey in 2006. Overall, 52.1% of the participants were of ages less than 15 years, 51.8% were males, 42.8% reported having some pocket money in a month, and 72.7% had at least a parent who was a smoker. Prevalence of current cigarette smoking was 35.7%. Males were more likely to be smokers than females (59.0% versus 19.3%). Further description of the sample is presented in Table 1.

Table 1. Characteristics of study participants in the East Timor Global Youth Tobacco Survey 2006

Factor	Total	Male	Female
	n* (%)†	n* (%)†	n* (%)†
Age (years)			
<15	960 (52.1)	421 (45.5)	503 (57.4)
15+	815 (47.9)	476 (54.5)	330 (42.6)
Gender			
Male	899 (51.8)		-
Female	836 (48.2)		
Pocket money received (US$)			
>5	212 (12.7)	120 (14.4)	81 (10.5)
1-5	161 (9.2)	93 (10.8)	64 (7.5)
<1	376 (20.9)	205 (22.5)	160 (19.2)
None	1026 (57.2)	472 (52.3)	528 (62.8)
Parents smoked			
None	454 (27.3)	224 (26.5)	213 (27.6)
Both	253 (16.2)	126 (15.9)	121 (16.9)
Father only	867 (51.8)	455 (53.6)	392 (50.4)
Mother only	74 (4.6)	33 (4.0)	38 (5.2)
Close friends smoked			
None of them	622 (33.8)	231 (26.0)	378 (42.9)
Some of them	398 (22.4)	208 (22.3)	184 (23.0)
Most of them	325 (19.0)	194 (21.7)	117 (15.5)
All of them	419 (24.8)	255 (30.0)	148 (18.5)

	Total	Male	Female
Frequency of media messages seen on anti-smoking program			
A lot	856 (49.4)	424 (48.3)	410 (50.9)
A few	380 (21.1)	198 (22.4)	166 (19.1)
None	508 (29.4)	253 (29.3)	243 (30.1)
Frequency of cigarette brand names seen when watched sports events or other programs on television (TV)			
Never watched TV	486 (27.5)	226 (25.1)	246 (29.8)
A lot	564 (31.5)	297 (33.0)	252 (30.1)
Sometimes	343 (20.0)	183 (21.2)	151 (18.8)
Never	358 (20.9)	173 (20.7)	175 (21.3)
Frequency of cigarette advertisements seen on billboard			
A lot	725 (41.6)	384 (44.2)	328 (39.6)
A few	414 (24.4)	211 (24.3)	185 (23.4)
None	566 (34.0)	265 (31.4)	288 (37.0)
Frequency of cigarette advertisements or promotion seen in magazines			
A lot	713 (40.5)	380 (43.1)	315 (38.0)
A few	465 (26.5)	231 (26.8)	219 (25.9)
None	562 (33.0)	259 (30.1)	286 (36.1)
Currently smoking			
Yes	611 (40.3)	457 (59.0)	128 (19.3)
No	979 (59.7)	339 (41.0)	620 (80.7)

* Unweighted frequency.

† Weighted percent.

Of the current smokers, 24.1% reported they usually bought their cigarettes in a store, and 41.2% who bought cigarettes in a store had never been refused purchase because of their age. Altogether, 21.9% of the smokers had ever been offered ‘free’ cigarettes by cigarette company representative. Current smokers also reported having bought cigarettes from peddlers (32.4%), someone bought for them (16.7%), got from someone older (13.7%), borrowed (13.3%), and stole (3.4%).

We also assessed whether the selected predictor variables were associated with self-reported history of cigarette smoking. In a multivariate analysis, we found that parental smoking, peer smoking, increasing age, male gender, exposure to cigarette promotion media in magazines, and exposure to anti-smoking media messages were independently associated with being a current cigarette smoker (see Table 2).

Table 2. Factors associated with currently smoking among in-school adolescents in East Timor, 2006

Factor	Adjusted OR (95%CI)*
Age (years)	
<15	0.70 (0.68, 0.72)
15+	1
Gender	
Male	2.52 (2.45, 2.60)
Female	1
Pocket money received (US$)	
>5	1.79 (1.67, 1.93)
1-5	0.73 (0.67, 0.79)
<1	1.51 (1.43, 1.60)
None	1
Parents smoked	
None	0.56 (0.53, 0.60)
Both	1.00 (0.93, 1.07)
Father only	0.85 (0.81, 0.89)
Mother only	1
Close friends smoked	
None of them	0.43 (0.41, 0.46)
Some of them	1.04 (0.99, 1.10)
Most of them	1.02 (0.97, 1.08)
All of them	1
Frequency of media messages seen on anti-smoking program	
A lot	1.16 (1.11, 1.20)
A few	1.17 (1.12, 1.23)
None	1
Frequency of cigarette brand names seen when watched sports events or other programs on television (TV)	
Never watched TV	0.64 (0.60, 0.67)
A lot	0.87 (0.83, 0.91)
Sometimes	1.74 (1.64, 1.84)
Never	1
Frequency of cigarette advertisements seen on billboard	
A lot	0.73 (0.70, 0.77)
A few	1.38 (1.31, 1.44)
None	1
Frequency of cigarette advertisements or promotion seen in magazines	
A lot	1.10 (1.05, 1.15)
A few	1.06 (1.01, 1.11)
None	1

OR (95%CI)* adjusted estimates for all the factors in the Table in a Backward logistic regression analysis.

DISCUSSION

We have reported an overall prevalence of current cigarette smoking of 40.3% among in-school adolescents in East Timor in 2006. The prevalence of smoking among adolescents in East Timor is probably among the highest in the world. Rudatsikira et al. (10) have reported prevalence of cigarette smoking of 4.5%, 1% among male and female adolescents, respectively, in Ethiopia. Kyrlesi et al. (14) reported a prevalence of current cigarette smoking of 16.2% among Greek in-school adolescents. Singh and Gupta (15) have reported current cigarette smoking of 2.1% and 1.7% among 13 to 18 year old males and females respectively in Jaipur, India. Among 7 to 9 graders in Thailand, Assanangkornchai et al. (16) have reported prevalence of current cigarette smoking of between 8.8% and 14.6%.

There are at least two possible reasons for the high prevalence of smoking among adolescents in East Timor. Firstly, the proximity and free flow of persons between East Timor and Indonesia, where smoking is prevalent. Male smoking in Indonesia range from 50% to about 83% (17). As the Indonesian government has been developing policy aimed to prevent smoking in the last few years, the tobacco companies in Indonesia have started to pay more attention to East Timor as their target customer. This will make it a more challenging situation if East Timor does not have strong policy and political will to tobacco control. Secondly prolonged periods of liberation fighting had compromised the public health infrastructure to enable concerted public health effort to prevent adolescent smoking.

We found that boys were more likely to have been smokers than girls. Another study in another setting has reported this observation (10). We believe the gender disparity could result from societal tolerant attitudes towards male smoking compared to female smoking. We also observed that having parents who smoked or having close friends who were smokers were independently associated with smoking in the adolescents. The association between having a close friend who smoke and adolescent's own smoking may suggest that an adolescent who is a smoker may be more likely to choose other smokers as friends. Alternatively, having a friend who smokes may be an influence in initiating smoking. Livaudais et al. (18) have reported that having friends who were smokers at baseline was associated with eventually becoming a smoker among Latino adolescents in the United States. Simmons-Norton (19) has reported on the socialization selection effects among adolescents regarding peer smoking.

The association between having a parent who is a smoker and adolescent's own smoking may be an indication of parental tolerance to smoking or easy availability and accessibility of cigarettes within the home. Adolescents who have parents who smoke may also have higher acceptability of smoking.

We also found that if the adolescent reported having been exposed to cigarette advertisements or promotion in magazines then, he or she was more likely to be a current smoker than if the adolescent was not exposed. However we also found that exposure to anti-smoking advertisements was associated with being a smoker, while more exposure to cigarette brand names and promotional billboard were associated with lower likelihood of being a smoker. That exposure to pro-tobacco advertisements is associated with adolescent smoking has been reported elsewhere (20).

The apparent paradoxical finding where exposure to anti-smoking was associated with increased likelihood of being a smoker is not a new finding. Henriksen et al. (21) have reported that tobacco-industry supported anti-tobacco messages may have the opposite effect on adolescent smoking. Weiss et al. (20) and Straub et al. (22) have also reported that anti-smoking or anti-tobacco messages may not be adequate to prevent smoking among adolescents. It would appear that in our study, exposure to anti-tobacco messages in fact had the opposite effect on adolescents. This calls for evaluation of tobacco messages targeted towards adolescents.

We also found that adolescents who received more than US$ 5 as pocket money in a month and those who got less than US$ 1 were more likely to be smokers. Unger et al. (23) have suggested that limiting the amount of pocket money among adolescents who receive more money may be a reasonable intervention. We do not know why even those who received less than a dollar had higher likelihood of smoking than those in the middle-income group. This could be a spurious finding. In an environment where smoking is prevalent, adolescents may also access cigarettes from friends, borrow from someone, having their cigarettes bought by someone (without them having to pay for them) and stealing from their own parents. It may also be an indication that there may have been another confounder that was not measured.

Our study has a number of important limitations. Firstly data were obtained only from in-school adolescents. To the extent that out of school adolescents are different from in-school adolescents in their smoking habits, our results may not be extrapolated to the entire adolescent population in East Timor. Data were also collected from those adolescents who were present on the day of the survey. Those students who were absent were never followed up. We do however believe that any biases that may have been introduced as a result of non availability of study participants was likely to be minimal as the response rate was high i.e., 81.1%. Furthermore our analysis took into consideration the non-response rate by weighting the analysis. Thirdly, data were self-reported. Like in all surveys that rely on self-reported data, there is always a possibility of both inadvertent and deliberate miss reporting. An evaluation of a similar methodology to the GYTS in the United States however has reported high reliability of adolescents reports (24).

In conclusion, the prevalence of smoking appears to be among the highest in the world. Exposure to anti-smoking messages did not appear to be associated with lower likelihood of being a smoker. Our findings suggest that health education or improving knowledge will be less effective to prevent smoking behavior without significant involvement or support from other aspects such as supportive environment, strong policy support, and community participation. There will be need for involvement and partnership from different stakeholders and community.

ACKNOWLEDGMENTS

We are grateful to the Centers for Disease Control (CDC), Atlanta, Georgia, United States of America for making the data set available for our analysis. We are also thankful to all the students who participated in the East Timor Global-Leste Youth Tobacco Survey 2006.

This chapter is a revised version of an original paper published in the Indian Pediatrcicsn (Siziya S, Muula AS, Rudatsikira E. Prevalence and correlates of current cigarette smoking among in-school adolescents in East Timor-Leste. Indian Pediatric 2008;45:963-968) and the authors have obtained the permission from the Indian Pediatrics to use this material.

REFERENCES

[1] Mathers CD, Loncar D. Projections of global mortality and burden of disease from 2002 to 2030. PLoS Med 2006;3:e442.

[2] Warren CW, Riley L, Asma S, Eriksen MP, Green L, Blanton C, et al. Tobacco use by youth: a surveillance report from the Global Youth Tobacco Survey project. Bull World Health Organ 2000;78:868-76.

[3] Gilliland FD, Islam T, Berhane K, Gauderman WJ, McConnell R, Avol E, et al. Regular smoking and asthma incidence in adolescents. Am J Respir Crit Care Med 2006;174:1094-1100.

[4] Rudatsikira E, Siziya S, Kazembe LN, Muula AS. Prevalence and associated factors of physical fighting among school-going adolescents in Namibia. Ann Gen Psychiatry 2007;6:18.

[5] Dierker LC, Sledjeski EM, Botello-Harbaum M, Ramirez RR, Chavez LM, Canino G. Association between psychiatric disorders and smoking stages within a representative clinic sample of Puerto Rican adolescents. Compr Psychiatry 2007;48:237-44.

[6] Francis K, Katsani G, Sotiropoulou X, Roussos A, Roussos C. Cigarette smoking among Greek adolescents: behavior, attitudes, risk, and preventive factors. Subst Use Misuse 2007;42:1323-36.

[7] Poortinga W. The prevalence and clustering of four major lifestyle risk factors in an English adult population. Prev Med 2007;44:124-8.

[8] Global Youth Tobacco Survey. URL: http://www.searo.who.int/en/Section1174/section1462/pdfs/GYTS_Fact sheets/TLS_factsheet%202006.pdf. Accessed August 20, 2007).

[9] Chalela P, Velez LF, Ramirez AG. Social influences, and attitudes and beliefs associated with smoking among border Latino youth. J Sch Health 2007;77:187-95.

[10] Rudatsikira E, Abdo A, Muula AS. Prevalence and determinants of adolescent tobacco smoking in Addis Ababa, Ethiopia. BMC Public Health 2007;7:176.

[11] Unger JB, Sun P, Johnson CA. Socioeconomic correlates of smoking among an ethnically diverse sample of 8th grade adolescents in Southern California. Prev Med 2007;44:323-7.

[12] Otten R, Engels RC, van de Ven MO, Bricker JB. Parental smoking and adolescent smoking stages: the role of parents' current and former smoking, and family structure. J Behav Med 2007;30:143-54.

[13] Andreeva TI, Krasovsky KS, Semenova DS. Correlates of smoking initiation among young adults in Ukraine: a cross-sectional study. BMC Public Health 2007; 7:106.

[14] Kyrlesi A, Soteriades ES, Warren CW, Kremastinou J, Papastergiou P, Jones NR, et al. Tobacco use among students aged 13-15 years in Greece: the GYTS project. BMC Public Health 2007;7:3.

[15] Singh V, Gupta R. Prevalence of tobacco use and awareness of risks among school children in Jaipur. J Assoc Physicians India 2006; 54:609-12.

[16] Assanangkornchai S, Pattanasattayawong U, Samangsri N, Mukthong A. Substance use among high-school students in Southern Thailand: trends over 3 years (2002-2004). Drug Alcohol Depend 2007;86:167-74.

[17] Reynolds C: The fourth largest market in the world. Tob Control 1999; 8:89-91.

[18] Livaudais JC, Napoles-Springer A, Stewart S, Kaplan CP.Understanding Latino adolescent risk behaviors: parental and peer influences. Ethn Dis 2007;17:298-304.

[19] Simons-Morton B. Social influences on adolescent substance use. Am J Health Behav 2007;31:672-84.

[20] Weiss JW, Cen S, Schuster DV, Unger JB, Johnson CA, Mouttapa M, et al. Longitudinal effects of pro-tobacco and anti-tobacco messages on adolescent smoking susceptibility. Nicotine Tob Res 2006; 8:455-65.

[21] Henriksen L, Dauphinee AL, Wang Y, Fortmann SP. Industry sponsored anti-smoking ads and adolescent reactance: test of a boomerang effect. Tob Control 2006;15:13-8.
[22] Straub DM, Hills NK, Thompson PJ, Moscicki AB. Effects of pro- and anti-tobacco advertising on nonsmoking adolescents' intentions to smoke. J Adolesc Health 2003;32:36-43.
[23] Unger JB, Sun P, Johnston CA. Socioeconomic correlates of smoking among ethnically diverse sample of 8th grade adolescents in Southern California. Prev Med 2007;44:323-7.
[24] Brener ND, Kann L, McManus T, Kinchen SA, Sundberg EC, Ross JG. Reliability of the 1999 youth risk behavior survey questionnaire. J Adolesc Health 2002;31: 336-42.

In: Smoking and Adolescence ISBN: 978-1-63484-311-9
Editors: M. L. Mazabam, S. Siziya et al. © 2016 Nova Science Publishers, Inc.

Chapter 20

Prevalence, Correlates of and Perceptions toward Cigarette Smoking among Adolescents in South Korea

Emmanuel Rudatsikira*[1], *MD, MPH, DrPH,
Adamson S Muula*[2,*], *MBBS, MPH, PhD,
and Seter Siziya*[3], *BA (Ed), MSc, PhD

[1]Departments of Biostatistics and Epidemiology and Global Health, Loma Linda University, School of Public Health, Loma Linda, California, USA

[2]Department of Community Health, University of Malawi, College of Medicine, Blantyre, Malawi

[3]Department of Community Medicine, University of Zambia, School of Medicine, Lusaka, Zambia

In this chapter we estimate the prevalence of current smoking, correlates of smoking and assess exposure to and perceptions towards smoking by gender. We used data from the South Korea Global Youth Tobacco Survey (GYTS). Frequencies of selected characteristics and their 95% confidence were obtained. Current cigarette smoking was defined as having smoked, even a single puff, within the last 30 days. Logistic

[*] Correspondence: Professor Adamson S Muula, Department of Community Health, University of Malawi, College of Medicine, Chichiri, Blantyre, Malawi. E-mail: amuula@medcol.mw.

regression analysis was conducted to assess the factors that were considered to be associated with current cigarette smoking in bivariate and multivariate analyses. Of the 5,615 respondents, 7.4% males and 5.0% females reported being current smokers (p = 0.003). Having smoked friends who was strongly associated with smoking after controlling for age, gender, parental smoking status, exposure to anti-smoking media messages, and perception of risks of smoking (OR=69.92; 95% CI [41.24, 118.57] for most friends and OR=11.86; 95% CI [7.26, 19.36] for some friends). Male gender and having one or both smoking parents were associated with smoking (OR=1.43; 95% CI [1.09, 1.89] and OR=1.29; 95% CI [1.00-, 1.71] respectively). Exposure to antismoking media messages was negatively associated with smoking (OR=0.52; 95% CI [0.36, 0.77]. Prevalence of smoking among adolescents in South Korea is lower than in many other Asian countries. There is however, need to strengthen anti-tobacco messages especially among adolescents.

INTRODUCTION

Tobacco use is a leading cause of deaths among non-communicable diseases globally (1). In the past 20 years mortality from lung and other tobacco-related cancers in Korea has increased, having largely been preceded by increase in prevalence of smoking (2-4). Many adults initiate smoking as adolescents, therefore prevention of cigarette smoking among adolescents is of paramount importance.

While many of the adverse health effects of cigarette smoking are experienced later in the life of the smoker, adolescent smoking has also short term untoward implications. Adolescent smokers have high incidence of asthma (5), exacerbation of asthma (6) and wheezing (7). Smoking in adolescents may also be a marker of other problem behaviors and unhealthy lifestyles (8). Park et al. have reported that smoking was associated with suicidal ideation among adolescents in Korea (9, 10). Shin et al. have reported that snoring in class was associated with being a smoker among adolescents in Korea (11). Elliot et al. have reported that adolescent females who used anabolic steroids were also likely to smoke cigarette in the United States (12). There is a growing literature on the prevalence of adolescent cigarette smoking in Korea. Many of the studies have reported mainly on demographic factors associated with being a smoker. Few studies have documented whether there are differences in the perceptions of smoking between boys and girls. The present study was carried out to assess the socio-demographic correlates of current smoking; compare exposure to tobacco-related messages/media by gender and compare perceptions towards cigarette smoking between boys and girls.

OUR STUDY

This study is based on secondary analysis of data from the South Korean Global Youth Tobacco Survey conducted in 2004. The survey was school based. The school population was students that were registered with the Ministry of Education, South Korea. A total of 75 schools within grades 1 to 3 and classes having at least 40 students were selected. The first-stage of sampling consisted of all the schools which had the eligible grades. The schools were selected with probability proportional to their enrollment size. The second sampling stage consisted of systematic sampling (with a random start) of classes from each school that participated in the survey. All classes in the selected schools were included in the sampling. All students in the selected classes were eligible to participate in the survey regardless of their ages. The overall response rate was 87.7%, with 92.0% (69 of the 75 sampled schools) school response rate. The student response rate was 95.3% (5,940 of the 6,234 eligible sampled students participated).

Questionnaires were completed anonymously in the classroom by the study participants within one class session. Students recorded their response directly on a computer scannable answer. Field researchers were trained in September 2004 in each of regions where they were instructed on standard procedure to assure comparability on data collection. The present study had approval from both the Ministry of Health and Ministry of Education. Letters from these ministries were sent to all the Principals of the 75 selected schools, inviting them to participate in the GYTS. All 75 schools agreed to participate. Data collection was carried out during October and November 2004. Ten trained enumerators were involved in administering the questionnaire.

Data analysis was performed using SUDAAN software (Research Triangle Institute, Research Triangle Park, North Carolina, United States of America). Current cigarette smoking (the main outcome) was defined as having smoked a cigarette, even a single puff, in the last 30 days preceding the survey. The predictor variables were obtained from the literature as factors that have been previously reported as being associated with adolescent smoking in other settings. These factors include: smoking in close friends (13, 14); gender (8) parental smoking (15) and exposure to tobacco related messages or advertisements (16). A weighting factor was used in the analysis to reflect the likelihood of sampling each student and to reduce bias by compensating for differing patterns of non-response. The weight used for estimation is given by the following formula:

W = W1 * W2 * f1 * f2 *f3 *f4

where W1 = the inverse of the probability of selecting the school
W2 = the inverse of the probability of selecting the classroom within the school
fl = a school-level non response adjustment factor calculated by school size category (small, medium, large)
f2= a class-level non response adjustment factor calculated for each school
f3 = a student-level non response adjustment factor calculated by class
f4 = a post stratification adjustment factor calculated by grade

We obtained frequencies as estimation of prevalence. We conducted logistic regression analysis to estimate the association between relevant predictor variables and current cigarette smoking for both bivariate (unadjusted odds ratios) and multivariate (adjusted odds ratios) analyses.

FINDINGS

A total of 5,615 students participated in the study of whom 3,006 (51.2%) were females. The median age was 13 (Q1 = 11-12, Q3 = 14) years, range 11 to 17 years.

Of the 5,615 participants, 7.4% (95% CI [6.4, 8.6]) males and 5.0% (95% CI [4.2, 6.0]) females reported being current smokers (p = 0.003). Having smoking friends was very strongly associated with smoking after controlling for age, gender, parental smoking status, exposure to anti-smoking media messages, and perception of hazards caused by smoking. Participants, who had most of their friends as smokers, were more likely to smoke than those who had no smoking friends (OR = 69.92; 95% CI [41.24, 118.57]). Adolescents who had some friends as smokers were also likely to be smokers themselves (OR = 11.86; 95% CI [7.26, 19.36]). Males were more likely to smoke than females (OR = 1.43; 95% CI [1.09, 1.89]). Compared to subjects with non-smoking parents, those whose parents smoked were 1.29 more likely to smoke (OR = 1.29; 95% CI [1.00, 1.71]). Exposure to anti-smoking media messages were negatively associated with smoking (OR = 0.52; 95% CI [0.36, 0.77] (see Table 1).

Table 1. Factors associated with current smoking among in-school adolescents

Characteristics	Percent of smokers	Unadjusted odds ratios (95% CI)	Adjusted odds ratios (95% CI)
Age (years)			
11-12	7.8	1.00	1.00
13	4.4	0.75 (0.59, 1.37)	1.03 (0.62, 1.72)
14	8.7	1.13 (0.81, 1.58)	1.52 (0.91, 2.54)
15	8.5	1.10 (0.77, 1.56)	1.32 (0.80, 2.19)
16-17	12.6	1.70 (0.39, 7.44)	2.01 (0.20, 20.19)
Gender			
Female	5.0	1.00	1.00
Male	7.4	1.51 (1.18, 1.93)	1.43 (1.09, 1.89)
Parental smoking status			
None	43.7	1.00	1.00
One or both parents	56.4	1.59 (1.24, 2.02)	1.29 (1.00, 1.71)
Best friend smokes			
None	55.9	1.00	1.00
Some	37.4	11.06 (7.23, 16.93)	11.86 (7.26, 19.36)
Most or all	6.7	63.96 (40.53, 100.97)	69.92 (41.24, 118.57)
Perception that smoking is harmful			
No	11.1	1.00	1.00
Yes	6.8	0.59 (0.36, 0.95)	1.06 (0.46, 2.43)
Seen anti-smoking media messages			
No	10.2	1.00	1.00
Yes	6.3	0.59 (0.43, 1.80)	0.52 (0.36, 0.77)

Table 2 indicates the participants were exposed to tobacco advertisement through newspapers/magazine (50.8%), and TV (95.5%). Altogether 7.8% respondents reported having an item with cigarette brand logo on it. Compared to females, males had lower estimates of exposure to cigarette advertisement on TV and in the newspapers/magazines (p=0.040 and p=0.020) respectively).

Table 2. Exposure to tobacco advertisements among adolescents

Characteristics	Number of participants	Percent of total (95% CI)	p value
Seen cigarette brand name on TV in past 30 days			
All	5412	95.5 (94.9, 96.1)	0.040
Males	2474	94.9 (93.9, 95.8)	
Females	2938	96.6 (95.7, 97.3)	
Seen tobacco adverts in newspapers/magazines in past 30 days			
All	5524	50.8 (49.4, 52.2)	0.020
Males	2567	48.3 (46.3, 50.4)	
Females	2957	52.8 (50.7, 54.8)	
Has item with cigarette brand logo on it			
All	5446	7.8 (7.1, 8.7)	0.129
Males	2536	8.1 (7.0, 9.3)	
Females	2910	7.7 (6.6, 8.9)	

Table 3. Attitudes towards tobacco smoking distributed by gender

Characteristics	Number of participants	Percent of totals (95% CI)	p values
Felt that boys who smoke have more friends			
All	2429	30.5 (28.6, 32.5)	<0.001
Males	1290	23.7 (21.3, 26.3)	
Females	1139	37.4 (34.3, 40.6)	
Felt that girls who smoke have more friends			
All	2711	17.3 (15.3, 19.7)	0.940
Males	1413	17.3 (15.3, 19.5)	
Females	1298	17.4 (15.3, 19.8)	
Felt that boys who smoke are attractive			
All	3562	14.6 (13.4, 15.9)	0.002
Males	1612	12.6 (11.0, 14.5)	
Females	1950	15.7 (14.0, 17.6)	
Felt that girls who smoke are attractive			
All	3978	5.8 (5.0, 6.6)	0.001
Males	1815	6.3 (5.2, 7.5)	
Females	2163	4.4 (3.5, 5.5)	
Felt that tobacco smoking is harmful to health			
All	5588	95.6 (95.0, 96.2)	0.001
Males	2592	94.5 (93.5, 95.4)	
Females	2996	97.3 (96.6, 97.9)	

Table 3 indicates that the vast majority (95.6%) of the respondents felt that smoking is harmful. About 1 in 3 respondents (30.5%) thought that male smokers had more friends while 17.3% thought so for females. Furthermore, 14.6% of the participants felt that boys who smoke are attractive and 5.8% felt the same for girls who smoke.

DISCUSSION

The present study found prevalence of current cigarette smoking of 7.4% and 5.0% among boys and girls, with median age of 12 years in South Korea. Kim (17) has reported prevalence of current cigarette smoking of 26% among in-school adolescents in grades 7th to 12th in Korea. We found just as had been reported by Kim (17) that males were more likely to be smokers than females. In 1995, Juon et al. (18) reported that among 7th and 11th graders in 1995, overall prevalence of current cigarette smoking was 8.5% (15.4% and 1.3% among males and females respectively). The prevalence of current smoking we found is similar to that estimated for Kampala (Uganda) and Lilongwe (Malawi) where prevalence was 5.6% and 6.2% respectively (19). In the present study female's estimate is higher than that estimated by Juon et al. 918) in 1995. However, the Juon et al. (18) study was over a decade ago and so the estimates may no longer be relevant at the present time. Kyrlesi et al. (20) reported an overall prevalence among Greek in-school adolescents of 10.2%. Boys were also more likely to be smokers compared to girls. The male predominance in smoking habit may be a reflection of socio-cultural acceptability of smoking among male Koreans, and this has been reported in many other settings (21).

The present study found that increasing age, having a parent or closest friend as smoker were positively associated with being a smoker. On the other hand, adolescents who reported having been exposed to antismoking messages were less likely to have been smokers. Perception that smoking was harmful to health was negatively associated with being a smoker in bivariate analysis. However, after controlling for potential confounders, there was no association between the variables.

The association between parental smoking or peer smoking and adolescent smoking has been described elsewhere (14, 15, 22). The relation between having a friend who smokes and adolescent's own smoking could be because an adolescent smoker is likely to choose other smokers as friends or that having a friend who smoke, could influence an adolescent into picking up the habit. However, due to the cross sectional nature of the current study, it is not possible to determine which of the two mechanisms is more likely. We do however believe that both of these explanations may be operational in this study setting.

The present study found that at least 95.5% of both males and females reported having seen tobacco brand names on television in the past 30 days. About half of the study participants reported seeing tobacco-related advertisements in magazines in past 30 days and 7.8% reported having an item with tobacco brand logo. Compared to male study participants, females were more likely to have seen pro-tobacco related advertisements in the media. Males were more likely to own an item with a tobacco brand logo. Although the present study found statistical differences between males and females with regard to the above characteristics, we also recognize that the actual differences are small. That adolescents in South Korea have high exposure to pro-tobacco advertisements on television and magazines, should be cause for concern. Andreeva et al. (16) have reported a higher likelihood of smoking initiation among adolescents who had been exposed to pro-tobacco media in magazines in Ukraine. The finding that pro-tobacco media is associated with smoking adolescents has been reported in many other setting (23).

When we assessed perceptions or attitudes toward smoking, girls were also more likely to believe that smoking is harmful to health than boys. Studies from elsewhere have documented that adolescents who have positive perception of smoking are likely to be smokers (24). Primack et al. (25) have reported that students' perceptions of smoking among the successful/elite and disapproval by parents/peers were independently associated with susceptibility to future smoking in the United States.

Park (9) has reported that school-based anti-smoking programs in Korea have had limited impact towards adolescent smoking. Park suggests that there is need to change the focus of school-based intervention programs from mere knowledge development to a skill training approach. The author also suggests an interactive delivery method be implemented to have better effects on smoking prevention. Kim et al. (26) have reported an experimental study on cessation program of adolescents smoking as being efficacious in preventing adolescent smoking. Current smoking status was determined by biomarkers in this study consisted of 9 sessions with content on enhancement of self-efficacy, stress management, correction of distorted thoughts, consciousness raising, and assertiveness training.

The current study shares limitations with all other studies conducted within the GYTS. Many of these limitations have been reported elsewhere (8,

20, 27, 28). The GYTS recruited in-school students and therefore excluded adolescents who were not enrolled in school. To the extent that in-school adolescents differed from out of school adolescents in the smoking habits. In the present study findings may not be applicable to all adolescents in Korea. However, school enrolment in Korea is high such that out of school children are a small minority. The GYTS collects data only from students who are present on the day of the survey. No follow-up of absent of truant students is done. There is data to suggest that truant adolescents are likely to be smokers and also to engage in other unhealthy lifestyle. To the extent that this may be the case also in Korea, the present study findings may be under-estimates. The data on current smoking status was obtained through self-reports. Adolescents may not have reported accurately their own history of smoking either due to failure to recall or intentionally. Adolescents who are not regular smokers for instance may fail to remember whether they had smoked within the past 30 days. Although there are these concerns, evidence from the United States using a similar data collection methodology as the GYTS found a high level of reliability of the data collection method (29). The findings from the GYTS are also limited by the fact that current smoking status was not verified through assessment of tobacco-related biomarkers such as exhaled carbon monoxide and blood, saliva or urine cotinine (30-32).

In conclusion, the present study has estimated the prevalence of current cigarette smoking among in-school adolescents in Korea, which is lower than in many other Asian countries. There is need to intensify adolescent targeted public health interventions programs as prevalence of smoking appears to be a major health concern in Korea.

ACKNOWLEDGMENTS

We are grateful to the Centers for Disease Prevention and Control (Atlanta, Georgia, United States of America) and the World Health Organization, Geneva, Switzerland for making the dataset available to us for analysis. The CDC and WHO had no part in the analysis, or decision to publish the findings from the study.

This chapter is a revised version of an original paper published in the Indian Journal of Pediatrics (Rudatsikira E, Muula AS, Siziya S. Prevalence, correlates of and perceptions toward cigarette smoking among adolescents in South Korea. Indian J Pediatr 2009;76:505-510) and the authors have obtained the permission from the Indian Journal of Pediatrics to use this material.

REFERENCES

[1] Ezzati M, AD Lopez AD, Rodgers A, Vander Hoorn S, Murray CJL, Comparative Risk Assessment Collaborating Group. Selected major risk factors and global and regional burden of disease. Lancet 2002;360:1347–60.

[2] Bae JM, Lee MS, Shin MH, Kim DH, Li ZM, Ahn YO. Cigarette smoking and risk of lung cancer in Korean men: the Seoul Male Cancer Cohort Study. J Korean Med Sci 2007;22:508-12.

[3] Choi Y, Kim Y, Hong YC, Park SK, Yoo KY. Temporal changes of lung cancer mortality in Korea. J Korean Med Sci 2007;22:524-8.

[4] Lee H, Yoon SJ, Ahn HS. Measuring the burden of major cancers due to smoking in Korea. Cancer Sci 2006;97:530-4.

[5] Frank P, Morris J, Hazell M, Linehan M, Frank T. Smoking, respiratory symptoms and likely asthma in young people: evidence from postal questionnaire surveys in the Wythenshawe Community Asthma Project (WYCAP). BMC Pulm Med 2006;6:10.

[6] Annesi-Maesano I, Oryszczyn MP, Raherison C, Kopferschmitt C, Pauli G, Taytard A, et al. Increased prevalence of asthma and allied diseases among active adolescent tobacco smokers after controlling for passive smoking exposure. A cause for concern? Clin Exp Allergy 2004;34:1017-23.

[7] Miedinger D, Chhajed PN, Karli C, Lupi GA, Leuppi JD. Respiratory symptoms and smoking behaviour in Swiss conscripts. Swiss Med Wkly 2006;136:659-63.

[8] Rudatsikira E, Abdo A, Muula AS. Prevalence and determinants of adolescent tobacco smoking in Addis Ababa, Ethiopia. BMC Public Health 2007;7:176.

[9] Park E. School-based smoking prevention programs for adolescents in South Korea: a systematic review. Health Educ Res 2006;21:407-15.

[10] Park HS, Koo HY, Schepp KG. Predictors of suicidal ideation for adolescents by gender. Taehan Kanho Hakhoe Chi 2005;35:1433-42.

[11] Shin C, Joo S, Kim J, Kim T. Prevalence and correlates of habitual snoring in high school students. Chest 2003;124:1709-15.

[12] Elliot DL, Cheong J, Moe EL, Goldberg L. Cross-sectional study of female students reporting anabolic steroid use. Arch Pediatr Adolesc Med 2007;161:572-7.

[13] Lee E, Tak Y. Peer and parental influences on adolescent smoking. Taehan Kanho Hakhoe Chi 2005;35:694-700.

[14] Scragg R, Laugesen M. Influence of smoking by family and best friend on adolescent tobacco smoking: results from the 2002 New Zealand national survey of year 10 students. Aust NZ J Public Health 2007;31:217-23.

[15] Otten R, Engels RC, van de Ven MO, Bricker JB. Parental smoking and adolescent smoking stages: the role of parents' current and former smoking, and family structure. J Behav Med 2007;30:143-54.

[16] Andreeva TI, Krasovsky KS, Semenova DS. Correlates of smoking initiation among young adults in Ukraine: a cross sectional study. BMC Public Health 2007;7:106.

[17] Kim YH. Korean adolescents' smoking behavior and its correlation with psychological variables. Addict Behav 2005;30:343-50.

[18] Juon HS, Shin Y, Nam JJ. Cigarette smoking among Korean adolescents: prevalence and correlates. Adolescence 1995;30:631-42.

[19] Muula AS, Mpabulungi L. Cigarette smoking prevalence among school-going adolescents in two African capital cities: Kampala Uganda and Lilongwe Malawi. Afr Health Sci 2007;7:45-9.

[20] Kyrlesi A, Soteriades ES, Warren CW, Kremastinou J, Papastergiou P, Jones NR, et al. Tobacco use among students aged 13-15 years in Greece: the GYTS project. BMC Public Health 2007;7:3.

[21] Ando M, Asakura T, Ando S, Simons-Morton BG. Psychosocial factors associated with smoking and drinking among Japanese early adolescent boys and girls: Cross sectional study. Biopsychosoc Med 2007 J4;1:13.

[22] Livaudais JC, Napoles-Springer A, Stewart S, Kaplan CP. Understanding Latino adolescent risk behaviors: parental and peer influences. Ethn Dis 2007;17:298-304.

[23] Lovato C, Linn G, Stead LF, Best A. Impact of tobacco advertising and promotion on increasing adolescent smoking behaviours. Cochrane Database Syst Rev 2003;4:CD003439.

[24] Castrucci BC, Gerlach KK, Kaufman NJ, Orleans CT. The association among adolescents' tobacco use, their beliefs and attitudes, and friends' and parents' opinions of smoking. Matern Child Health J 2002;6: 159-67.

[25] Primack BA, Switzer GE, Dalton MA. Improving measurement of normative beliefs involving smoking among adolescents. Arch Pediatr Adolesc Med 2007;161:434-9.

[26] Kim S, Nam KA, Seo M, Lee HH. Effectiveness of a smoking cessation program for adolescents. Taehan Kanho Hakhoe Chi 2004;34:646-54.

[27] Centers for Disease Control and Prevention (CDC). Tobacco use among students aged 13-15 years—Kurdistan Region, Iraq, 2005. MMWR 2006;55:556-9.

[28] Global Youth Tobacco Survey Collaborative Group. Tobacco use among youth: a cross country comparison. Tob Control 2002;11:252-70.

[29] Brener ND, Kann L, McManus T, Kinchen SA, Sundberg EC, Ross JG. Reliability of the 1999 youth risk behavior survey questionnaire. J Adolesc Health 2002;31:336-42.

[30] Hung J, Lin CH, Wang JD, Chann CC. Exhaled carbon monoxide level as an indicator of cigarette consumption in a workplace cessation program in Taiwan. J Formos Med Assoc 2006;105: 210-3.

[31] Jenkins RA, Counts RW. Personal exposure to environmental tobacco smoke: salivary cotinine, airborne nicotine, and nonsmoker misclassification. J Expo Anal Environ Epidemiol 1999;9:352-63.

[32] Low EC, Ong MC, Tan M. Breath carbon monoxide as an indication of smoking habit in the military setting. Singapore Med J 2004;45:578-82.

In: Smoking and Adolescence ISBN: 978-1-63484-311-9
Editors: M. L. Mazabam, S. Siziya et al. © 2016 Nova Science Publishers, Inc.

Chapter 21

CIGARETTE SMOKING AND ADOLESCENTS IN JAMAICA

Adamson S Muula[1,*], MBBS, MPH, PhD, Seter Siziya[2], BA(Ed), MSc, PhD, and Emmanuel Rudatsikira[3], MD, MPH, DrPH

[1]Department of Community Health, University of Malawi, College of Medicine, Blantyre, Malawi

[2]Department of Community Medicine, University of Zambia, School of Medicine, Lusaka, Zambia

[3]Departments of Biostatistics and Epidemiology and Global Health, Loma Linda University, School of Public Health, Loma Linda, California, USA

In this chapter we estimate the correlates of current cigarette smoking among in-school adolescents in Jamaica 2006 and compare prevalence of smoking and associated factors between 2000 and 2006. In 2006, 1854 participated of whom 49.5 were males and 50.5% females. Altogether 1752 adolescents, 48.8% male and 51.2% females participated in the 2000 survey. Between 2000 and 2006, the prevalence of smoking among Jamaican school-going adolescents went up slightly from 15.2% to 16.7% but this was not statistically significant ($p = 0.222$). The perception that smoking is not harmful increased from 10.9% to 15.9% while parental

* Correspondence: Adamson S Muula, Department of Community Health, University of Malawi, College of Medicine, Blantyre, Malawi. E-mail: muula@email.unc.edu.

smoking decreased from 39.4% to 35.5%. There was a decrease in the rates of adolescents exposed to tobacco adverts on billboards (p-value = 0.037) and in newspapers/magazine (p-value < 0.001). The percentage of adolescents who reported having an item with a tobacco brand logo on it increased from 13.9% to 16.4%. The perception that boys and girls who smoked had more friends increased between 2000 and 2006 (p-values = 0.016 and 0.004 respectively). Current smoking was associated with male gender (OR = 1.55; 95% CI [1.09–2.19]), having smoking parents (OR = 1.75; 95% CI [1.23–2.50]), and smoking friends (OR = 14.94; 95% CI [8.61–25.92] for most or all friends smokers and OR = 4.38; 95% CI [2.93–6.56] for some friends smokers)). Results from this study indicate smoking was positively associated with male gender, having smoking friends or parents. We observed a slightly non-significant increase in the prevalence of smoking between 2000 and 2006 among adolescents in Jamaica. Although there was a decrease in the rates of adolescents exposed to advertisement, the percentage of those who had an item with a tobacco brand logo had increased. The possible impact of the Jamaica's ratification of the Framework Convention on Tobacco control remains to be observed.

INTRODUCTION

Tobacco use is a leading cause of preventable morbidity and mortality from non-communicable diseases (1-3). Adolescent smoking is of public health significance as many adult smokers initiated the smoking habit as adolescents. Adolescent smoking is also important as it is associated with short-term health effects such as incident and exacerbation of asthma (4). Smoking in adolescents may also be a marker of other unhealthy lifestyles or social problems such as alcohol use, illicit drug use, sedentary lifestyle, unprotected sex and truancy (5-9).

Globally, studies to estimate the prevalence of adolescent smoking and associated factors have been spurred by the Global Youth Tobacco Survey (GYTS) (10, 11). The GYTS was established by the World Health Organization (WHO) and Centers for Disease Control and Prevention's (CDC's) Office on Smoking and Health to track tobacco use among young people across countries using a standard methodology and core questionnaire. The aim of the GYTS surveillance system is to enhance the capacity of countries to design, implement, and evaluate tobacco control and public health prevention programs. Many of the published reports on Global Youth Tobacco Survey have been single year prevalence reports. However, as repeat surveys are conducted within the same settings (countries), there is opportunity to track the changes in prevalence of smoking and associated factors. In the case of Jamaica, the first round of the GYTS was conducted in 2000 and a repeat survey done in 2006. We therefore have two time points when data on adolescent smoking were obtained using nationally representative survey methods and common methodology. We therefore carried this study to estimate the prevalence of current cigarette smoking among in-school adolescents in Jamaica and associated factors using GYTS methodology in 2000 and 2006. Furthermore, we also conducted regression analysis to estimate the size of effect of association between current cigarette smoking and a list of explanatory variables. Data from the Jamaica GYTS were selected because this country has had a repeat GYTS, with the second survey having conducted just a few years following ratification of the Framework Convention on Tobacco Control (FCTC).

OUR STUDY

We conducted secondary analysis of the Jamaican Global Youth Tobacco Survey (GYTS) implemented in 2000 and 2006. A full description of the data collection methods in the GYTS has been reported elsewhere (11). Current cigarette smoking was defined as having smoked a cigarette, even a single puff, within the last 30 days preceding the survey. We were also interested to explore if the differences in the prevalence of smoking between the 2000 and 2006 survey. Data were analysed using SUDAAN software version 9 (Research Triangle Institute, Research Triangle Park, North Carolina, United States of America). Chi-square tests were used to compare differences between proportions.

FINDINGS

Altogether 1,752 adolescents, 48.8% male and 51.2% females participated in the 2000 survey. In 2006, 1,854 participated of whom 49.5 were males and 50.5% females. Table 1 indicates the prevalence of smoking among Jamaican school-going adolescents went up from 15.2% in 2000 to 16.7% in 2006, but this was not statistically significant ($p = 0.222$). The perception that smoking is not harmful increased 5% (from 10.9% to 15.9%). Reported parental smoking decreased from 39.4% to 35.5% in the same period of time.

Table 1. Prevalence of smoking among Jamaican adolescents in 2000 and 2006

Characteristic	Year 2000	Year 2006	P value
	% (95% CI)	% (95% CI)	
Age (years)			0.942
Total	15.2 (13.4–17.3)	16.7 (12.9–18.6)	
<14	11.6 (9.8–14.3)	15.5 (12.9–18.6)	
14	15.8 (9.2–25.7)	15.2 (12.2–18.7)	
15	20.9 (16.9–25.3)	18.2 (14.6–22.5)	
16+	22.9 (18.5–26.5)	21.7 (16.3–28.3)	
Gender			0.859
Females	11.7 (9.8–13.9)	12.0 (10.0–14.3)	
Males	19.3 (16.1–23.0)	21.8 (18.9–25.0)	
Parental smoking status			0.782
None	60.8 (57.8–64.5)	64.4 (61.8–66.4)	
One or both parents smokers	27.0 (22.7–31.0)	35.5 (33.1–38.4)	
Perception that smoking is harmful			0.890
Yes	10.9 (7.9–12.7)	15.9 (13.1–18.5)	
No	89.1 (86.5–91.7)	84.1 (81.9–86.3)	

Table 2 compares the rates of exposure to adverts between 2000 and 2006. There was a significant decrease in the prevalence of adolescents exposed to tobacco adverts on billboards ($p = 0.037$) and in newspapers/magazine ($p < 0.001$). The percentage of adolescents who reported having an item with a tobacco brand logo on it increased from 13.9% to 16.4%.

Table 3 indicates that the perception that boys and girls who smoked had more friends increased significantly between 2000 and 2006 ($p = 0.016$ and 0.004 respectively). There was no significant difference in the perception that boys or girls who smoked were attractive.

Table 2. Exposure to tobacco advertisements among Jamaican adolescents in 2000 and 2006

Characteristic	Year 2000	Year 2006	P value
	% (95% CI)	% (95% CI)	
Seen cigarette brand name on TV in past 30 days	76.9 (74.6–79.0)	67.4 (65.0–69.7)	0.080
Males	76.4 (72.6–79.7)	66.0 (62.5–69.3)	
Females	77.4 (74.6–80.0)	68.7 (65.5–71.8)	
Has item with cigarette brand logo	13.9 (12.2–15.8)	16.4 (14.6–18.3)	0.296
Males	15.7 (12.8–19.0)	19.4 (16.6–22.4)	
Females	12.2 (10.3–14.4)	13.5 (11.4–15.9)	
Seen tobacco adverts on billboards in past 30 days	66.0 (66.5–68.4)	62.9 (60.5–65.2)	0.037
Males	64.9 (60.8–68.7)	63.0 (59.5–66.3)	
Females	67.0 (64.0–9.9)	62.8 (59.5–66.0)	
Seen tobacco adverts in newspapers/magazines in past 30 days	61.4 (58.8–63.8)	56.5 (54.1–58.9)	<0.001
Males	61.7 (57.6–65.6)	56.2 (52.7–59.8)	
Females	61.1 (58.0–64.1)	56.8 (53.4–60.1)	

Table 3. Attitudes towards tobacco smoking distributed among Jamaican adolescents in 2000 and 2006

Characteristic	Year 2000	Year 2006	P value
	% (95% CI)	% (95% CI)	
Felt that boys who smoke have more friends	49.4 (45.4–51.5)	69.6 (66.7–72.3)	0.016
Males	44.8 (39.5–48.0)	64.4 (60.0–68.6)	
Females	54.3 (48.6–57.1)	75.0 (71.2–78.5)	
Felt like girls who smoke had more friends	25.2 (22.6–27.9)	35.9 (33.2–38.8)	0.004
Males	24.9 (21.0–29.3)	34.9 (30.9–39.0)	
Females	25.4 (22.3–29.0)	37.1 (33.2–41.2)	
Felt that boys who smoke are attractive	10.6 (8.9–12.6)	14.8 (13.0–16.9)	0.175
Males	13.8 (10.8–17.5)	17.9 (14.9–21.4)	
Females	7.8 (6.2–9.9)	12.2 (10.0–14.7)	
Felt that girls who smoke are attractive	8.9 (7.4–10.7)	11.1 (9.5–12.9)	0.327
Males	11.7 (9.1–15.1)	13.6 (11.0–16.4)	
Females	6.3 (4.8–8.2)	8.9 (7.0–11.2)	

Table 4. Factors associated with current smoking among Jamaican adolescents in 2006

Characteristics	Unadjusted odds ratios (95% CI[1])	Adjusted odds ratios (95% CI)
Age (years)		
<14	1	1
14	0.97 (0.69, 1.37)	0.79 (0.50, 1.25)
15	1.21 (0.86, 1.71)	1.08 (0.68, 1.73)
16+	1.51 (1.00, 2.29)	0.92 (0.53, 1.62)
Gender		
Female	1	1
Male	2.04 (1.56, 2.68)	1.55 (1.09, 2.19)
Parental smoking status		
None	1	1
One or both parents smokers	2.38 (1.80, 3.16)	1.75 (1.23, 2.50)
Best friend smokers		
None	1	1
Some	5.38 (3.80, 7.61)	4.38 (2.93, 6.56)
Most or all	21.99 (13.99, 34.57)	14.94 (8.61, 25.92)
Perception that smoking is harmful		
No	1	1
Yes	0.83 (0.57, 1.23)	0.95 (0.57, 1.58)

Table 4 presents results from bivariate and multivariate analyses (2006). In bivariate analysis, current smoking was positively associated with male gender (OR = 2.04; 95% CI [1.56–2.68]), having smoking parents (OR = 2.38; 95% CI [1.80–3.16]), and smoking friends (OR = 21.99; 95% CI [13.99–34.57] for most or all friends smokers and OR = 5.38; 95% CI [3.80–7.61] for some friends smokers). The perception that smoking is harmful was associated with a non-significant decrease in the odds of smoking (OR = 0.83; 95% [0.57–1.23]). Results from the multivariate analysis were weaker than in bivariate analysis but with the same inference.

DISCUSSION

The prevalence of current cigarette smoking among in-school adolescents in 2000 and 2006 were 15.2% and 16.7% respectively, with no statistically significant change. The male and females GYTS prevalence estimates of current cigarette smoking among in-school adolescent were: 7.6% and 6.4% in Barbados (2002); 6.2% and 3.7% in Bahamas (2004); 18.9% and 10.4% in Belize (2002); 14.1% and 13.8% in Haiti (2005); 11.5% and 7.9% in St Lucia (2000) and 16.0% and 7.6% in Trinidad and Tobago (2000) (12). Furthermore the prevalence of current cigarette smoking in-school adolescents had been reported at 1%–4.5% in Ethiopia, (10), 3.0% in Blantyre-Malawi (13), and 17.5% overall prevalence in the Americas (14).

We also observed that the proportion of adolescents who reported having a parent who was a smoker reduced, so did adolescents who reported having been exposed to pro-tobacco advertisements through billboards and magazines. However the proportion of adolescents who reported owning an item with a tobacco brand logo increased. It is difficult to determine the reasons for increases in some of the characteristics while there are increased in other pro-tobacco measures.

One observation regarding the Jamaican tobacco landscape is that the country signed into the World Health Organization's Framework Convention on Tobacco Control (FCTC) on 24 September 2003 and adoption followed on 7 July 2005. Currently, Jamaica has banned tobacco advertisements on local television and radio programs but advertisements from international programs have not been banned. There are also tobacco cessation programs at some health facilities with nicotine replacement therapy available. However, more still needs to be done as advertisements in local newspapers, magazines, billboards, tobacco brand logos on items not related to tobacco, public environmental tobacco smoking have not been banned. There are however, national tobacco control objectives and a dedicated agency for the control of tobacco (12).

We also found that current smoking among the adolescents was associated with having closest friends who were smokers, parental smoking and male gender. Perception that smoking was harmful to health was associated with reduced likelihood of smoking.

Previous studies on adolescent smoking conducted elsewhere have also reported positive relationship between peer smoking, parental smoking, male gender and smoking (10). Parental smoking may influence adolescent smoking by facilitating the ready availability of cigarettes in the home and moderating parental attitudes towards adolescent smoking. Peer smoking could influence adolescent attitudes and smoking in a similar way as has been described for parental smoking. It is also possible that adolescents who are smokers may be more likely to choose other smokers as closest friends. However due to the cross sectional nature of data collection over the two surveys, it is not possible to assign any of the factors as causes of adolescent smoking. Furthermore, for non-time varying factors such as gender, we cannot really say that male gender is the cause of smoking but rather that being male may be associated with other intermediate factors that may explain male predominance of smoking.

We found that adolescents who perceived that smoking was harmful were less likely to smoke and those who perceived that smoking made youth attractive were less likely to smoke. According to the PRECEED/PROCEED model of health promotion individuals are likely to adopt a healthy behavior if they have the appropriate knowledge and attitude, are exposed to reinforcing and enabling factors such as friends, family and health workers (15). We therefore suggest that intervention programs should aim to change adolescent behavior by highlighting the harmful effects of smoking. There is need to ensure that adolescents are not exposed to images that glamorize smoking. Negative attitudes towards smoking may influence eventual avoidance of smoking among adolescents.

It is however interesting to note that exposure to pro-tobacco advertisement on television, magazines and newspapers and billboards declined from 2000 to 2006. However, ownership of item with tobacco brand logo increased over the period under review. Whether the decline in prevalence of exposure to advertisement was related to bans on local television programs remain to be seen. Paradoxically, the proportion of adolescents with favorable perception towards smoking increased.

In a study of high school forms 4 and 5 and Jamaica, Siyobo and Lee (16) reported prevalence of cigarette smoking at 16.6%. Males, urban residents and adolescents whose parents were skilled professionals were more likely to smoke than rural, female and children of less skilled parents. A comparison of the Soyibo and Lee report (16) and our findings from the current study (years 2000 and 2006 surveys), suggest stability of the prevalence of cigarette smoking among adolescents in Jamaica.

The limitations of the GYTS have been reported previously elsewhere (10). Firstly data from the Global Youth Tobacco Survey are obtained through self-reports. As is the case with essentially all study methods where study participants self-report, there may be under-reporting as well as over-reporting. The GYTS aims to minimize such misreporting for emphasizing the collection of data through anonymous questionnaires. The possibility of mis-reporting cannot be entirely removed just by emphasizing anonymity although it can be reduced substantially.

Data from the GYTS are obtained only from students who are available in school that the survey is administered in the particular school. Students who are absent from school due to any reason are not followed up. Slonim-Nevo and Mukuka have reported that out of school adolescent were more likely to engage in unhealthy behaviours compared to in-school peers (17). If this were also the case in Jamaica, then our results would be under-estimates. We however do not know whether this was the case or not; although it is important for the reader to keep this possibility in mind.

As the GYTS only recruits students that are enrolled in school, the findings may not be applicable to all adolescents in Jamaica as out of school adolescents may have prevalence estimates substantially different from adolescents who were enrolled in school. However, primary and secondary school enrolment ratios in Jamaica are 90% and 88% with 97% and 92% attendance ratios (18). Any biases that may result because of non-enrolment and nonattendance at school are likely to be minimal. Our results can be described as fairly representative of the adolescent population in Jamaica.

Traditionally, trend analysis requires at least assessment of the prevalence at three different time points. Our study is based in two time points. However, even with the slight increase, a third reading that will show that trend is up may be more meaningful, a downward future prevalence will suggest inconclusive findings. We await future GYTS or similarly designed studies to assess whether there is a trend in prevalence of cigarette smoking among in school adolescents in Jamaica. In these future studies, it should be possible to use ARIMA (autoregressive integrated moving average) analysis to identify real changes having separated out noise from the results (19).

In conclusion, we have demonstrated that the prevalence of current cigarette smoking among in school adolescents in Jamaica has risen slightly but not statistically significant. In fact the prevalence is relatively similar to previous estimate in the late 1990's. Predictors of smoking such as male gender and smoking status of parents or friends have either decreased on remained stable over the years. The recent signing in of Jamaica to the WHO's Framework Convention on Tobacco Control may provide the socio-political environment for significant reduction of tobacco use among adolescents in Jamaica.

ACKNOWLEDGMENTS

The authors are grateful to the Centers for Disease Control and Prevention (Atlanta, Georgia, United States of America) and the World Health Organization, Division of Non- communicable Diseases for making the data available for our analysis. Funding for the GYTS is provided by the Canadian Public Health Association, National Cancer Institute, United Nations Children Emergency Fund, and World Health Organization – Tobacco Free Initiative. The authors are not associated in any way with the funding agencies of the GYTS. We are thankful to the in-school adolescents who had participated in the survey.

This paper is a revised version of a publication in the BMC Research Notes (Muula AS, Siziya S, Rudatsikira E. Cigarette smoking and associated factors among in-school adolescents in Jamaica: comparison of the Global Youth Tobacco Surveys 2000 and 2006. BMC Res Notes 2008;1:8) and the authors have obtained the permission from BMC Research Notes to use this material.

REFERENCES

[1] Mannino DM, Buist AS. Global burden of COPD: risk factors, prevalence, and future trends. Lancet 2007;370:765-73.

[2] Mathers CD, Loncar D. Projections of global mortality and burden of disease from 2002 to 2030. PLoS Med 2006;3:e442.

[3] He J, Gu D, Wu X, Reynolds K, Duan X, Yao C, et al. Major causes of death among men and women in China. N Engl J Med 2005;353:1124-34.

[4] Gilliland FD, Islam T, Berhane K, Gauderman WJ, McConnell R, Avol E, et al. Regular smoking and asthma incidence in adolescents. Am J Respir Crit Care Med 2006;174:1094-100.

[5] Larson NI, Story M, Perry CL, Neumark-Sztainer D, Hannan PJ. Are diet and physical activity patterns related to cigarette smoking in adolescents? Findings from Project EAT. Prev Chronic Dis 2007;4:A51.

[6] Ando M, Asakura T, Ando S, Simons-Morton BG. Psychosocial factors associated with smoking and drinking among Japanese early adolescent boys and girls: Cross-sectional study. Biopsychosoc Med 2007;1:13.

[7] Best D, Manning V, Gossop M, Gross S, Strang J. Excessive drinking and other problem behaviours among 14–16 year old schoolchildren. Addict Behav 2006;31:1424-35.

[8] Licanin I, Redzic A. Alcohol abuse and risk behavior among adolescents in larger cities in Bosnia and Herzegovina. Med Arh 2005;59:164-7.

[9] Bachman JG, Johnston LD, O'Malley PM. Smoking, drinking, and drug use among American high school students: correlates and trends, 1975–1979. Am J Public Health 1981;71:59-69.

[10] Rudatsikira E, Abdo A, Muula AS. Prevalence and determinants of adolescent tobacco smoking in Addis Ababa, Ethiopia. BMC Public Health 2007;7:176.

[11] Centers for Disease Control and Prevention (CDC). Global Tobacco Surveillance System (GTSS): purpose, production, and potential. J Sch Health 2005;75:15-24.

[12] World Report on the Global Tobacco Epidemic 2008. Geneva: World Health Organization, 2008.

[13] Muula AS. Prevalence and determinants of cigarette smoking among adolescents in Blantyre City, Malawi. Tanzan Health Res Bull 2007;9:48-51.

[14] Centers for Disease Control and Prevention (CDC). Use of cigarettes and other tobacco products among students aged 13– 5 years – worldwide, 1999-2005. MMWR 2006;55:553-6.

[15] Green LW, Kreuter MW. Health promotion planning: An educational and environmental approach, 2nd ed. Palo Alto, CA: Mayfield, 1991.

[16] Soyibo K, Lee MG. Use of alcohol, tobacco and non-prescription drugs among Jamaican high school students. West Indian Med J 1997;464:111-4.

[17] Slonim-Nevo V, Mukuka L. AIDS-related knowledge, attitudes and behavior among adolescents in Zambia. AIDS Behav 2005;9:223-31.

[18] UNICEF: State of the World's Children 2008. URL: http://www.unicef.org/sowc08/statistics/tables.php.

[19] The United States Census Bureau. The X-12-ARIMA Seasonal Adjustment Program. URL: http://www.census.gov/srd/www/x12a/.

In: Smoking and Adolescence ISBN: 978-1-63484-311-9
Editors: M. L. Mazabam, S. Siziya et al. © 2016 Nova Science Publishers, Inc.

Chapter 22

TOBACCO AND ADOLESCENTS IN HIMACHAL PRADESH, INDIA

Jayakaran S Job[1,2], MD, DrPH, Adamson S Muula[3,*], MPH, MBBS, Seter Siziya[4], BA(Ed), MSc, PhD, and Emmanuel Rudatsikira[1,2], MD, MPH, DrPH

[1]Department of Global Health, School of Public Health, Loma Linda University, Loma Linda, California, USA
[2]Department of Epidemiology and Biostatistics, Loma Linda University, Loma Linda, USA
[3]Department of Public Health, Division of Community Health, College of Medicine, University of Malawi, Blantyre, Malawi
[4]Department of Community Medicine, School of Medicine, University of Zambia, Lusaka, Zambia

In this chapter we estimate the prevalence and associated factors of tobacco use among school-going adolescents in Himachal Pradesh, India. Data was used from the Global Youth Tobacco Survey (GYTS) 2004 to determine tobacco use prevalence, determinants, attitudes, and exposure to tobacco advertisements among adolescents. Frequencies and their 95% confidence intervals (CI) were calculated. Odds ratios (unadjusted and

* Correspondence: Adamson S Muula, MBBS, MPH, PhD, Department of Public Health, Division of Community Health, College of Medicine, University of Malawi, Private Bag 360, Chichiri, Blantyre 3, Malawi. E-mail: adamsonmuula@yahoo.com.

adjusted) and their 95% CI were obtained using logistic regression analysis. Of the 1,976 respondents whom gender was identified, 6.4% males and 3.9% females reported current tobacco use (p = 0.021). After controlling for age, gender, parental tobacco use status, and perception of risks of tobacco use, 'having some friends who were tobacco users' was associated with tobacco use (OR = 4.65; 95% CI [2.85, 7.59], the association being stronger if all their friends were tobacco users OR=11.78; 95% CI [4.84, 28.63]. Participants reported high exposure to tobacco advertisements on billboards (71.0%), magazine (100%) and television (53.3%). Nearly one in seven respondents (14.7%) reported possessing an item with tobacco brand on it. The proportion of males who felt that tobacco use was harmful was higher than that for females (p=0.002). Findings from this study emphasize the critical role of friends, parents and the media in influencing adolescent tobacco use behaviours and the need for considering social and domestic environments in planning gender-specific interventions for this vulnerable population subgroup.

INTRODUCTION

Tobacco use is a leading cause of non-communicable diseases such as chronic obstructive pulmonary disease, cardiovascular conditions and a range of cancers (1). There is growing evidence that while tobacco use has stabilised or is in decline in western industrialised nations, there is increased prevalence of use in resource-limited settings and emerging economies (2). A list of reasons why this situation has arisen include: aggressive marketing by tobacco firms; limited public health interventions, and a pre-occupation with communicable diseases that has overstretched public heath efforts (3-6). Furthermore, the global proliferation of various mass media, may also have contributed to the "globalisation" of tobacco use (7, 8).

While data on tobacco use, especially data on cigarette smoking and associated factors among adolescents in many states in India has been reported, data from some areas are limited. Data is also currently available on the factors that are associated with tobacco use among adolescents in other international settings (9-12). Public health program planners are likely to benefit from data generated from their own geographical areas when considering options to determine the most efficient allocation of often scarce public intervention resources for example, by targeting factors that are strongly associated with tobacco use based on the effect measures. Furthermore, in the absence of published data, it may be difficult to raise the social profile and concerns associated with tobacco use among researchers and policy makers. Finally, meta-analysis of data on the factors that are associated with tobacco use can only be carried out using available published information.

A publication by Sinha et al. (13) aimed at linking tobacco control policies and data on tobacco use in India considered the prevalence of the following attributes among 13 to 15 year olds in India: smoking; cessation experience; exposure to second-hand smoke; access to, and availability of tobacco and exposure to advertisements. Not only is this publication restricted to ages 13 to 15 years, as is the focus of the GYTS (Global Youth Tobacco Survey), but only prevalence estimates and not an assessment of the association between tobacco use and those explanatory variables were reported. The reader therefore is left to speculate whether those exposures are in fact associated with tobacco use. Furthermore, Sinha et al. (13) aggregated data from all states in the country and average India estimates were obtained and no individual state estimates were reported.

The India Tobacco Control Act (ITCA) was signed into law in 2003 with the goal to reduce tobacco consumption and protect citizens from exposure to secondhand smoke (SHS). In 2005, the Indian government ratified the World Health Organization Framework Convention on Tobacco Control (WHO FCTC). Among the many provisions of the ITCA are sections prohibiting smoking in public places, prohibiting direct or indirect advertisement of cigarettes and other tobacco products on billboards and in all media excluding point of sale, and prohibiting the sale of tobacco products to persons less than 18 years of age that is the focus of the GYTS. Data used in this article were collected in 2004, possibly before the ITCA had enough time to effect meaningful changes regarding tobacco use practices among adolescents in India. In this paper we attempt to estimate the prevalence and associated factors of tobacco use among in-school adolescents in Himachal Pradesh, India. Previous reports from this setting have not been able to demonstrate which factors may be associated and therefore important in the prevention of smoking.

OUR STUDY

The present study was a secondary analysis of publicly available data from the Centers for Disease Control and Prevention (CDC) on the 2004 Global Health Survey for the State of Himachal Pradesh, India. The survey was conducted according to the Global Tobacco Surveillance System (GTSS) as has been described elsewhere (14). The GYTS used a standard survey questionnaire with core questions (the same in all geographical settings) and country-specific questions that countries can add to cover research questions considered pertinent by country cooperating partners as critical for that particular setting.

The GYTS recruited in-school adolescents in classes with the majority of its students who are between the ages 13 and 15 years. A two-stage clustered sampling survey approach is used in which the primary sampling units (PSUs) are schools with students in the eligible age group (13-15 years). At the second stage of sampling, eligible classes (classes with the majority of students of ages 13 to 15 years) within the selected schools are randomly selected. All the students within the selected classes are eligible to participate in the study, regardless of their actual ages. Only students who are present on the day the survey is administered in a particular school are surveyed and no replacement of absent students is attempted. While all students eligible and present are invited to participate, the students are informed that they are free to elect not to participate and also free not to answer any question with which they feel uncomfortable. Surveys using the same methodology have been conducted in other settings (13).

The GYTS questionnaire is administered and anonymously self-completed within a single class period. Information collected include the following variables: age, gender, current smoking status, parental smoking, having friends who smoked, perception that smoking is harmful to health, exposure to tobacco advertisements, and approval of smoking among boys and girls.

Data were obtained from the CDC and analyzed using SUDAAN software 9.0 (Research Triangle Institute, Research Triangle Park, North Carolina, United States). Frequencies and 95% confidence intervals of relevant variables such as demographics, approval of smoking among boys and girls, and exposure to tobacco advertisements were generated and are reported. To assess the associations between a selected list of variables identified from the literature as possibly associated with current cigarette smoking, logistic regression analysis was conducted both at bivariate and multivariate level. These explanatory variables were: gender; age; smoking by the best friend, and parental smoking.

The bivariate logistic regression analysis was conducted to obtain unadjusted odds ratios with current tobacco use (Yes or No) as the outcome of interest. Tobacco use was defined as having used tobacco in any form (smoking, chewing or applying tobacco) during the past 30 days.

Each of the following variables was considered as explanatory variables: age; gender; peer smoking; parental smoking; and perception that smoking is harmful. Further multivariable models were also fitted to obtain adjusted odds ratios.

FINDINGS

Of the 1,976 students whom gender was reported, 41.8% were females. The median age for the sample was 15 (Q1= 16-17, Q3=14) years. The prevalence of current tobacco use was 6.4% (95% CI [5.1, 8.0]) among males and 3.9% (95% CI [2.8, 5.5]) among females.

Table 1 indicates that in bivariate analysis, males were more likely to use tobacco than females (OR=1.66; 95% CI [1.08, 2.56]). Compared to participants whose parents did not use tobacco, those with parents who were tobacco users were more likely to use tobacco (OR=1.85; 95% CI [1.23, 2.79]). Those with most or all friends who used tobacco were 14 times more likely to use tobacco than those who had no friends who used tobacco (OR=14.36; 95% CI [6.77, 30.46]). Participants who perceived that tobacco use was harmful were less likely to use tobacco than those who did not perceive tobacco as harmful to health (OR=0.56; 95% CI [0.37, 1.00]).

Table 1 also indicates that in multivariate analysis, having close friends who used tobacco was very strongly associated with tobacco use after controlling for age, gender, parental tobacco use, and perception of hazards caused by tobacco use. Those who had most or all friends who used tobacco were more than 11 times likely to use tobacco than those who had no friends who used tobacco (OR=11.71; 95% CI [4.79, 28.64]). Those who had some friends who used tobacco were more than four times likely to use tobacco than those who had no friends who used tobacco (OR=4.65; 95% CI [2.85, 7.58]).

Table 2 indicates that participants were exposed to tobacco advertisements through magazine (100%), billboards (71.0%), and television (53.3%). More than one in ten respondents (14.7%) reported possessing an item with tobacco brand logo on it. There was no gender difference in rates of those who reported having an item with tobacco brand logo (p =0.851) nor on prevalence of exposure to tobacco advertisements on hoardings (p=0.149) and television (p=0.474).

Table 1. Factors associated with current tobacco use in Himachal Pradesh, India

Characteristic	Percentage of smokers	Unadjusted Odds ratio (95% Confidence Interval)	Adjusted Odds ratio (95% Confidence Interval)
Age (years)			
11–12	3.8	1.00	1.00
13	6.4	1.71 [0.71, 4.08]	1.29 [0.49, 3.34]
14	3.9	1.03 [0.44, 2.45]	0.87 [0.34, 2.21]
15	4.8	1.27 [0.55, 2.94]	0.98 [0.39, 2.47]
16–17	7.1	1.93 [0.86, 4.31]	1.15 [0.46, 2.84]
Gender			
Female	3.9	1.00	1.00
Male	6.4	1.66 [1.08, 2.56]	1.21 [0.73, 1.99]
Parental tobacco use			
None	4.1	1.00	1.00
One or both parents smokers	7.3	1.85 [1.23, 2.79]	1.30 [0.81, 2.07]
Best friends tobacco users			
None	3.1	1.00	1.00
Some	12.7	4.63 [2.99, 7.16]	4.65 [2.85, 7.58]
Most or all	31.2	14.36 [6.77, 30.46]	11.71 [4.79, 28.64]
Perception that tobacco use is harmful			
No	7.2	1.00	1.00
Yes	4.7	0.56 [0.37, 1.00]	0.87 [0.46, 1.63]
Family member discussed harmful effects of tobacco use			
No	5.9	1.00	1.00
Yes	4.9	0.84 [0.56, 1.28]	0.84 [0.51, 1.39]

Table 2. Exposure to tobacco advertisements distributed by gender among adolescents in Himachal Pradesh, India

Characteristics	Number of participants	% of total and 95% CI [p value]*
		[P=0.474]
Seen tobacco brand name on TV in past 30 days	1973	53.3 [51.0,55.5]
Males	1140	54.0 [51.1, 56.9]
Females	833	52.2 [48.7, 55.6]
Has item with tobacco brand logo	1969	14.7 [13.2, 16.4]

Characteristics	Number of participants	% of total and 95% CI [p value]*
Males	1136	14.8 [12.8, 17.1]
Females	833	14.6 [12.3, 17.1]
		[P=0.149]
Seen tobacco adverts on hoardings in past 30 days	1973	71.0 [68.9, 73.0]
Males	1140	72.3 [69.6, 74.9]
Females	833	69.1 [65.8, 72.2]

* p value comparing levels of exposure between males and females.

Table 3. Attitudes towards tobacco use distributed by gender among adolescents in Himachal Pradesh, India

Characteristic	Number of participants	% of total and 95% CI [p value]*
Felt that boys who use tobacco have more friends	1701	100
Males	1000	100
Females	701	100
		[P<0.001]
Felt like girls who use tobacco have more friends	1647	12.5 [10.9, 14.3]
Males	959	15.5 [13.3, 18.0]
Females	688	8.3 [6.4, 10.6]
		[P=0.673]
Felt that boys who use tobacco are attractive	1337	26.7 [24.3, 29.1]
Males	789	27.9 [24.8, 21.2]
Females	548	24.9 [21.5, 28.7]
Felt that girls who use tobacco are attractive	1675	24.7 [22.7, 26.9]
Males	978	27.7 [24.9, 30.6]
Females	697	20.5 [16.7, 23.7]
		[P=0.002]
Felt that tobacco use is harmful to health	1772	84.8 [83.0, 86.4]
Males	1028	87.1 [84.8, 89.0]
Females	744	81.6 [78.6, 84.3]

* p value comparing levels of exposure between males and females.

Table 3 indicates that the majority (84.8%) of respondents felt that tobacco use was harmful to health. All participants thought that male smokers had more friends compared to 12.5% who felt that females who used tobacco had more friends. About 1 in 4 respondents thought that males and females who used tobacco were attractive (26.7% and 24.7% respectively). The proportion of males (87.1%) who felt that tobacco use was harmful was significantly higher (p=0.002) than that for females (81.6%).

DISCUSSION

We report an overall current tobacco use of 6.4% (95% CI [5.1, 8.0]) among males and 3.9% (95% CI [2.8, 5.5]) among females (p = 0.021). We found male predominance (but not statistically significant) of tobacco use. The male predominance has been reported with regard to cigarette smoking in other settings (16-18). However, this finding is not universal. For instance, in the United States of America, cigarette smoking rates are similar among male and female adolescents (19), while in other countries like Turkey, the gender gap is closing (20). We suggest that the acceptability of smoking among males compared to females may be responsible for the higher rates found in males in Himachal Pradesh. We found in the current study that tobacco use among boys was perceived as more favourable compared to use in females.

As also reported in other studies, we found that the odds of being a tobacco user were higher among adolescents whose friends used tobacco, and among those who had parents who used tobacco, and among males. This was not significant at multivariate analysis. Although there was higher tobacco use among adolescents 16-17 years old (7.1%) compared to those 11-12 years (3.8%), the difference was not statistically significant. When designing specific anti-tobacco intervention programs, these study findings suggest the importance of focusing efforts directed at friends who use tobacco.

In a cross sectional study, and when data on the temporal sequence of events are not available, it is not possible to determine if a factor is causally associated with the outcome (tobacco use) (21, 22). In the context of this study analysis, it is not possible to assess whether befriending a smoker is a cause of tobacco use or if tobacco users themselves are more likely to befriend other tobacco users. Perhaps, both mechanisms may be at work. Another explanation for this observation may be that tobacco users are more likely to influence others to initiate and continue this behaviour.

We did not find that adolescents who believed that tobacco is harmful to health were less or more likely to use tobacco. While we posit that adolescent education about the effects of education is a worthwhile exercise although it may not necessarily result in significant behavioural change. This is not surprising as knowledge alone has been found to be insufficient to effect positive behavioural change (24).

We report in the present study levels of exposure to tobacco advertisement in various forms of media. We consider the study results as baseline findings to assess the potential impact of the India Tobacco Control Act (which was signed into law the same year of the survey) and the WHO FCTC efforts to prevent tobacco advertisement in India.

Despite the inherent strengths of this study (such as, obtaining a cross state sample and using a standardized questionnaire), the present study has several limitations. Firstly, as data were collected by a cross sectional survey, the effect measures reported (odds ratios) are only indicative of associations between the variables. Hence, one cannot ascribe any causation. Secondly, self-reported data is based on the subject's memory and honesty. To the extent that study participants intentionally misreported or failed to recall any of the variables, our results may be biased. Thirdly, no attempt was done to verify or validate current tobacco use with tobacco metabolites laboratory analysis of specimens such as saliva or urine (25). Finally, the data were collected from adolescents attending school and available on the day their school was visited by the data collection team. If out of school adolescents and students who were absent differ from other students in their tobacco use, our results may not be representative of all adolescents in Himachal Pradesh.

CONCLUSION

Using data from the 2003 Himachal Global Youth Tobacco Survey, we report a prevalence of all forms of tobacco at 6.4% among males and 3.9% in females. Adolescent tobacco use was associated with tobacco use among friends and parents. The proportion of males who felt that tobacco use was harmful was significantly higher than that for females. These findings call for consideration of the adolescents' social and domestic environments in the design, implementation and evaluation of gender-specific interventions to prevent tobacco use.

ACKNOWLEDGMENTS

The authors declare that they have no financial disclosures or competing interests. We are grateful to the Centers for Disease Control and Prevention (CDC), Atlanta, Georgia, United States, for making the data available for our analysis. The CDC however did not influence the decision to analyse the data or submission of manuscript for publication. We also thank the students who participated in the Himachal Pradesh GYTS conducted in 2004.

REFERENCES

[1] Mathers CD, Loncar D. Projections of global mortality and burden of disease from 2002 to 2030. PLoS Med 2006;3:e442.

[2] Lopez AD, Mathers CD. Measuring the global burden of disease and epidemiological transitions: 2002-2030. Ann Trop Med Parasitol 2006;100:481-99.

[3] Haddock CK, Hoffman K, Taylor JE, Schwab L, Poston WS, Lando HA. An analysis of messages about tobacco in the Military Times magazines. Nicotine Tob Res 2008;10:1191-7.

[4] Suzuki S, Itano D, Yamamoto LG. Prime-time television exposure to high priority school-aged social-developmental issues. Hawaii Med J 2008;67:74-5, 83.

[5] Belstock SA, Connolly GN, Carpenter CM, Tucker L. Using alcohol to sell cigarettes to young adults: a content analysis of cigarette advertisements. J Am Coll Health 2008;56:383-9.

[6] Braun S, Mejia R, Ling PM, Pérez-Stable EJ. Tobacco industry targeting youth in Argentina. Tob Control 2008;17:111-7.

[7] Yach D, Bettcher D. Globalisation of tobacco industry influence and new global responses. Tob Control 2000;9:206-16.

[8] Beaglehole R, Yach D. Globalisation and the prevention and control of non-communicable disease: the neglected chronic diseases of adults. Lancet 2003;362:903-8.

[9] Rudatsikira E, Muula AS, Siziya S, Mataya RH. Correlates of cigarette smoking among school-going adolescents in Thailand: findings from the Thai global youth tobacco survey 2005. Int Arch Med 2008;1:8.

[10] Rudatsikira E, Dondog J, Siziya S, Muula AS. Prevalence and determinants of adolescent cigarette smoking in Mongolia. Singapore Med J 2008;49:57-62.

[11] Unger JB, Palmer PH, Dent CW, Rohrbach LA, Johnson CA. Ethnic differences in adolescent smoking prevalence in California: are multi-ethnic youth at higher risk? Tob Control 2000;9(Suppl 2):II9-14.

[12] Alexander C, Piazza M, Mekos D, Valente T. Peers, schools, and adolescent cigarette smoking. J Adolesc Health 2001;29:22-30.

[13] Sinha DN, Gupta PC, Reddy KS, Prasad VM, Rahman K, et al. Linking Global Youth Tobacco Survey 2003 and 2006 data to tobacco control policy in India. J Sch Health. 2008;78:368-73.

[14] The Global Tobacco Surveillance System Collaborating Group. The global tobacco surveillance system (GTSS): purpose, production and potential. J Sch Health 2005;75:15-24.

[15] Warren CW, Jones NR, Peruga A, Chauvin J, Baptiste JP, et al. Centers for Disease Control and Prevention (CDC). Global youth tobacco surveillance, 2000-2007. MMWR Surveill Summ 2008;57:1-28.

[16] Siziya S, Rudatsikira E, Muula AS. Antismoking messages and current cigarette smoking status in Somaliland: results from the Global Youth Tobacco Survey 2004. Confl Health 2008;2:6.

[17] Centers for Disease Control and Prevention (CDC). Tobacco use among students aged 13-15 years--Sri Lanka, 1999-2007. MMWR Morb Mortal Wkly Rep 2008;57:545-9.

[18] Gururaj G, Girish N. Tobacco use amongst children in Karnataka. Indian J Pediatr 2007;74:1095-8.

[19] Centers for Disease Control and Prevention (CDC). Cigarette use among high school students--United States, 1991-2007. MMWR Morb Mortal Wkly Rep 2008;57: 686-8.

[20] Erguder T, Soydal T, Uğurlu M, Cakir B, Warren CW. Tobacco use among youth and related characteristics, Turkey. Soz Praventivmed 2006;51:91-8.

[21] Kaufman JS, Poole C. Looking back on "causal thinking in the health sciences." Annu Rev Public Health 2000;21:101-19.

[22] Rothman KJ, Greenland S. Causation and causal inference in epidemiology. Am J Public Health 2005;95(Suppl 1):S144-50.

[23] Glanz K, Lewis FM, Rimer BK. Health behavior and health education: Theory, research and practice, 3rd ed. San Francisco: Jossey-Bass, 2002.

[24] Lubin JH, Caporaso N, Hatsukami DK, Joseph AM, Hecht SS. The association of a tobacco-specific biomarker and cigarette consumption and its dependence on host characteristics. Cancer Epidemiol Biomarkers Prev 2007;16:1852-7.

In: Smoking and Adolescence ISBN: 978-1-63484-311-9
Editors: M. L. Mazabam, S. Siziya et al. © 2016 Nova Science Publishers, Inc.

Chapter 23

ADOLESCENT CIGARETTE SMOKING IN THE WEST BANK (JUDEA AND SAMARIA)

Emmanuel Rudatsikira*[1], *MD, MPH, DrPH,
Adamson S Muula*[2,*], *MBBS, MPH, PhD,
and Seter Siziya*[3], *BA (Ed), MSc, PhD

[1]Departments of Biostatistics and Epidemiology and Global Health, Loma Linda University, School of Public Health, Loma Linda, California, USA

[2]Department of Community Health, University of Malawi, College of Medicine, Blantyre, Malawi

[3]Department of Community Medicine, University of Zambia, School of Medicine, Lusaka, Zambia

While our knowledge on the prevalence and associated factors of cigarette smoking continues to grow, there are limited data from the conflict regions of the Middle East. We therefore conducting a secondary analysis of the Global Youth Tobacco Survey (2005) from the West Bank (Judea and Samaria) to assess the prevalence and social correlates of smoking. Methods: Data from the Global Youth Tobacco Survey (GYTS) 2005 were used to determine current cigarette smoking prevalence and associated factors, attitudes, and exposure to, tobacco advertisements among adolescents. Current cigarette smoking was defined as having

---

[*] Correspondence: Adamson S Muula, Department of Community Health, University of Malawi, College of Medicine, Blantyre, Malawi. E-mail: muula@email.unc.edu.

smoked even a single puff within the last 30 days preceding the survey. Data were analyzed using SUDAAN software 9.0. Results: Of the 2,182 respondents, 28.7% males and 9.6% females reported being current smokers ($p < 0.01$). Having smoking friends was strongly associated with smoking after controlling for age, gender, parental smoking status, and perception of risks of smoking (OR = 9.79; 95% CI [6.75, 14.22] for most friends and OR = 4.68; 95% CI [3.36, 6.52] for some friends). Male gender and having one or both smoking parents were associated with smoking (OR = 2.29; 95% CI [1.70, 3.09] and OR = 1.85; 95% CI [1.41, 2.42] respectively). Conclusions: We report that overall about 1 in 5 school-going adolescents in the West Bank were current cigarette smokers in 2005. Factors associated with smoking were having parents or peer who was smoker and feelings that smoking was harmful was protective. Many adolescents are exposed to pro-tobacco advertisements. In general, males who smoked were perceived positively than females.

INTRODUCTION

Tobacco use is the single most common cause of preventable morbidity and mortality from non-communicable disease (1-3). Many adults who smoke initiated the habit of tobacco use as adolescents (4, 5). While many of the health effects of tobacco are experienced later in life, some health problems such as incident and exacerbation of asthma are observed in the short term (6, 7).

Several authors have also reported on the clustering of unhealthy behaviours among adolescents who smoke [8-10]. These authors report that adolescent smokers are also likely to use illicit drugs, alcohol, be truant from school. Thus cigarette smoking may be a marker of many other public health concerns that affect adolescents.

The West Bank (Judea and Samaria) is administratively located in the Eastern Mediterranean Region (EMR) of the World Health Organization (WHO). Warren et al. (11) have reported that prevalence of current cigarette smoking among in-school adolescents in the Eastern Mediterranean region as 6.7% and 3.2% for males and females. In 2001, prevalence of current cigarette smoking among 13 to15 year old adolescents ranged from 13.9% to 14.7% in this region (12). While the Tobacco Youth Survey Collaborative Group (12) reported on the prevalence of tobacco use in West Bank, the report did not report on the correlates of cigarette smoking. The Tobacco Youth Survey Tobacco Group also only reported prevalence of tobacco use among 13 years to 15 years olds. Prevalence data, while useful may be limited as these on their own may fail to inform the design and evaluation of interventions aimed to prevent adolescent smoking. We therefore conducted secondary analysis of the West Bank GYTS-2005 to examine the prevalence and associated factors to cigarette smoking among in-school adolescents.

OUR STUDY

The current study involved secondary analysis of existing data available from the Centers for Disease Control and Prevention (CDC), Atlanta, Georgia, United States of America on West Bank Global Youth Tobacco Survey GYTS) conducted in 2005. Comprehensive description of the GYTS purpose and methodology has been reported elsewhere (13-16). In brief however, the GYTS is a school-based survey of students aged 13–15 years. It is a cross-sectional study utilizing a multistage sample design with schools selected proportional to enrollment size. Within a selected school, classrooms are chosen randomly. All the students within the selected classes are eligible for participation regardless of their actual ages. A questionnaire is self-completed anonymously by the students and this takes between 30 to 40 minutes. The GYTS core questionnaire aims to collect the following information: prevalence of cigarette smoking and other tobacco use among young people; knowledge and attitudes of young people towards cigarette smoking; role of the media and advertising on young people's use of cigarettes; access to cigarettes; tobacco-related school curriculum; exposure to environmental tobacco smoke (ETS) and cessation of cigarette smoking.

The West Bank GYTS used a two-stage probability sampling technique. In the first stage, primary sampling units were schools which were selected with a probability proportional to their enrolment size. In the second step of sampling, a systematic sample of classes in the selected school was obtained. All students in the selected classes were eligible to participate. A self-completed questionnaire was used and completed within one class session. Response rate in the West Bank GYTS was 96.5%. For the purpose of this study, only data related to estimation of prevalence of smoking and associated factors are reported.

Data analysis was performed using SUDAAN software version 9.0 (Research Triangle Institute, Research Triangle Park, NC, United States of America) (17) to calculate weighted prevalence estimates and 95% CIs. The main outcome was current cigarette smoking which was defined as having smoked cigarettes, even a single puff within the past 30 days of the preceding the date of completion of questionnaire. This is the standard definition that has been used within the Global Youth Tobacco Survey (13-16, 18). Differences in estimates were judged as statistically significant at the $p < 0.05$ level. We also conducted logistic regression analysis to estimate the association between relevant predictor variables and current smoking.

FINDINGS

2,182 students participated in the study of whom 1002 (50.7%) were female, and 1094 (49.3%) were males. The median age was 15 years, range 11 to 17 years.

Table 1. Factors associated with current smoking in West Bank, Palestine

Characteristics	Percent of smokers	Unadjusted odds ratios with 95% CI	Adjusted odds ratios with 95% CI
Age (years)			
11-12	18.4	1.00	1.00
13	12.4	**0.63 [0.41, 0.96]**	0.93 [0.55, 1.57]
14	20.0	1.11 [0.77, 1.60]	1.34 [0.83, 2.16]
15	21.3	1.20 [0.84, 1.72]	1.50 [0.93, 2.42]
16-17	23.4	**1.43 [1.01, 2.03]**	1.53 [0.95, 2.45]
Gender			
Combined	18.9		
Female	9.6	1.00	1.00
Male	28.7	**3.81 [2.93, 4.96]**	**2.29 [1.70, 3.09]**
Parental smoking status			
None	31.3	1.00	1.00
One or both parents smokers	68.7	**2.01 [1.58, 2.55]**	**1.85 [1.41, 2.42]**
Best friend smokers			
None	6.8	1.00	1.00
Some	29.9	**5.89 [4.38, 7.92]**	**4.68 [3.36, 6.52]**
Most or all	49.6	**13.57 [9.71, 18.97]**	**9.79 [6.75, 14.22]**
Perception that smoking is harmful			
No	17.4	1.00	1.00
Yes	82.6	**0.66 [0.43, 1.02]**	0.79 [0.47, 1.32]

Table 1 presents the prevalence rates and factors associated with smoking. Of the 2,182 participants, 18.9 were current smokers (28.7% of males and

9.6% of females) reported being current smokers ($p < 0.001$). Having smoking friends was strongly associated with smoking after controlling for age, gender, parental smoking status, and perception of hazards caused by smoking. Subjects who had smoking friends were more likely to smoke than those who had no smoking friends (OR = 9.79; 95% [6.75, 14.22] for most friends smokers and OR = 4.68; 95% CI [3.36, 6.52] for some smoking friends). Males were more than twice likely to smoke as females (OR = 2.29; 95% [1.70, 3.09]). Compared to subjects with non smoking parents, those whose parents smoked were 1.85 more likely to smoke (OR = 1.85; 95% CI [1.41, 2.42]).

Table 2. Exposure to tobacco advertisements among adolescents in West Bank, Palestine

Characteristics	**Number of participants**	**% of total and 95% CI**
		P = 0.289
Seen cigarette brand name on TV in past 30 days	1571	49.4 [46.8, 51.9]
Males	864	51.4 [48.0, 54.9]
Females	707	47.2 [43.4, 50.9]
		P < 0.001
Has item with cigarette brand logo	1985	19.7 [18.0, 21.6]
Males	1035	23.2 [20.6, 25.9]
Females	950	16.3 [14.0, 18.9]
		P < 0.001
Seen tobacco adverts on billboards in past 30 days	2036	77.8 [69.7, 73.7]
Males	1056	76.7 [73.9, 79.2]
Females	980	67.1 [64.0, 70.0]
		P < 0.001
Seen tobacco adverts in newspapers/magazines in past 30 days	2015	
Males	1049	71.1 [68.2, 73.8]
Females	966	59.2 [56.0, 62.3]

Table 2 indicates the participants were exposed to tobacco adverts through billboards (77.8%), magazine (65.0%), and TV (49.4%). Almost one in five respondents (19.7%) reported having an item with cigarette brand logo on it. Compared to females, males had higher rates of those who reported having an item with cigarettes logo (p = 0.001) and being exposed to tobacco adverts on billboards and magazine compared to females (p < 001).

Table 3 indicates that the vast majority (92.1%) of the respondents felt that smoking is harmful. 53.3% thought that male smokers had more friends while 33.4% thought so for females. 28.8% felt that boys who smoke are attractive and 22.7% felt the same for girls who smoke.

Table 3. Attitudes towards tobacco smoking distributed by gender in West Bank, Palestine

Characteristic	**Number of participants**	**% of total and 95% CI**
		P=0.231
Felt that boys who smoke have more friends	1459	53.3 [50.7, 55.9]
Males	823	54.5 [51.0, 58.0]
Females	636	51.8 [47.9, 55.8]
		P = 0.130
Felt like girls who smoke had more friends	1512	33.4 [31.0, 35.9]
Males	824	31.4 [28.2, 34.8]
Females	688	35.5 [31.9, 39.2]
		P = 0.842
Felt that boys who smoke are attractive	1531	28.9 [26.6, 31.3]
Males	809	28.7 [25.6, 32.0]
Females	722	29.1 [25.8, 32.6]
		P = 0.487
Felt that girls who smoke are attractive	1645	22.7 [20.3, 24.8]
Males	873	23.1 [20.4, 26.2]
Females	772	22.2 [19.3, 25.3]
		P = 0.079
Felt that tobacco smoking is harmful to health	1833	92.1 [90.7, 93.3]
Males	944	90.6 [88.4, 92.4]
Females	889	93.6 [91.7, 95.0]

DISCUSSION

Our study of in-school adolescents in West Bank found an overall prevalence of current cigarette smoking at 18.9%. This is higher than prevalence estimates of 13.9% to 14.7% reported for 2001 among adolescents 13 to 15 years in the same area (12). This difference could be due to a number of reasons. Firstly, in the 2001 study only study participants aged 13 to 15 years were reported. As age is associated with history of smoking, our inclusion of much older adolescents could partly explain this difference. The other possible reason is that the socio-political environment of the West Bank has changed over the years since 2001. The increased social disruptions experienced in the area may facilitate increasing smoking among adolescents. Also compared to the overall prevalence of adolescents' cigarette smoking in the Eastern Mediterranean region (6.7% and 3.2% for males and females), our finding suggest a higher prevalence of current cigarette smoking in the West Bank. The prevalence of smoking in this study is slightly higher than 16.6% reported from Jordan (12).

We found that males were likely to be smokers than females (OR = 3.81, 95% CI, 2.93, 4.96). We believe this due to cultural acceptability of cigarette smoking amongst males than females. Rudatsikira et al. (19) have reported male predominance of smoking among adolescents in Ethiopia. However, the Global Youth Tobacco Survey Collaborating Group has reported that overall, considering all the many settings that they have conducted the GYTS, there was little gender differences in cigarette smoking (20). This does not suggesting that local differences do not occur; just the general picture does not support marked gender disparities.

We also found that having parents or friends who smoked was positively associated with the adolescents being a smoker. Believing that smoking was harmful to health was negatively associated with being a current smoker. The association between having smoking parents or friends and adolescents' own smoking has been demonstrated in many other studies (19, 21-23). Mercken et al. have reported that social selection and social influence play an important role in explaining similarity of smoking behaviour among friends (24). Mercken et al. (24) have also reported that although parental smoking was important in influencing adolescent smoking, sibling smoking was much more influential. De vries et al. (25) have reported also that adolescents' own attitudes towards smoking may influence them in the selection of friends i.e., adolescents with favourable attitudes towards smoking are more likely to choose smokers as friends.

We also assessed exposure of study participants to pro-tobacco advertisements through mass media. Overall as shown in Table 2, exposure to cigarette brand names on television, having an item with a tobacco brand logo, having seen billboard with tobacco advertisement was high. Males were more likely to have been exposed to these advertisements than females. As tobacco advertisements have been known to influence adolescents smoking (26-28), the higher prevalence of smoking among males compared to females could in part be explained by the higher exposure to pro-tobacco advertisements among the males.

While we found that there was a gender difference in exposure to pro-tobacco advertisements, there was no gender difference in attitudes towards smoking (Table 3). Over 90% of both males and females thought that smoking was harmful to health. Overall 53.3% thought boys who smoke had more friends, while 33.4% thought girls who smoked had more friends. 28.9% thought that boys who smoked were more attractive while 22.7% thought girls who smoked were more attractive. The fact that more study participants felt boys who smoked had more friends or were more attractive most likely exhibits societal attitudes that smoking is more acceptable among males than females.

Limitations of the study

Our study has a number of limitations. We used self-reported information on current smoking status. Data on smoking status within the GYTS methodology are not validated with a biomarker such as exhaled carbon monoxide or cotinine levels (29-30). The degree of potential reporting bias was not assessed. However data from the United States using similar methodology have shown good test-retest reliability (31). Huerta et al. have also reported high reliability of smoking history among Israel youths (32). However these authors noted that as years pass from date since smoked, data become less reliable. Our study is based on smoking history within the last 30 days and so should be reasonable reliable.

The data used obtained from the survey were collected from school-going adolescents. To the extent that the smoking prevalence and associated factors between in-school and out-of school adolescents, our finding may not be generalized to the whole adolescent population in West Bank.

Data were also collected from adolescents who were present at school on the day of the survey. These absent students may have different characteristics from those who are present. Michaud et al. (32) have reported in a survey of adolescents in Switzerland that higher proportion of absent students were sexually active, used tobacco, alcohol, and cannabis more often than did present students. Thus to the extent that absent students are different from present peers in West Bank, bias may have been introduced. However the with a response rate of 96.5%, any bias that may have resulted because of absenteeism is likely to have been minimal.

CONCLUSION

We have reported that overall about 1 in 3 school-going adolescents in the West Bank were current cigarette smokers in 2005. Factors associated with smoking were having parents or peer who was smoker and feelings that smoking was harmful was protective. Many adolescents in the West Bank are exposed to pro-tobacco advertisements. In general, males who smoked were perceived positively than females.

Conflict of interest

The authors declare they have no competing interests. Authors' contribution: ER designed analysis plan, led data analysis and participated in drafting of manuscript, SS participated in the interpretation of findings and drafting of manuscript and ASM participated in the interpretation of findings and drafting of manuscript.

ACKNOWLEDGMENTS

The authors thank the Centers for Disease Control and Prevention (CDC), Atlanta, Georgia, United States of America, for making the data used in this study available for our analysis. However, the CDC took no part in the decision of the models used and any other data analysis or the decision to publish this paper. We also thank the students who participated in the survey.

REFERENCES

[1] Ezzati M, Lopez AD, Rodgers A, Vander Hoorn S, Murray CJL and the Comparative Risk Assessment Collaborating Group. Selected major risk factors and global and regional burden of disease. Lancet 2002; 360:1347-60.

[2] Peto R, Lopez AD, Boreham J, Thun, Heath Jr C. Mortality from smoking in developed countries 1950–2000: indirect estimation from National Vital Statistics. Oxford: Oxford University Press, 1994.
[3] WHO IARC. Monographs on the evaluation of carcinogenic risks to humans, vol 83: tobacco smoke and involuntary smoking. Lyon: IARC Press, 2004.
[4] Brook JS, Balka EB, Ning Y, Brook DW. Trajectories of cigarette smoking among African Americans and Puerto Ricans from adolescence to young adulthood: associations with dependence on alcohol and illegal drugs. Am J Addict 2007;16:195-201.
[5] White HR, Violette NM, Metzger L, Stouthamer-Loeber M. Adolescent risk factors for late-onset smoking among African American young men. Nicotine Tob Res 2007;9:153-61.
[6] Gilliland FD, Islam T, Berhane K, Gauderman WJ, McConnell R, Avol E, Peters JM. Regular smoking and asthma incidence in adolescents. Am J Respir Crit Care Med 2006;174:1094-100.
[7] Annesi-Maesano I, Oryszczyn MP, Raherison C, Kopferschmitt C, Pauli G, Taytard A, et al. Increased prevalence of asthma and allied diseases among active adolescent tobacco smokers after controlling for passive smoking exposure. A cause for concern? Clin Exp Allergy 2004; 34:1017-23.
[8] Dierker LC, Sledjeski EM, Botello-Harbaum M, Ramirez RR, Chavez LM, Canino G. Association between psychiatric disorders and smoking stages within a representative clinic sample of Puerto Rican adolescents. Compr Psychiatry 2007;48:237-44.
[9] Rhee D, Yun SC, Khang YH. Co-occurrence of problem behaviors in South Korean adolescents: findings from Korea Youth Panel Survey. J Adolesc Health 2007;40:195-7.
[10] Ohene SA, Ireland M, Blum RW. The clustering of risk behaviors among Caribbean youth. Matern Child Health J 2005;9:91-100.
[11] Warren CW, Jones NR, Eriksen MP, Asma S. Global Tobacco Surveillance System (GTSS) collaborative group: Patterns of global tobacco use in young people and implications for future chronic disease burden in adults. Lancet 2006;367:749-53.
[12] The Global Youth Tobacco Survey Collaborative Group: Tobacco use among youth: a cross country comparison. Tobacco Control 2002;11: 252-270.
[13] Warren CW, Riley L, Asma S, Eriksen MP, Green L, Blanton C, et al. Tobacco use by youth: a surveillance report from the Global Youth Tobacco survey project. Bull World Health Organ 2000;78(7):868–76.
[14] The Global Youth Tobacco Survey Collaborative Group. Tobacco use among youth: a cross country comparison, Tob Control 2002;11:252-70.
[15] The Global Youth Tobacco Survey Collaborative Group. Differences in worldwide tobacco use by gender: findings from the Global Youth Tobacco Survey. J Sch Health 2003;73:207–215.
[16] Global Tobacco Surveillance System Collaborating Group. Global Tobacco Surveillance system (GTSS): purpose, production, and potential. J Sch Health 2005;75:15–24.

[17] Shah BV, Barnwell BG, Bieler GS. SUDAAN: software for the statistical analysis of correlated data. User's manual, release 7.5. Research Triangle Institute, Research Triangle Park, 1997.

[18] Kyrlesi A, Soteriades ES, Warren CW, Kremastinou J, Papastergiou P, Jones NR, et al. Tobacco use among students aged 13-15 years in Greece: the GYTS project. BMC Public Health 2007;7:3.

[19] Rudatsikira E, Abdo A, Muula AS. Prevalence and determinants of adolescent tobacco smoking in Addis Ababa, Ethiopia. BMC Public Health 2007;7:176.

[20] Global Youth Tobacco Survey Collaborating Group. Differences in worldwide tobacco use by gender: findings from the Global Youth Tobacco Survey. J Sch Health 2003;73:207-15.

[21] Jindal SK, Aggarwal AN, Gupta D, Kashyap S, Chaudhary D. Prevalence of tobacco use among school going youth in North Indian States. Indian J Chest Dis Allied Sci 2005;47:161-6.

[22] Scragg R, Laugesen M. Influence of smoking by family and best friend on adolescent tobacco smoking: results from the 2002 New Zealand national survey of year 10 students. Aust NZ J Public Health 2007; 31:217-23.

[23] Livaudais JC, Napoles-Springer A, Stewart S, Kaplan CP. Understanding Latino adolescent risk behaviors: parental and peer influences. Ethn Dis 2007;17:298-304.

[24] Mercken L, Candel M, Willems P, de Vries H. Disentangling social selection and social influence effects on adolescent smoking: the importance of reciprocity in friendships. Addiction 2007;102:1483-93.

[25] de Vries H, Candel M, Engels R, Mercken L. Challenges to the peer influence paradigm: results for 12-13 year olds from six European countries from the European Smoking Prevention Framework Approach study. Tob Control 2006;15:83-9.

[26] Andreeva TI, Krasovsky KS, Semenova DS. Correlates of smoking initiation among young adults in Ukraine: a cross-sectional study. BMC Public Health 2007;7:106.

[27] Peters RJ, Kelder SH, Prokhorov A, Springer AE, Yacoubian GS, Agurcia CA, Amos C: The relationship between perceived exposure to promotional smoking messages and smoking status among high school students. Am J Addict 2006;15:387-91.

[28] DiFranza JR, Wellman RJ, Sargent JD, Weitzman M, Hipple BJ, Winickoff JP. Tobacco Consortium, Center for Child Health Research of the American Academy of Pediatrics: Tobacco promotion and the initiation of tobacco use: assessing the evidence for causality. Pediatrics 2006;117:e1237-48.

[29] Thaqi A, Franke K, Merkel G, Wichmann HE, Heinrich J. Biomarkers of exposure to passive smoking of children: frequency and determinants. Indoor Air 2005;15:302-10.

[30] Breland AB, Kleykamp BA, Eissenberg BA. Clinical laboratory evaluation of potential reduced exposure products for smokers. Nicotine Tob Res 2006;8:727-38.

[31] Brener ND, Colins JL, Kann L, Warren CW, Williams BT. Reliability of the Youth Risk Behavior Survey Questionnaire. Am J Epidemiol 1995; 141:575-80.

[32] Huerta M, Chodick G, Balicer RD, Davidovitch N, Grotto I. Reliability of self-reported smoking history and age at initial tobacco use. Prev Med 2005;41:646-50.

[33] Michaud PA, Delbos-Piot I, Narring F. Silent dropouts in health surveys: are nonrespondent absent teenagers different from those who participate in school-based health surveys? J Adolesc Health 1998;22:326-33.

In: Smoking and Adolescence ISBN: 978-1-63484-311-9
Editors: M. L. Mazabam, S. Siziya et al. © 2016 Nova Science Publishers, Inc.

Chapter 24

CIGARETTE SMOKING, CLOSE FRIENDSHIP, SEXUAL INTERCOURSE AND ADOLESCENTS IN MAURITANIA

David Mulenga[1*], BSc, MPH, Mazyanga L Mazaba[2,3], BSc, MSc, Olusegun Babaniyi[3], MBBS, MPH, MSc, and Seter Siziya[1], BA(Ed), MSc, PhD

[1]Copperbelt University, School of Medicine, Ndola, Zambia
[2]University Teaching Hospital, Lusaka, Zambia
[3]EPI Unit, World Health Organization, Lusaka, Zambia

There are undesirable consequences of early commencement of sexual activity among adolescents which include human immunodeficiency virus infection and unwanted pregnancy. In this chapter we determine associations of cigarette smoking and close friendships with ever having had sexual intercourse among school-going adolescents in Mauritania. Secondary analysis of 2010 Mauritania Global School-based Health Survey data was conducted. Associations were established using weighted logistic regression analysis. A total of 2,063 students participated in the survey of which 43.5% were males. A third (33.2%) of students reported ever had sexual intercourse. Compared to female adolescents, males were 15% (AOR=1, 15, 95% CI [1.13, 1.17]) more

[*] Corresponding: David Mulenga, BSc, MPH, Copperbelt University, School of Medicine, PO Box 71191, Ndola, Zambia. Email: mulengingo@yahoo.co.uk.

likely to report having had sexual intercourse. Overall, adolescents who smoked cigarettes were more likely (AOR = 2.01, 95% CI [1.96, 2.06]) to report having had sexual intercourse compared to non-smokers. Having close friends was negatively associated with sexual intercourse (AOR = 0.64, 95% CI [0.62, 0.67]). Future work is needed to develop and employ measures that would prevent early sexual intercourse using the factors identified in the current study.

INTRODUCTION

Issues of reproductive health and sexuality are very important fundamental aspects of our day to day living (1) and yet not much has been documented on the prevalence and correlates of sexual behaviour among adolescents (2, 3). There are undesirable consequences of sexual activity among school going adolescents which include human immunodeficiency virus infection and unwanted pregnancy (4). School going adolescents may also engage in substance use risk behaviours (5), which have an impact on their sexual behaviour, for instance researchers have documented that sexual risk taking and heavy alcohol use coexist in many communities of young people (6, 7). Zabin (8) in the study that sought to explore the association between smoking and sexual behaviour among teens in US contraceptive clinics, noted that smoking may be representative of a cluster of behaviours which are especially problematical when initiated outside the normative schedule of such behaviours. Therefore, accurate and up-to-date information on sexual behaviour and its correlates of this particular group is crucially important.

According to Biddlecom et al. (9), parents have an influence on the sexual and reproductive health of adolescents that they can help to develop necessary skills on safe sexual life and good reproductive health. According to Gevers et al. (10) in South Africa, it is illegal for adolescents under age 16 years to engage in any sexual behaviour whether kissing, petting, or penetrative sex, regardless of consent. Feleke et al. (11) also noted that the utilization of reproductive health services is an important component in preventing adolescents from different sexual and reproductive health problems.

Sexual and reproductive health problems among adolescents are not only in African countries like Mauritania, but even developed countries experience similar challenges. It has been reported by Hellerstedt et al. (12) that half of the students in grades 9 to 12 in the United States reported that they had sexual intercourse at least once. They also reported that about 80% of pregnancies among those aged 15 to 19 years which made up to a quarter of all US unintended pregnancies were not planned. In Canada, where reports indicate that while less than 50% of teenagers reported having had sexual intercourse before the age 18, more than two-thirds would have had sexual intercourse by the age of 20 (13).

In most African countries, in-school adolescents engage in sexual activities in their teens. In a study by Oljira et al. (14), it was reported that a significant proportion of in-school adolescents in Eastern Ethiopia were engaged in sexual relationships. In another study done in two major universities of Ethiopia, Wasie et al. (15) observed that a significant number of students had history of sexual intercourse. In Mauritania, sexual behaviour of school going adolescents is not different from many parts of Africa. The 2010 Global School-based Health Survey (Mauritania 2010 fact sheet) reported that among students who ever had sexual intercourse, the percentage that had sexual intercourse for the first time before age 14 years was as high as 73.7%. In another study done by Ndiaye et al. (16) in Nouakchott in the Islamic Republic of Mauritania, it was noted that there was multiplication of sexually-transmitted diseases, including HIV, among the pupils due to insufficient condom use among sexually active students. Therefore, research in this area of study will yield a lot of information to correct the situation by informing preventive strategies. Hence, the objective of the study was to determine associations of cigarette smoking and close friendship with ever had sexual intercourse among school-going adolescents in Mauritania in order to inform interventions to prevent early sexual intercourse.

OUR STUDY

Analysis was based on data obtained from the 2010 Mauritania Global School-based Student Health Survey (GSHS) that is available on a World Health Organization web site (http://www.who.int/chp/gshs/mauritaniadataset/en/). The focus of the GSHS is on students aged 13-15 years, and grades with the majority of students were selected. In Mauritania, the majority of these students were in year 1 to 4 of high school. Drawing of the sample involved sampling schools proportional to their enrolment size. This was followed by randomly selecting classes and all students in the selected classes were requested to participate in the survey. The school response rate was 96% and that of the students was 74%, giving an overall response rate of 70%.

A questionnaire found on a web site for Centers for Disease Control and Prevention (http://www.cdc.gov/gshs/countries/africa/mauritania.htm) with many modules among which was on sexual behaviour and Tobacco use was used to collect data. The questionnaire was self-administered by the students. They responded to questions on a computer scannable answer sheet.

Variables that were considered in this manuscript are those that were significantly associated with ever had sexual intercourse in the literature. The exposure variables were Smoked cigarettes and Had close friend. The variable Smoked cigarettes was obtained from the question: "During the past 30 days, on how many days did you smoke cigarettes? Responses were 0 days, 1 or 2 days, 3 to 5 days, 6 to 9 days, 10 to 19 days, 20 to 29 days and all 30 days. At analysis, the variable was recoded as 1 for having smoked cigarettes for at least 1 day and 0 for not having smoked cigarettes in the past 30 days. The other explanatory variable Had close friends was obtained by asking the question: "How many close friends do you have?" Responses were 0, 1, 2, 3 or more. This variable was recoded as either 0 for having no close friends or 1 if had at least one close friend. The outcome variable: Ever had sexual intercourse was obtained by asking the question: "Have you ever had sexual intercourse?" Responses were Yes or No.

FINDINGS

A total of 2,063 students participated in the survey of which 54.5% were males. Among all students, 17.5% of them (17.9% of males and 16.4% of females) smoked cigarettes. About a third (33.2%) of all students (35.6% of males and 29.3% females) reported ever had sexual intercourse. These results are shown in Table 1.

Associations between smoking cigarettes and possible confounding factors with having had sexual intercourse are shown in Tables 2 and 3. Age, gender, smoking cigarettes and having close friends were associated with sexual intercourse. In both males and females, adolescents aged less than 14 years were less likely to report having ever had sexual intercourse compared to those aged 16 years or older. While male adolescents aged 14 or 15 years were less likely to have had sexual intercourse compared to males adolescents age 16 years or older, female adolescents aged 14 or 15 years were more likely to have had sexual intercourse compared with females adolescents of age 16 years or older. Compared to female adolescents, male adolescents were 15% (AOR = 1,15, 95% CI [1.13, 1.17]) more likely to report having had sexual intercourse.

Table 1. Sample description for 2010 Mauritania Global School-based Health Survey

Factor	Total	Males	Females
	n* (%)**	n* (%)**	n* (%)**
Age (years)			
<14	312 (15.6)	157 (16.4)	148 (14.2)
14	410 (20.0)	185 (19.5)	220 (20.5)
15	595 (28.9)	256 (27.3)	334 (31.0)
16+	711 (35.6)	348 (36.8)	356 (34.3)
Gender			
Male	964 (43.5)	-	-
Female	1069 (45.5)		
Smoked cigarettes			
Yes	339 (17.5)	161 (17.9)	167 (16.4)
No	1594 (82.5)	732 (82.1)	845 (83.6)
Had close friends			
Yes	1862 (92.6)	872 (92.9)	967 (92.5)
No	151 (7.4)	71 (7.1)	77 (7.5)
Ever had sexual intercourse			
Yes	550 (33.2)	282 (35.6)	254 (29.3)
No	1134 (66.8)	509 (64.4)	618 (70.7)

n* - Unweighted frequency (%)** - Weighted percent.

Totals may not all up due to missing data.

Table 2. Factors associated with sexual intercourse in bivariate analyses

Factor	Total	Males	Females
	OR* (95% CI**)	OR* (95% CI**)	OR* (95% CI**)
Age (years)			
<14	0.81 (0.78, 0.85)	0.86 (0.81, 0.90)	0.67 (0.62, 0.71)
14	0.86 (0.83, 0.89)	0.80 (0.76, 0.83)	1.02 (0.97, 1.07)
15	1.06 (1.02, 1.09)	1.01 (0.96, 1.05)	1.15 (1.10, 1.20)
16+	1	1	1
Gender			
Male	1.16 (1.14, 1.18)	-	-
Female	1		
Smoked cigarettes			
Yes	2.06 (2.01, 2.11)	2.37 (2.29, 2.45)	1.63 (1.57, 1.69)
No	1	1	1
Had close friends			
Yes	0.65 (0.62, 0.67)	0.72 (0.68, 0.75)	0.59 (0.56, 0.62)
No	1	1	1

OR* - Unadjusted odds ratio.

CI** - Confidence interval.

Adolescents who smoked cigarettes were more likely (AOR = 2.01, 95% CI [1.96, 2.06]) to report having had sexual intercourse (AOR = 2.45, 95% CI [2.36, 2.54] among males and AOR=1.58, 95% CI [1.53, 1.65] among females). Adolescents who had close friends were less likely (AOR=0.64, 95% CI [0.62, 0.67]) to report having had sexual intercourse (AOR=0.68, 95% CI [0.65, 0.72] among males and AOR=0.58, 95% CI [0.55, 0.62] among females).

Table 3. Factors associated with sexual intercourse in multivariate analyses

Factor	Total AOR* (95% CI**)	Males AOR* (95% CI**)	Females AOR* (95% CI**)
Age (years)			
<14	0.76 (0.72, 0.79)	0.84 (0.80, 0.89)	0.62 (0.58, 0.67)
14	0.93 (0.89, 0.96)	0.84 (0.80, 0.89)	1.09 (1.03, 1.15)
15	1.00 (0.97, 1.04)	0.91 (0.87, 0.95)	1.14 (1.09, 1.20)
16+	1	1	1
Gender			
Male	1.15 (1.13, 1.17)	-	-
Female			
Smoked cigarettes			
Yes	2.01 (1.96, 2.06)	2.45 (2.36, 2.54)	1.58 (1.53, 1.65)
No	1	1	1
Had close friends			
Yes	0.64 (0.62, 0.67)	0.68 (0.65, 0.72)	0.58 (0.55, 0.62)
No	1	1	1

AOR* - Adjusted odds ratio; CI** - Confidence interval.

Discussion

The current study has established that cigarette smoking and close friendships are related to ever have had sexual intercourse among school-going adolescents in Mauritania. Age and gender were also associated with ever had sexual intercourse. While male adolescents aged 14 or 15 years were less likely to have had sexual intercourse compared to male adolescents aged 16 years or older, female adolescents aged 14 or 15 years were more likely to have had sexual intercourse compared with female adolescents of age 16 years or older. This finding suggests that adolescent girls may have been engaging in sexual intercourse with males who were older than themselves. More male adolescents reported ever had sexual intercourse compared to the female counterparts and this may be due to the explorative nature of young males. This finding is common in many other studies looking at sexual behaviour among school going adolescents (17).

The current study has demonstrated the coexistence of sexual risk behaviour and cigarette smoking. Adolescents who smoked cigarettes were more likely to report ever had sexual intercourse compared to those who did not smoke cigarettes. This accords the findings by Zabin (8) which showed that the relationship of smoking and early coitus appeared among both Blacks and Whites despite strong racial differentials. Zabin (8) further noted that the evidence clearly suggested that those who initiated sexual activity in early adolescence demonstrated levels of smoking well beyond the norm not only for their age groups but even for adult populations.

Both male and female adolescents who had close friends were less likely to report having ever had sexual intercourse in the present study. This might be that these adolescents spent more time with their close ordinary friends than with those who might have wanted to engage in sexual intercourse with them.

This study is unique in its attempt to determine associations of cigarette smoking and close friendship with sexual experience among Mauritanian school going adolescents via a population-based survey. However, the study was not designed to examine the specific experiences of Mauritanian School going adolescents and, thus, we were not able to describe the cultural assets or traditional behaviours that are known to positively affect the sexual and reproductive health of Mauritanian school going adolescents. Because family and cultural ties are important to the health of African school going adolescents, further work is needed to specifically identify salient community and family ties that are associated with health-promoting behaviours and attitudes. Future work is needed to develop and employ measures that would prevent early sexual intercourse using the factors identified in the current study.

ACKNOWLEDGMENTS

We thank the World Health Organization for availing the data set in a public domain, and Centers for Disease Control and Prevention for the questionnaire. We extend our gratitude to the students for their participation in the survey.

This paper is a revised version of the original publication in the *International Journal of Child and Adolescent Health* (Mulenga D, Mazaba-Liwewe ML, Babaniyi O, Siziya S. Associations of cigarette smoking and close friendship with sexual intercourse among school-going adolescents in Mauritania. Int J Child Adolesc Health 2015;8:299-304) and the authors have obtained the permission from the International Journal of Child and Adolescent Health to use this material.

REFERENCES

[1] Shiferaw K, Getahun F, Asres G. Assessment of adolescents' communication on sexual and reproductive health matters with parents and associated factors among secondary and preparatory schools' students in Debremarkos town, North West Ethiopia. Reprod Health 2014;11(1):2.

[2] Chi X, Yu L, Winter S. Prevalence and correlates of sexual behaviors among university students: a study in Hefei, China. BMC Public Health 2012;12:972.

[3] De Rosa CJ, Ethier KA, Kim DH, Cumberland WG, Afifi AA, Kotlerman J, Loya RV, Kerndt PR. Sexual intercourse and oral sex among public middle school students: prevalence and correlates. Perspect Sex Reprod Health 2010;42(3):197-205.

[4] Ishida K, Stupp P, McDonald O. Prevalence and correlates of sexual risk behaviors among Jamaican adolescents. Int Perspect Sex Reprod Health 2011;37(1):6-15.

[5] Kang M, Rochford A, Skinner SR, Mindel A, Webb M, Peat J, Usherwood T. Sexual behaviour, sexually transmitted infections and attitudes to chlamydia testing among a unique national sample of young Australians: baseline data from a randomised controlled trial. BMC Public Health 2014;14:12.

[6] Connor J, Psutka R, Cousins K, Gray A, Kypri K. Risk drinking, risky sex: a national study of New Zealand University students, Alcohol Clin Exp Res 2013;37(11):1971-8.

[7] Siziya S, Muula AS, Kazembe LN, Rudatsikira E. Harmful lifestyles' clustering among sexually active in-school adolescents in Zambia. BMC Pediatr 2008;8:6.

[8] Zabin LS. The Association between smoking and sexual behavior among teens in US contraceptive clinics. Am J Public Health 1984;74(3):261-3.

[9] Biddlecom A, Awusabo-Asare K, Bankole. A Role of parents in adolescent sexual activity and contraceptive use in four African countries. Int Perspect Sex Reprod Health 2009;35(2):72-81.

[10] Gevers A, Mathews C, Cupp P, Russell M, Jewkes R. Illegal yet developmentally normative: a descriptive analysis of young, urban adolescents' dating and sexual behaviour in Cape Town, South Africa. BMC Int Health Hum Rights 2013;13:31.

[11] Feleke SA, Koye DN, Demssie AF, Mengesha ZB. Reproductive health service utilization and associated factors among adolescents (15--19 years old) in Gondar town, Northwest Ethiopia. BMC Health Serv Res 2013;13(1):294.

[12] Hellerstedt WL, Peterson-Hickey M, Rhodes KL, Garwick A. Environmental, social, and personal correlates of having ever had sexual intercourse among American Indian youths. Am J Public Health 2006;96(12):2228–34.

[13] Rotermann, M. Sexual behaviour and condom use of 15- to 24-year-olds in 2003 and 2009/2010. Health Rep 2012;23(1):1-5.

[14] Oljira L, Berhane Y, Worku A. Pre-marital sexual debut and its associated factors among in-school adolescents in Eastern Ethiopia. BMC Public Health 2012;12:375.

[15] Wasie B, Belyhun Y, Moges B, Amare B. Effect of emergency oral contraceptive use on condom utilization and sexual risk taking behaviours among university students, Northwest Ethiopia: a cross- sectional study. BMC Res Notes 2012;5:501.

[16] Ndiaye P, Abdallahi el HO, Diedhiou A, Tal-Dia A, Lemort JP. Evaluation of condom use among students of the El Mina middle school in Nouakchott in the Islamic Republic of Mauritania. Sante 2005;15(3):189-94.

[17] Leigh BC, Morrison DM, Trocki K, Temple MT. Sexual behavior of American adolescents: results from a U.S. national survey. J Adolesc Health 1994;15(2): 117-25.

In: Smoking and Adolescence ISBN: 978-1-63484-311-9
Editors: M. L. Mazabam, S. Siziya et al. © 2016 Nova Science Publishers, Inc.

Chapter 25

A SUMMARY: SMOKING AND ADOLESCENCE

Mazyanga L Mazaba[1,*], BSc, MSc,
Seter Siziya[2], BA (Ed), MSc, PhD,
and Joav Merrick[3-7], MD, MMedSci, DMSc

[1]World Health Organization, Lusaka, Zambia
[2]School of Medicine, Copperbelt University, Ndola, Zambia
[3]National Institute of Child Health and Human Development, Jerusalem, Israel
[4]Office of the Medical Director, Health Services, Division for Intellectual and Developmental Disabilities, Ministry of Social Affairs and Social Services, Jerusalem, Israel
[5]Division of Pediatrics, Hadassah Hebrew University Medical Center, Mt Scopus Campus, Jerusalem, Israel
[6]Kentucky Children's Hospital, University of Kentucky College of Medicine, Lexington, Kentucky, USA
[7]Center for Healthy Development, School of Public Health, Georgia State University, Atlanta, USA

[*] Correspondence: Mazyanga L Mazaba, Plot 4609 UN Annex Building, Corner Andrew Mwenya/Beit Road, Roadspark, POBox 32346, Lusaka, Zambia, E-mail: mazmazli@yahoo.com; liwewema@who.int.

INTRODUCTION

A total of 22 studies have been reported in the preceding chapters. Two studies were conducted within five years in each of the following countries: Jamaica, Jordan and Zambia (Lusaka). There appears to have been a reduction in the prevalence of smoking in two of those studies. In one study in Zambia, the prevalence of smoking was higher in rural than urban areas, suggesting a negative association between economic development with smoking, with urban areas reporting the lowest prevalence.

Three countries had prevalence of smoking of less than 5%: Kilimanjaro in Tanzania (2.2%) and Malawi (2.55) and Punjab in India (3.3%). Malawi being one of the major producers of tobacco, but with low prevalence of smoking, prevalence of smoking cannot be accounted for only by availability of tobacco. Mongolia, South Korea, India (Pradesh) and Zambia (Kafue) had prevalence of 5-9%. Jamaica, Greece, Iraq (Kurdistan), Jordan, Cote d'Ivoire, Somaliland, Zambia, Mauritania, Thailand and West Bank had prevalence of smoking of 10-19%. Countries with prevalence of smoking of 20% or higher were East Timor-Leste and Lithuania.

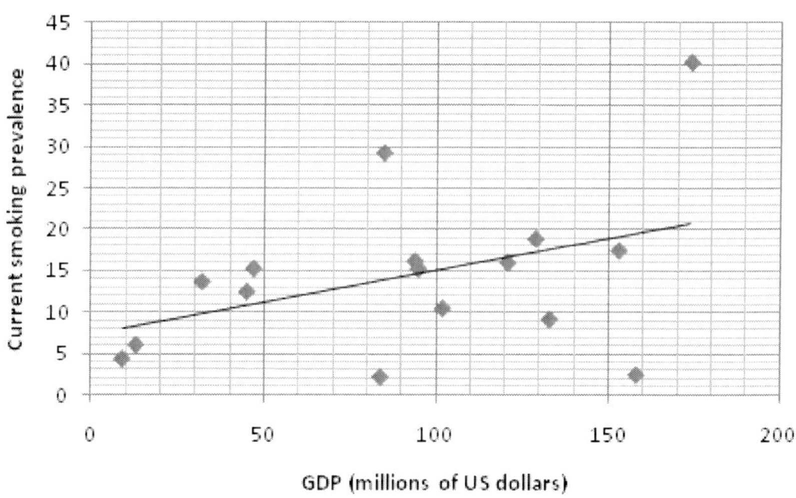

Figure 1. Linear relationship between prevalence of smoking and Gross Domestic Product (GDP).

The association between gender and smoking has not been consistent. Analysis of the association between gender and smoking was conducted in 16 studies out of which no significant associations were found in four studies, and significant associations were observed in the remaining 12 studies. In all of these 12 studies, males were more likely to smoke than females. Table 1 shows smoking prevalence by study site and gender. No significant linear relationship (see figure 1) was observed between prevalence of smoking and Gross Domestic Product (slope=0.077, SE=0.046, p=0.120), suggesting that economic development may not be associated with prevalence of smoking.

Table 1. Smoking prevalence by study site and gender

Country	Year	Sample size	Overall	Male	Female	Adjusted Odds Ratio 95% Confidence Interval
Jamaica	2000	1752	15.2			
Jamaica	2006	1854	16.7			1.55 (1.09, 2.19)
South Korea	2004	5615	6.1[a]	7.4	5.0	1.43 (1.09, 1.89)
East Timor-Leste	2006	1790	40.3	59.0	19.3	2.52 (2.45, 2.60)
Mongolia	2003	4105	9.2	15.4	4.4	3.22 (2.45, 4.24)
Thailand	2005	18368	13.7[a]	22.0	5.2	3.64 (2.72, 4.86)
Punjab, India	2003	2014	3.3			1.18 (1.16, 1.20)
Lithuania	2005	1822	29.3[a]	35.8	27.1	1.31 (1.03, 1.66)
Greece	2005	6141	12.5	13.3	11.8	1.62 (1.08, 3.08)
Kurdistan, Iraq	2006	1989	15.3	25.1	2.7	2.21 (2.15, 2.27)
Jordan	1999	3912	16.9	26.9	12.4	Not done
Jordan	2003	6313	15.5	20.0	10.1	Not done
Cote d'Ivoire	2003	2694	15.3	23.0	6.2	Not done
Somaliland	2004	1563	15.8	10.3	11.1	Not significant
Malawi	2005	5135	2.5	3.2	1.8	1.07 (1.04, 1.10)

Table 1. (Continued)

Country	Year	Sample size	Overall	Male	Female	Adjusted Odds Ratio 95% Confidence Interval
Kilimanjaro, Tanzania	2003	2323	2.2[a]	3.0	1.4	Not done
Zambia	2007	2378	10.5	9.3	12.1	Not significant
Chongwe, Zambia	2002	1845	27.0[b]			Not done
Kafue, Zambia	2002	1872	8.2	10.4	6.2	Not done
Lusaka, Zambia	2002	1241	9.2[c]	9.4	8.7	0.99 (0.95, 1.03)
Lusaka, Zambia	2007	1362	6.8[c]	6.7	6.8	Not done
Lusaka, Zambia	2007	2376	10.5			Not done
Kafue, Zambia	2007	2927	11.1			Not done
Chongwe, Zambia	2007	1377	13.5			Not done
Mauritania	2010	2063	17.5	17.9	16.4	1.15 (1.13, 1.17)
West Bank	2005	2182	18.9	28.7	9.6	2.29 (1.70, 3.09)
Pradesh, India	2004	1976	5.4[a]	6.4	3.9	1.21 (0.73, 1.99)

[a]Computed using weighted mean.
[b]prevalence of ever smoked.
[c]prevalence for 13-15-year-olds.

Table 2 lists factors that were identified to be associated with adolescence smoking in the studies presented in this book. A total of 13 papers published results on the association between parental smoking and adolescence smoking. In 12 of these papers, adolescents with parents who smoked were more likely to smoke as well. Meanwhile, all 14 papers that reported on an association between best friend smoking status and adolescence smoking found that adolescents with best friends who smoked were also more likely to smoke. In 6 of the 7 papers, adolescents who stated that cigarette smoking is harmful to health were more likely to smoke.

Table 2. Factors associated with smoking among school-going adolescents

Factor associated with smoking	Number of studies	
	More likely	Less likely
Parents smoke	12	1
Best friends smoke	14	0
Cigarette smoking is harmful to health	1	6
Has an item with a cigarette logo on it	4	2
A lot of media messages seen on anti-smoking program	1	1
A lot of cigarette brand names seen at sports events	2	1
A lot of cigarette advertisements seen on billboards	2	4
A lot of cigarette advertisements or promotion seen in print media	2	4
Smoking makes one gain weight	2	0
Girls who smoke are less attractive	0	2
Boys who smoke are less attractive	1	1
Girls who smoke have more friends	1	1
Boys who smoke have more friends	2	0
Adolescents who receive pocket money	1	0
A lot seeing actors smoke on television	3	0
A lot of antismoking messages seen at social gathering	3	1
Seen actors smoking on television	2	1
Family member discussed harmful effects of smoking	0	2
A lot of antismoking messages seen at sports events	1	0
Taught smoking makes teeth yellow, bad breath	0	2
Taught that your peers do not smoke	0	1
Religious organizations discourage young people to smoke	1	1
Received pocket money	3	0
Youth group discourages young people from smoking	0	1
Taught dangers of smoking	1	0
Advertisement messages at sports events	1	0
Seen a lot of advertisement at social gathering	2	0
Favoured banning smoking in public places	0	1
Offered free cigarettes by sales representative	0	1

Six studies reported an association between having an item with a cigarette logo and adolescence smoking. Four of these six studies found that adolescents who had an item with a cigarette logo on it were more likely to smoke. The finding that adolescents who had seen cigarette advertisements on billboards or in print media were less likely to smoke was reported in four of the six studies. Three of the four studies reported that adolescents who had seen a lot of antismoking messages at social gathering were more likely to smoke.

The notion that the smoking epidemic is reducing in developed countries and on an increase in developing countries may not be generalized to all countries in different economic developmental stages. Inconsistencies were observed in factors associated with adolescence smoking, except for the association between best friend smoking status and adolescence smoking. Site specific factors for adolescence smoking must be identified to be used in designing interventions to curtail prevalence of adolescence smoking in those sites.

Section two: Acknowledgments

In: Smoking and Adolescence ISBN: 978-1-63484-311-9
Editors: M. L. Mazabam, S. Siziya et al. © 2016 Nova Science Publishers, Inc.

Chapter 26

ABOUT THE EDITORS

Mazyanga L Mazaba, BSc, MSc, graduated from the University of Zambia, School of Medicine. She specialises in the areas of virology and public health (vaccines and preventable diseases). She is currently a National Professional Officer-laboratory scientist and data manager with the World Health Organization under the Expanded Program on Immunisation (EPI), particularly, polio, measles, rubella, influenza, rota virus and yellow fever surveillance and involved in laboratory diagnosis and training laboratory and surveillance personnel in sample collection and management. She has vast experience in immunology, virology, various diagnostic methods, data management, outbreak investigations and field epidemiology. She has published in a variety of peer reviewed journals and presented papers at international and national conferences in the field of virology and epidemiology. She is now working in the field of epidemiology as she pursues a DSc in epidemiology. E-mail: liwewema@who.int.

Seter Siziya, BA(Ed), MSc, PhD, born in Lusaka, Zambia, is a professor of medical biostatistics with the Copperbelt University in the School of Medicine, Ndola Central Hospital in Zambia. He was recognized as one of the Hot 100 authors worldwide for the BioMedCentral Journals in 2007; awarded a certificate of achievement by the Copperbelt University for outstanding achievement in research at the Copperbelt University School of Medicine in 2012; Received a Vice-Chancellor's award for excellence for the years in 2013 at the Copperbelt University; and received a meritorious award for excellence in research and academic development from the Zambia Medical Association in 2013. He previously worked for the Tropical Diseases Research Centre, Ndola, Zambia; University of Zimbabwe and the University of Zambia. He has been teaching biostatistics, epidemiology and research methods to both undergraduate and postgraduate students in the universities he has worked in. He has been a reviewer, editorial member and associate editor for international journals. He has published numerous papers on tobacco smoking, HIV, Integrated management of childhood illnesses, immunization, measles, non-communicable diseases, suicide, bullying, alcohol and occupational health. He is a member of the Health Professions Council of Zambia and chairs its Education committee. E-mail: ssiziya@gmail.com.

Joav Merrick, MD, MMedSci, DMSc, born and educated in Denmark is professor of pediatrics, child health and human development, Division of Pediatrics, Hadassah Hebrew University Medical Center, Mt Scopus Campus, Jerusalem, Israel and Kentucky Children's Hospital, University of Kentucky, Lexington, Kentucky United States and professor of public health at the Center for Healthy Development, School of Public Health, Georgia State University, Atlanta, United States, the medical director of the Health Services, Division for Intellectual and Developmental Disabilities, Ministry of Social Affairs and Social Services, Jerusalem, the founder and director of the National Institute of Child Health and Human Development in Israel. Numerous publications in the field of pediatrics, child health and human development, rehabilitation, intellectual disability, disability, health, welfare, abuse, advocacy, quality of life and prevention. Received the Peter Sabroe Child Award for outstanding work on behalf of Danish Children in 1985 and the International LEGO-Prize ("The Children's Nobel Prize") for an extraordinary contribution towards improvement in child welfare and well-being in 1987. E-mail: jmerrick@zahav.net.il.

In: Smoking and Adolescence ISBN: 978-1-63484-311-9
Editors: M. L. Mazabam, S. Siziya et al. © 2016 Nova Science Publishers, Inc.

Chapter 27

About the World Health Organization in Zambia

The mission of World Health Organization (WHO) is the attainment by all peoples of the highest possible level of health. The WHO came into force on 7th April 1948 including 150 countries separated into six regional offices. The primary role is to direct and coordinate international health with the United Nations' system. The main areas of work include health systems; promoting health through the life-course; non-communicable diseases; cooperate services; and preparedness, surveillance and response (1). Among its functions are (a) To act as the directing and co-ordinating authority on international health work; (b) To assist Governments, upon request, in strengthening health services and (c) To stimulate and advance work on the prevention and control of epidemic, endemic and other diseases. WHO also proposes conventions (2) such as the WHO Framework Convention on Tobacco Control (FCTC) that was adopted on 21st May 2003 and came into force on 27th February 2005. There are 47 WHO country offices in the WHO African region (3). Zambia became a member of the WHO in 1965, a year after attaining its independence.

WHO Reforms

WHO is reforming to be better equipped in addressing the increasingly complex challenges of health in the 21st century. The reform has three aims, which are programmatic reform to improve people's health, governance reform, to increase coherence in global health and managerial reform in pursuit of organizational excellence. The priority areas for the WHO Africa region identified by the current Regional Director for Africa, Dr. Moeti Matshidiso, are improving health security; strengthening national health systems; sustaining focus on the health-related Millennium Development Goals/Sustainable Development Goals (MDGs/SDGs); addressing the social determinants of health; and transforming WHO Africa region. In line with the WHO reforms, Regional Director for Africa has put in place a programme, the Transformation Agenda (TA) 2015-2020. This programme is accelerating the implementation of WHO reform within the WHO Africa region. It is a vision and strategy for change aimed to facilitate the emergence of "the WHO that staff and stakeholders wants." Its objective is to ensure that the WHO Secretariat in the Africa region evolves into the primary leader in health development in Africa. The TA is bold, ambitious and seeks to engender a regional health organization that is foresighted, proactive, responsive, transparent, and accountable and a result driven organization (4). The TA is aimed at enhancing the implementation of WHO reform within the WHO Africa region. The focus areas for the agenda are pro-results values; smart technical focus; responsive strategic operations; and effective communications and partnerships. Under each of these focus areas are a set of strategic actions that are closely aligned with the global reforms of WHO (5).

Mission of the WHO Zambia country office

Emanating from the WHO mission, the mission of the WHO Country Office (WCO) Zambia is to promote the attainment of the highest sustainable level of health by all people living in Zambia through collaboration with the government and other partners in health development and the provision of technical and logistic support to country programs. The WHO Country Cooperation Strategy (CCS) articulates WHO's strategic priorities for supporting the national and developmental agenda, which are (i) To support the universal scale up of priority essential health interventions in routine and emergency situations at the household, community and national levels; (ii) To advocate for policies and strategies to address determinants of health; (iii) To support governance and facilitate the strengthening of Health systems for universal and equitable access to quality health services; and (iv) To provide technical leadership in matters of health and promote partnership and networking (6).

Adolescent health remains a national health priority in the National Health Strategic Plan (NHSP) 2011-2016. WCO Zambia remains committed to this important priority and supports various aspects related to adolescent health including advocating for documentation, availability and accessibility of adolescent health services through its Child and Adolescent health unit. In line with the TA, WCO Zambia shall endeavor to build upon achievements thus far and attend to challenges identified, ensuring improved and more effective support to the health sector. The focus on WCO Zambia will be to ensure that Zambia achieves its national health objectives and MDGs/SDGs (7).

REFERENCES

[1] World Health Organization. About WHO. URL: http://www.who.int/about/en/.

[2] World Health Organization. Healthy documents. World alliance for breastfeeding action. People's Health Assembly. URL: http://healthydocuments.org/

[3] World Health Organization. WHO country offices in the WHO African region. URL: http://www.afro.who.int/en/countries.html.

[4] Mathidiso Moeti. URL: http://www.who.int/about/who_reform/change_at_who/issue6/matshidiso-moeti/en/.

[5] World Health Organization Regional Office for Africa. URL: http://www.afro.who.int/en/rdo/transformation-agenda.html.

[6] World Health Organization. The mission of the WHO Zambia Country Office. URL: http://www.zm.one.un.org/node/115.

[7] World Health Organization. WHO Zambia 2014 annual report. Luzaka: WHO, 2015.

Contacts

Dr. Jacob Mufunda

WHO Representative Zambia
Plot 4609 UN Annex Building, Corner Andrew Mwenya/Beit Road
Roadspark, PO Box 32346, Lusaka Zambia
E-mail: mufundaj@who.int

Mazyanga L Mazaba

NPO Laboratory Sciences
Plot 4609 UN Annex Building, Corner Andrew Mwenya/Beit Road
Roadspark, PO Box 32346, Lusaka Zambia
E-mail: mazmazli@yahoo.com; liwewema@who.int

In: Smoking and Adolescence ISBN: 978-1-63484-311-9
Editors: M. L. Mazabam, S. Siziya et al. © 2016 Nova Science Publishers, Inc.

Chapter 28

About the School of Medicine, Copperbelt University in Ndola, Zambia

The Copperbelt University School of Medicine (CBU SOM) was approved by the Senate of the Copperbelt University and inaugurated by the President of the republic of Zambia in June 2011, and the Zambia Health Professions Council approved the commencement of training in Dentistry and Medicine. The school admitted its inaugural class on the 14th November 2011. The school has three departments: Basic sciences, Clinical sciences (in which Public Health unit is housed) and Dental sciences. Copperbelt University School of Medicine is the second public Medical School in Zambia. It is the first Dental School in Zambia offering the Bachelors in Dental Surgery (BDS).

Mission

On establishment, the mission of the CBU SOM was to produce medical doctors and dentists who understand the health care context of the Zambian community, who will be able to convert their knowledge into solutions that will impact the care of the sick in Zambia. New programs have since been introduced including Bachelor of Science degree in clinical medicine, Master of Medicine in surgery, urology and obstetrics and gynaecology; Master of Science and Doctor of Science degrees by dissertation. Degrees by dissertation will produce senior and expert medical scientists who would manage academic research units and academic research departments or institutions within the university system or other similar institutions. This school's mission stems from the Copperbelt University mission which is "To contribute to the development and sustenance of the well-being of the people of Zambia and the world through the provision of flexible, innovative, entrepreneurial, inclusive programmes of teaching, learning, research and service." In view of the new programs that have been introduced, the school's mission would need to be recast to take into consideration these new programs.

CURRICULUM MODEL

The curriculum model is innovative. It is a modern approach to curriculum design which is open and integrative. It provides for vertical integration between the basic sciences and dental/medical practice, as well as horizontal integration of the basic sciences to each other. The curriculum allows for early exposure to dental/medical practice and continuous teaching in basic sciences throughout the programs. The curriculum uses a combination of delivery of curriculum of student centered and systems based learning to achieve a learning mix that produces the best in the student. Community based training is an integral part of the curriculum that runs throughout the programs and anchors the training within the context of the community. The model is open by breaking the subject specific system of training in favour of learning by concept system. During the MSc and DSc programs, students are exposed to non-examinable modules in medical sciences, research methods, leadership and administration.

RESEARCH ACTIVITIES

The school has a research coordinator. There are three research groups, namely: basic sciences, clinical sciences and public health. Under basic sciences, the study areas are tuberculosis, nutrition, anatomy organs and weight, and schistosomiasis; in the clinical group the topics are circumcision, and under public health group, the study areas are maternal and child health, non-communicable diseases, substance abuse among adolescents, integrated management of childhood diseases, infectious diseases and health systems.

LINKAGES AND PARTNERSHIPS

The CBU SOM collaborates with local research institutions that include the Tropical Diseases Research Centre and the School of Medicine of the University of Zambia. Internationally, it is part of two consortia, the Consortium of New Medical Schools (CONSAMS) that include the University of Namibia, University of Botswana, University of Lurio in Mozambique, University of Lesotho, Oulu University in Finland and the University of Vanderbilt in the USA. The other consortium is the Medical Education Initiative which consists of 13 Universities in Africa and is funded under a National Health Institute program of the USA government. The School recently commenced an international collaboration with the University of Tel Aviv in Israel, spearheaded mainly through teaching of the new MPH program to commence in 2016. The school is open to creating more linkages and partnerships worldwide to be part of the research and teaching communities in solving local and international health problems.

CONSULTANCY

The school has varied expertise reflected in the teaching programs. CBU SOM provides consultancies in line with and outside the research activities of the school. The School provides consultancies to several institutions including the Ministry of Health, the World Health Organization (National and International Office) and The National Science Research Council.

TARGETS

Building from the Copperbelt University vision of "to be an institution in which scholarship flourishes in an environment characterised by world class infrastructure and collaborative relations and supported by an accountable, transparent and efficient University governance system," the school hopes to produce sufficient doctors and dentist to meet the WHO recommendation of 1 doctor per 5,000 population, 1:10,000 and one specialist per 10,000 populations, 1:300,000 respectively. Through this to improve the health indices in Zambia to the level obtaining in developed countries. Through research collaboration with other institutions (locally and internationally), the school will become a centre of excellence in research.

Contacts

Mrs. Helen Mwenya Mukumba
Registrar, Copperbelt University
Jambo Drive, Riverside, PO Box 21692, Kitwe, Zambia
E-mail: registrar@cbu.ac.zm

Professor Seter Siziya
Clinical Sciences Department
School of Medicine
PO Box 71191, Ndola, Zambia
E-mail: ssiziya@gmail.com

In: Smoking and Adolescence ISBN: 978-1-63484-311-9
Editors: M. L. Mazabam, S. Siziya et al. © 2016 Nova Science Publishers, Inc.

Chapter 29

About the National Institute of Child Health and Human Development in Israel

The National Institute of Child Health and Human Development (NICHD) in Israel was established in 1998 as a virtual institute under the auspices of the Medical Director, Ministry of Social Affairs and Social Services in order to function as the research arm for the Office of the Medical Director. In 1998 the National Council for Child Health and Pediatrics, Ministry of Health and in 1999 the Director General and Deputy Director General of the Ministry of Health endorsed the establishment of the NICHD.

Mission

The mission of a National Institute for Child Health and Human Development in Israel is to provide an academic focal point for the scholarly interdisciplinary study of child life, health, public health, welfare, disability, rehabilitation, intellectual disability and related aspects of human development. This mission includes research, teaching, clinical work, information and public service activities in the field of child health and human development.

SERVICE AND ACADEMIC ACTIVITIES

Over the years many activities became focused in the south of Israel due to collaboration with various professionals at the Faculty of Health Sciences (FOHS) at the Ben Gurion University of the Negev (BGU). Since 2000 an affiliation with the Zusman Child Development Center at the Pediatric Division of Soroka University Medical Center has resulted in collaboration around the establishment of the Down Syndrome Clinic at that center. In 2002 a full course on "Disability" was established at the Recanati School for Allied Professions in the Community, FOHS, BGU and in 2005 collaboration was started with the Primary Care Unit of the faculty and disability became part of the master of public health course on "Children and society." In the academic year 2005-2006 a one semester course on "Aging with disability" was started as part of the master of science program in gerontology in our collaboration with the Center for Multidisciplinary Research in Aging. In 2010 collaborations with the Division of Pediatrics, Hadassah Hebrew University Medical Center, Jerusalem, Israel around the National Down Syndrome Center and teaching students and residents about intellectual and developmental disabilities as part of their training at this campus.

RESEARCH ACTIVITIES

The affiliated staff have over the years published work from projects and research activities in this national and international collaboration. In the year 2000 the International Journal of Adolescent Medicine and Health and in 2005 the International Journal on Disability and Human Development of De Gruyter Publishing House (Berlin and New York) were affiliated with the National Institute of Child Health and Human Development. From 2008 also the International Journal of Child Health and Human Development (Nova Science, New York), the International Journal of Child and Adolescent Health (Nova Science) and the Journal of Pain Management (Nova Science) affiliated and from 2009 the International Public Health Journal (Nova Science) and Journal of Alternative Medicine Research (Nova Science). All peer-reviewed international journals.

National Collaborations

Nationally the NICHD works in collaboration with the Faculty of Health Sciences, Ben Gurion University of the Negev; Department of Physical Therapy, Sackler School of Medicine, Tel Aviv University; Autism Center, Assaf HaRofeh Medical Center; National Rett and PKU Centers at Chaim Sheba Medical Center, Tel HaShomer; Department of Physiotherapy, Haifa University; Department of Education, Bar Ilan University, Ramat Gan, Faculty of Social Sciences and Health Sciences; College of Judea and Samaria in Ariel and in 2011 affiliation with Center for Pediatric Chronic Diseases and National Center for Down Syndrome, Department of Pediatrics, Hadassah Hebrew University Medical Center, Mount Scopus Campus, Jerusalem.

International Collaborations

Internationally with the Department of Disability and Human Development, College of Applied Health Sciences, University of Illinois at Chicago; Strong Center for Developmental Disabilities, Golisano Children's Hospital at Strong, University of Rochester School of Medicine and Dentistry, New York; Centre on Intellectual Disabilities, University of Albany, New York; Centre for Chronic Disease Prevention and Control, Health Canada, Ottawa; Chandler Medical Center and Children's Hospital, Kentucky Children's Hospital, Section of Adolescent Medicine, University of Kentucky, Lexington; Chronic Disease Prevention and Control Research Center, Baylor College of Medicine, Houston, Texas; Division of Neuroscience, Department of Psychiatry, Columbia University, New York; Institute for the Study of Disadvantage and Disability, Atlanta; Center for Autism and Related Disorders, Department Psychiatry, Children's Hospital Boston, Boston; Department of Pediatric and Adolescent Medicine, Western Michigan University Homer Stryker MD School of Medicine, Kalamazoo, Michigan, United States; Department of Paediatrics, Child Health and Adolescent Medicine, Children's Hospital at Westmead, Westmead, Australia; International Centre for the Study of Occupational and Mental Health, Düsseldorf, Germany; Centre for Advanced Studies in Nursing, Department of General Practice and Primary Care, University of Aberdeen, Aberdeen, United Kingdom; Quality of Life Research Center, Copenhagen, Denmark; Nordic School of Public Health, Gottenburg, Sweden, Scandinavian Institute of Quality of Working Life, Oslo, Norway;

The Department of Applied Social Sciences (APSS) of The Hong Kong Polytechnic University Hong Kong.

TARGETS

Our focus is on research, international collaborations, clinical work, teaching and policy in health, disability and human development and to establish the NICHD as a permanent institute at one of the residential care centers for persons with intellectual disability in Israel in order to conduct model research and together with the four university schools of public health/medicine in Israel establish a national master and doctoral program in disability and human development at the institute to secure the next generation of professionals working in this often non-prestigious/low-status field of work.

Contact

Joav Merrick, MD, MMedSci, DMSc
Professor of Pediatrics, Child Health and Human Development
Medical Director, Health Services,
Division for Intellectual and Developmental Disabilities,
Ministry of Social Affairs and Social Services,
POB 1260, IL-91012 Jerusalem, Israel.
E-mail: jmerrick@zahav.net.il

In: Smoking and Adolescence ISBN: 978-1-63484-311-9
Editors: M. L. Mazabam, S. Siziya et al. © 2016 Nova Science Publishers, Inc.

Chapter 30

ABOUT THE BOOK SERIES "PUBLIC HEALTH: PRACTICES, METHODS AND POLICIES"

Public health is a book series with publications from a multidisciplinary group of researchers, practitioners and clinicians for an international professional forum interested in the broad spectrum of public health issues. Books already published:

- Rubin IL, Merrick J, eds. Environment and public health: Environmental health, law and international perspectives. New York: Nova Science, 2014.
- Shek DTL, Siu AMH, Merrick J, eds. Tomorrow's leaders: Service leadership and holistic development in Chinese university students. New York: Nova Science, 2015.
- Siziya S, Mazaba ML, Merrick J, eds. Arbovirus: Public health experience from Zambia. New York: Nova Science, 2015.
- Obeng C, Obeng SG, Merrick J, eds. Health issues in diverse cultures. New York: Nova Science, 2015.
- Friedman BD, Merrick J, eds. Public health, social work and health inequalities. New York: Nova Science, 2015.

Contact

Professor Joav Merrick, MD, MMedSci, DMSc
Medical Director, Health Services, Division for Intellectual and Developmental Disabilities, Ministry of Social Affairs and Social Services
POBox 1260, IL-91012 Jerusalem, Israel. E-mail: jmerrick@zahav.net.il.

SECTION THREE: INDEX

INDEX

B

C

D

E

M

N

O

P

Q

R

S

T

U

V

W

Y

Z